SAFETY OF DIETARY SUPPLEMENTS FOR HORSES, DOGS, AND CATS

Committee on Examining the Safety of Dietary Supplements for Horses, Dogs, and Cats

Board on Agriculture and Natural Resources

Division on Earth and Life Studies

NATIONAL RESEARCH COUNCIL
OF THE NATIONAL ACADEMIES

THE NATIONAL ACADEMIES PRESS
Washington, D.C.
www.nap.edu

THE NATIONAL ACADEMIES PRESS 500 Fifth Street, N.W. Washington, DC 20001

NOTICE: The project that is the subject of this report was approved by the Governing Board of the National Research Council, whose members are drawn from the councils of the National Academy of Sciences, the National Academy of Engineering, and the Institute of Medicine. The members of the committee responsible for the report were chosen for their special competences and with regard for appropriate balance.

This study was supported by a grant from The Department of Health and Human Services (U.S. Food and Drug Administration) under Contract No. 223-01-2460/0031. Any opinions, findings, conclusions, or recommendations expressed in this publication are those of the author(s) and do not necessarily reflect the views of the organizations or agencies that provided support for the project.

Library of Congress Cataloging-in-Publication Data

National Research Council (U.S.). Committee on Examining the Safety of Dietary Supplements for Horses, Dogs, and Cats.
Safety of dietary supplements for horses, dogs, and cats / Committee on Examining the Safety of Dietary Supplements for Horses, Dogs, and Cats, Board on Agriculture and Natural Resources, Division on Earth and Life Studies, National Research Council of the National Academies.
p. cm. — (Animal nutrition series)
Includes bibliographical references and index.
1. Animal nutrition. 2. Dietary supplements. I. Title. II. Series: Animal nutrition series (Washington, D.C.)
SF95.N316 2008
636.08′52—dc22
2008042167

International Standard Book Number-13: 978-0-309-12570-3
International Standard Book Number-10: 0-309-12570-7

Additional copies of this report are available from the National Academies Press, 500 Fifth Street, N.W., Lockbox 285, Washington, DC 20055; (800) 624-6242 or (202) 334-3313 (in the Washington metropolitan area); Internet, http://www.nap.edu

Printed in the United States of America

THE NATIONAL ACADEMIES

Advisers to the Nation on Science, Engineering, and Medicine

The **National Academy of Sciences** is a private, nonprofit, self-perpetuating society of distinguished scholars engaged in scientific and engineering research, dedicated to the furtherance of science and technology and to their use for the general welfare. Upon the authority of the charter granted to it by the Congress in 1863, the Academy has a mandate that requires it to advise the federal government on scientific and technical matters. Dr. Ralph J. Cicerone is president of the National Academy of Sciences.

The **National Academy of Engineering** was established in 1964, under the charter of the National Academy of Sciences, as a parallel organization of outstanding engineers. It is autonomous in its administration and in the selection of its members, sharing with the National Academy of Sciences the responsibility for advising the federal government. The National Academy of Engineering also sponsors engineering programs aimed at meeting national needs, encourages education and research, and recognizes the superior achievements of engineers. Dr. Charles M. Vest is president of the National Academy of Engineering.

The **Institute of Medicine** was established in 1970 by the National Academy of Sciences to secure the services of eminent members of appropriate professions in the examination of policy matters pertaining to the health of the public. The Institute acts under the responsibility given to the National Academy of Sciences by its congressional charter to be an adviser to the federal government and, upon its own initiative, to identify issues of medical care, research, and education. Dr. Harvey V. Fineberg is president of the Institute of Medicine.

The **National Research Council** was organized by the National Academy of Sciences in 1916 to associate the broad community of science and technology with the Academy's purposes of furthering knowledge and advising the federal government. Functioning in accordance with general policies determined by the Academy, the Council has become the principal operating agency of both the National Academy of Sciences and the National Academy of Engineering in providing services to the government, the public, and the scientific and engineering communities. The Council is administered jointly by both Academies and the Institute of Medicine. Dr. Ralph J. Cicerone and Dr. Charles M. Vest are chair and vice chair, respectively, of the National Research Council.

www.national-academies.org

COMMITTEE ON EXAMINING THE SAFETY OF DIETARY SUPPLEMENTS FOR HORSES, DOGS, AND CATS

JIM E. RIVIERE, *Chair*, North Carolina State University, Raleigh
DAWN M. BOOTHE, Auburn University, Auburn, Alabama
GAIL L. CZARNECKI-MAULDEN, Nestle Purina PetCare PTC, St. Louis, Missouri
DAVID A. DZANIS, Dzanis Consulting & Collaborations, Santa Clarita, California
PATRICIA A. HARRIS, WALTHAM Centre for Pet Nutrition, Leicestershire, England
WOUTER H. HENDRIKS, Wageningen University, Wageningen, The Netherlands
CLAUDIA A. KIRK, University of Tennessee, Knoxville
LORI K. WARREN, University of Florida, Gainesville

Staff

AUSTIN J. LEWIS, Study Director
RUTHIE S. ARIETI, Senior Project Assistant

Acknowledgments

This report has been reviewed in draft form by persons chosen for their diverse perspectives and technical expertise in accordance with procedures approved by the National Research Council's Report Review Committee. The purpose of this independent review is to provide candid and critical comments that will assist the institution in making its published report as sound as possible and to ensure that the report meets institutional standards of objectivity, evidence, and responsiveness to the study charge. The review comments and draft manuscript remain confidential to protect the integrity of the deliberative process. We wish to thank the following for their review of this report:

Kevin L. Armbrust, Mississippi State University
John E. Bauer, Texas A&M University, College Station
William Bookout, National Animal Supplement Council, Valley Center, CA
George A. Burdock, The Burdock Group, Orlando, FL
Cynthia A Cole, IDEXX Pharmaceuticals, Greensboro, NC
Mark E. Cook, University of Wisconsin, Madison
David W. Freeman, Oklahoma State University, Stillwater
George A. Graber, Center for Veterinary Medicine, Food and Drug Administration (retired)
Robert H. Poppenga, University of California, Davis
Jennifer Radosevich, Kemin Nutrisurance, Des Moines, IA
Kelly S. Swanson, University of Illinois, Urbana-Champaign
Susan G. Wynn, Bells Ferry Veterinary Hospital, Acworth, GA

Although the reviewers listed above have provided many constructive comments and suggestions, they were not asked to endorse the conclusions or recommendations, nor did they see the final draft of the report before its release. The review of this report was overseen by George C. Fahey, Jr., University of Illinois. Appointed by the National Research Council, he was responsible for making certain that an independent examination of this report was carried out in accordance with institutional procedures and that all review comments were carefully considered. Responsibility for the final content of this report rests entirely with the author committee and the institution.

The committee wholeheartedly acknowledges the support of Dr. Austin Lewis, Program Officer for the committee, who did an outstanding job of both keeping our deliberations on track and focused on the final product. His gentle, but extremely insightful and effective, guidance during meetings and conference calls is largely responsible for the final product that emerged. The committee also owes its deep gratitude to Ruthie Arieti, Senior Project Assistant, who managed to keep track of both our committee's diverse schedules and inputs in a manner that resulted in a smooth flow for all activities associated with our work. Her active maintenance of the committee website greatly facilitated our research and writing, as well as fostering a camaraderie amongst staff and committee members that was crucial to allowing our committee to meet its objectives. We appreciate the efforts of Robin Schoen, Director of the Board on Agriculture and Natural Resources, for her encouragement and support in allowing us to complete the project in a manner and time frame both acceptable to us and our sponsor. The technical editing by Paula Whitacre, Full Circle Communications, was much appreciated. Finally, the committee wants to express its sincere thanks to the individuals listed in Appendix D who provided advice, data, and input into our deliberations. Several pet food companies also provided data (via the Pet Food Institute) that were included in the report, but the individual companies prefer to remain anonymous.

Contents

Tables, Figures, and Boxes

TABLES

FIGURES

BOXES

Summary

It has been estimated that between 10 and 33 percent of dogs and cats in the United States are fed an animal dietary supplement, with some of the same supplements also being fed to horses. For the purpose of this report, the committee defined an animal dietary supplement as "a substance for oral consumption by horses, dogs, or cats, whether in/on feed or offered separately, intended for specific benefit to the animal by means other than provision of nutrients recognized as essential or for provision of essential nutrients for intended effect on the animal beyond normal nutritional needs, but not including legally defined drugs." The growth in use of animal dietary supplements has raised several concerns. Among the issues involved are the safety of specific animal dietary supplements and the approaches that should be taken to determine the safety of animal dietary supplements in general. The passage of the Dietary Supplement Health and Education Act (DSHEA) in 1994 amended the way in which human dietary supplements are regulated, but the Center for Veterinary Medicine (CVM) of the Food and Drug Administration (FDA) indicated that the less restrictive regulatory approach of DSHEA should not apply to products intended for animals. Thus, dietary supplements for humans and dietary supplements for animals are subject to regulation under two different sections of the Federal Food, Drug, and Cosmetic Act (FFDCA), even though they may be the same substances, given in the same manner, for the same purpose. Currently FDA and other regulatory bodies are under pressure to resolve the public's desire to provide these products to their animals with the restrictions that exist within the current statutory and regulatory framework.

THE COMMITTEE'S TASK

The committee's assignment was to assess the safety of three dietary supplements (lutein, evening primrose oil, and garlic) offered for horses, dogs, and cats. During its review of the data for each of the three supplements, the committee was asked to examine general considerations that need to be taken into account in determining the safety of animal dietary supplements. The committee was to describe its findings and conclusions about the safety of the three supplements and provide recommendations for factors to consider in future analyses. It was made clear to the committee that the report should address only safety and that utility or efficacy of animal dietary supplements was not part of the task. Thus the committee did not assess the validity of utility or efficacy claims.

The study was requested and sponsored by the CVM of FDA. The report was intended to help form the basis of a more general framework for evaluating animal dietary supplement safety. The primary approach taken by the committee was to examine published scientific reports to assess whether feeding these three supplements to horses, dogs, or cats presents a significant adverse health effect that changes normal function in the animals. Additional information was also received directly from pet food and animal dietary supplement industry representatives. This information was also examined and included when appropriate. The knowledge gained from conducting these assessments allowed the committee to review and begin to define factors that should be considered when evaluating the safety of animal dietary supplements in general.

KEY FINDINGS

A consistent finding from the study of lutein, evening primrose oil, and garlic was that there are insufficient safety data of a quality normally required for animal drugs and animal food additives. Ideally, the committee would have liked to have the data to define a no observed adverse effect level (NOAEL), or at least a safe upper limit (SUL), for each of the three supplements. With the limited data currently available, the committee could only report historical safe intakes and estimate a presumed safe intake (PSI) for the three animal dietary supplements studied. The committee identified a number of data elements for consideration when constructing any framework for assessing animal dietary supplement safety that may be different from those routinely considered for drugs. Because most ingredients in animal dietary supplements are not proprietary substances, it is unlikely that the amount of target animal data will ever be sufficient for safety assessment, and research findings in other species provide important evidence about safety. Based on one of the specific animal dietary supplements studied (e.g., garlic, see Chapter 8), it is clear that safety of the same supplements in humans does not guarantee safety in animals. A number of factors were defined that might be considered when selecting appropriate surrogates for horses, dogs, and cats. Based on an analysis of the available data for animal dietary supplement safety, the committee developed a broad seven-point scale for assessing suitability of different data types.

There is a clear need for a comprehensive adverse event reporting system. Existing systems have limitations because of difficulties in defining dosages, active ingredients, or consistent adverse signals as well as issues with respect to compliance and ease of access. Finally, the absence of laws and regulations that specifically address animal dietary supplements causes considerable confusion to the industry and the public.[1] Clarification is required to enable a clear differentiation between an animal dietary supplement and a food additive or animal drug as well as factors that differentiate regulation of human and animal dietary supplements. The "generally recognized as safe (GRAS)"[2] designation of an ingredient is helpful but does not imply general safety for all species at all levels of intake.

SPECIFIC FINDINGS AND RECOMMENDATIONS

Insufficient Data of Adequate Quality to Quantitatively Establish the Safety of Lutein, Evening Primrose Oil, and Garlic

There are insufficient safety data for these supplements of a quality normally required for animal drugs and food additives, despite the fact that exposure to target populations may be greater. With the limited data currently available, the committee could only estimate a PSI for garlic, evening primrose oil, and lutein. The following factors are important considerations when constructing any framework for assessing animal dietary supplement safety:

- It is crucial to assess the quality and relevance of data used in studies not specifically defined to detect safety. It is important to keep the purpose of the original study in mind. At a minimum, studies require peer review or some level of documented quality assurance. The committee found it very difficult to evaluate the statistical power of the available studies to detect a significant adverse event. Assessment of studies was hampered by such factors as poor definition of signals, lack of sufficient animal numbers, or failure to evaluate for a well-known adverse signal.
- The detection of an actual adverse effect is difficult. In some studies, explanatory information is lacking for adverse events. Sometimes a single case report is all the evidence available for adverse events associated with an animal dietary supplement.
- Validated analytical methods and standards are often lacking. There is often lack of consensus for what the active compound actually is because "activity" is not clearly defined, making standardization by active compound, required for drug studies, impossible. Even if the active compound is known, an acceptable quality standard and validated matrix-appropriate assay for quantitation may not be available or used.
- There are a number of challenges associated with defining dosage of animal dietary supplements. Supplements are often dosed on the basis of intended use and employ units not directly correlated to putative active ingredients. The committee faced the dilemma that doses were neither consistent nor directly related to a common safety endpoint and often varied considerably across studies (e.g., flavor vs. health benefit for garlic).
- Dosage of some supplements (e.g., those not provided in specific dosage forms) is intrinsically different than that associated with drugs, which are dosed on a milligram per kilogram of body weight (BW) basis. However many supplements are incorporated as quantity per unit food. Lack of knowledge of the actual dose of biologically active ingredients given in the studies evaluated by this committee is a major factor that has prevented defining exposure levels associated with lack of adverse events.
- Dietary supplements may be given in combination with other supplements or dietary constituents (e.g., multiple vitamin and supplement preparations), making the attribution of a specific adverse effect to one specific supplement difficult.
- Contaminants and adulterants are a potential issue for all supplements.
- Processing techniques are crucial determinants of final composition and properties.

Use of Nontarget Animal Data

Because of the limited amount of data with target animals, research findings in other species provide important safety signals. Based on the three specific animal dietary supplements studied, it is clear that safety of the same supplements in humans does not guarantee safety in animals. The clearest example of this is with garlic, where excess intakes may cause hemolytic anemia in horses, dogs, and

[1]The report contains minor changes from the prepublication version to clarify that in the United States there are currently no laws and regulations that address animal dietary supplements as a specific group or entity.

[2]In the United States, the term GRAS has a specific legal meaning as discussed in Chapter 2.

cats, which is an adverse effect not described in humans. The committee has identified some factors that might be considered when selecting appropriate surrogates for horses, dogs, and cats:

- Nutritional, metabolic, pharmacokinetic, and natural dietary patterns are important when selecting appropriate animal model species.
- Supplements that are naturally occurring in a diet should be considered differently than those not natural for a given species (e.g., lutein for horses vs. cats).
- Information gleaned from a study of the evolutionary diets of wild and feral species vs. diets of domestic animals may provide some indications of normal intake.

Evaluation of the Suitability of Data for Assessing Animal Dietary Supplement Safety

As a result of conducting these reviews, the committee ranked the suitability of assessing acceptable and relevant data based on the following broad seven-class scale, with class 1 providing the highest degree of confidence. Within each of these classes, it is appropriate to give more credence to data addressing several populations at risk. It should be noted, that for the three supplements assessed by this committee, the highest rank of data found was class 2, with the majority of studies being in class 4, 5, or 6. The classes in the scale were defined as follows:

1. Safety studies conducted in the target species similar to that acceptable for animal drug safety determination.
2. Studies in the target species that specifically assess some marker of potential adverse effect. These studies could include clinical, epidemiological, or defined experimental models.
3. Safety studies in a nontarget species closely related biologically to a target species (e.g. wolf for dog, mink for cat, donkey for horse).
4. Nonsafety (e.g., efficacy or long-term feeding) studies in a target species.
5. Documented historical or common usage in target species; case reports; adverse event database.
6. Safety studies in a more distantly related species, including humans.
7. Ex vivo/in vitro studies.

The committee strongly recommends that animal dietary supplement efficacy studies monitor for specific adverse event signals. Efficacy studies should be accompanied by reasonable attempts to identify and evaluate the risk of potential adverse events. Furthermore, data that have been collected that support potential safety should be clearly described and reported. A simple statement that there were "no adverse effects/events" is of limited value.

Adverse Event Reporting System

There is a clear need for a comprehensive adverse event reporting system. Existing systems are deficient often for the factors discussed above related to difficulty of defining dosages, active ingredients, or consistent adverse signals. The committee's analysis of these supplements has not uncovered a system for adverse reporting that is similar to those in place for drugs. As a committee, we believe that lack of adverse events being reported to a manufacturer is weak evidence for a lack of adverse effects having actually occurred. Although major, life-threatening, adverse events will usually be reported, this may not be the case with less serious events that are not routinely tested for or could be confused with other problems. Similarly, extensive exposure without specifically monitoring biomarkers of adverse effects does not necessarily demonstrate safety.

An adverse event reporting system for animal dietary supplements would be very helpful. This system should be structured to capture the details of dietary exposure (e.g., dose, active ingredient, concomitant supplement, drug or chemical exposure, and disease) and open to public access.

Regulation of Animal Dietary Supplements

The absence of laws and regulations that specifically address animal dietary supplements causes considerable confusion to the industry and the public. Clarification is required to differentiate clearly the regulation of human and animal dietary supplements as well as factors that differentiate an animal dietary supplement from a food additive or animal drug. Any future animal dietary supplement regulations should take into account existing standards such as those of the Association of American Feed Control Officials, Codex, and the analytical standards of United States Pharmacopeia.

Lutein

For horses, the PSI of lutein is 8.3 mg/kg BW when eaten as forage or natural sources; no data exist to support recommendations regarding supplements. In dogs, the PSI of lutein is 1.8 mg/kg BW, with a historical safe intake of 0.45 mg/kg BW. In cats, the PSI of lutein is 7.2 mg/kg BW, with a historical safe intake of 0.85 mg/kg BW.

Evening Primrose Oil

The PSI for evening primrose oil in horses is set at 400 mg/kg BW. This PSI assumes the level of total fat will not exceed 23 percent of the diet by weight, including any quantity of evening primrose oil added. For dogs, the PSI is set at 424 mg/kg BW, which is the upper level used in clinical trials. Most likely the upper safe intake for evening primrose oil is quite a bit higher than this in dogs. For cats, the PSI is set at 391 mg/kg BW; however, it is likely that cats could tolerate higher levels. Because evening primrose oil does not contain adequate amounts of all the essential fatty acids (particularly arachidonic acid, α-linolenic acid, eicosapentaenoic acid, and docosahexaenoic acid) and the cat has limited Δ5- and Δ6-desaturase activities, the main concern when feeding high concentrations of evening primrose oil (particularly above the PSI level) is a deficiency of essential fatty acids.

Garlic

Although more data are needed, intake levels of 15 mg/kg BW/day of dried garlic powder on a long-term basis are unlikely to result in a risk of an adverse event in horses under normal circumstances. Levels up to 90 mg/kg BW/day may not be associated with any adverse events in healthy, nonexercising, nonoxidatively stressed adult horses. The threshold level above which the risk of an adverse event will increase significantly is likely to be between 15 and 200 mg/kg BW of dried garlic, more probably between 90 and 200 mg/kg BW, potentially depending on the health and oxidative status of the individual horse involved. In dogs, garlic has a long history of safe use as a supplement, with mean levels of $\approx$ 22 mg/kg BW being reported with apparently no serious adverse events. Levels of up to 56 mg/kg BW of garlic powder or garlic oil seem to have been included in foods for dogs with no apparent adverse events being reported. For cats, there are insufficient data to support a generic recommendation that covers all the types of garlic preparations. Mean intake levels of 17 mg/kg BW have been reported with apparently no serious adverse events, which is similar to the levels recommended for long-term use with no apparent problems. Currently, however, there seems to be less supportive data for the long-term feeding of cats with garlic-supplemented feeds above this level. This lack, coupled with the potential for an increased susceptibility in cats, means that more data are needed to support the safety of inclusion of garlic at levels above those historically used as a flavor. For these reasons it was not possible to establish a PSI of garlic for cats.

CONCLUSIONS

The committee could not identify data on lutein, evening primrose oil, or garlic that would allow for a quantitative upper limit of safety to be clearly defined (e.g., NOAEL or SUL). This shortage of data resulted in trying to estimate existing intake levels as those presumed to be safe. The committee believes these levels are conservative for lutein and evening primrose oil, but probably more on target for garlic because of the reporting of adverse events. However, for all of the study limitations outlined above, a more precise definition of safe intake levels would be conjecture. Cross-species extrapolations of safety are difficult. The human insensitivity to hemolytic effects of garlic clearly seen in horses, dogs, and cats illustrates this limitation. An adverse event reporting system is badly needed. The existence of such a system, properly constructed, monitored, and open to public scrutiny, might have aided the committee in quantifying safe intake levels. Finally, the absence of laws and regulations that specifically address animal dietary supplements causes considerable confusion to the industry and the public. Clear and precise regulations so that only safe animal dietary supplements are allowed on the market need to be established.

1

Introduction and Background

SIGNIFICANCE OF ANIMALS AND DIETARY SUPPLEMENTS

Horses, dogs, and cats are a major part of contemporary life in the United States and other countries worldwide and constitute a significant budget item of many families. According to the 2007–2008 National Pet Owners Survey conducted by the American Pet Products Manufacturers Association, 63 percent of U.S. households own a pet (APPMA, 2007). The survey indicates that there are 75 million owned dogs and 88 million owned cats in the United States. These numbers do not include the 6 to 8 million dogs and cats that enter shelters each year (HSUS, 2007) or the large numbers of stray animals. It has been estimated that there are 70 million feral cats in the United States (National Geographic, 2004).

The APPMA study also indicated that there are approximately 14 million owned horses in the United States, although the exact number is not known. Another study, conducted for the American Horse Council (AHC, 2005), indicated that there were 9.2 million owned horses in the United States and that 6.6 million of these were used for "showing" and "recreation." The government report Equine 2005, published by the U.S. Department of Agriculture (USDA) National Animal Health Monitoring System (NAHMS, 2007), lists a total equid (horses, ponies, mules, burros, and donkeys) inventory of about 3.75 million in 2002. This survey is limited to farms that include horses as part of a business (commercial) and does not include recreational horse owners.

Expenditures on dogs and cats increased from $21 billion in 1996 to $38.5 billion in 2006 (Figure 1-1), an increase of 43 percent after adjustment for inflation. The APPMA (2007) survey estimated that more than $40 billion would be spent on dogs and cats in the United States during 2007. This represents more than $550 for each household that owns a dog or cat. Feed accounts for 40 percent of these expenditures (Figure 1-2), followed by supplies (24 percent), and over-the-counter medicines and veterinary care (another 24 percent). Although the APPMA survey did not collect data on expenditures for dietary supplements, they are undoubtedly included in each of these three major categories (feed, supplies, and veterinary care). A recent survey among owners estimated that approximately 10 percent of owners administered dietary supplements to their dogs and cats (Freeman et al., 2006). Multivitamins (4.9 percent), chondroprotective agents (2 percent), and fatty acids (1.2 percent) were the most common dietary supplements used.

The AHC (2005) study estimated that the horse industry in the United States contributes $39 billion in direct economic impact to the U.S. economy and supports 1.4 million jobs on a full-time basis. Expenditures on dietary supplements for horses are unknown, but a USDA survey (NAHMS, 1998) found that 4.9 percent of horses on U.S. farms were fed herbal supplements and 3.7 percent were fed chondroitin sulfate.

A trade organization that represents many manufacturers and distributors of dietary supplements for animals is the National Animal Supplement Council (NASC, 2007). This organization has estimated that approximately one-third of horses, dogs, and cats receive a dietary supplement and that the total animal dietary supplement business is a $1.3-billion industry annually (approximately 50 percent for dogs and cats and 50 percent for horses). This value applies only to products sold in specific dosage forms which are similar to human dietary supplements (B. Bookout, personal communication, 2008).

REGULATION OF DIETARY SUPPLEMENTS

Dietary supplements for both humans and animals are subject to regulation under the Federal Food, Drug, and Cosmetic Act (FFDCA). Passage of the Dietary Supplement Health and Education Act (DSHEA) and its signature into law on October 15, 1994, amended the FFDCA to limit and proscribe the regulation of dietary supplements by the Food and Drug Administration (FDA). Although the language of

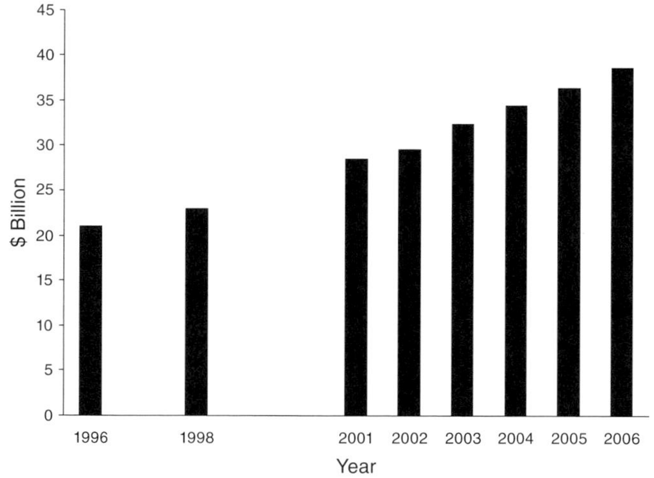

FIGURE 1-1 Annual expenditures on dogs and cats in the United States.
NOTE: Surveys were not conducted in 1997, 1999, and 2000.
SOURCE: Adapted from APPMA (2007).

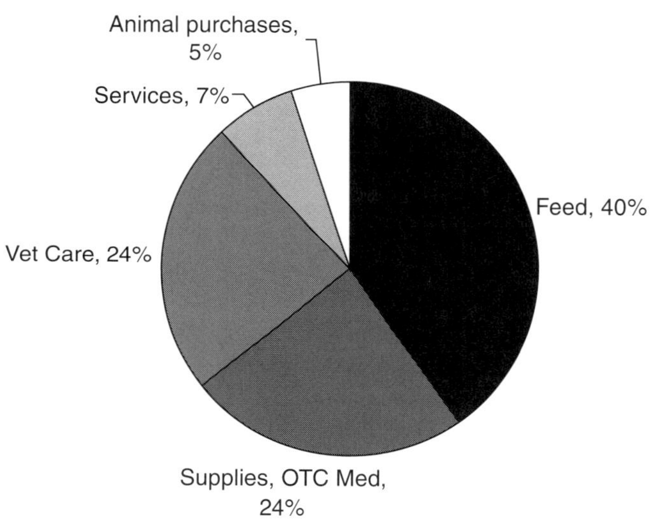

FIGURE 1-2 Categories of expenditures on dogs and cats in the United States in 2006.
NOTE: OTC Med is over-the-counter medicines, Vet Care is veterinary care, and Services include grooming and boarding.
SOURCE: Adapted from APPMA (2007).

DSHEA does not explicitly limit its applicability to supplements for humans, the FDA, in an April 22, 1996, Federal Register notice, stated that there was nothing in the legislative record to indicate that DSHEA should apply to animal products or that Congress believed the law should apply to animals. One of the major concerns of the FDA seems to have been that residues from animals fed dietary supplements could enter the human food chain.

Thus, dietary supplements for humans and dietary supplements for animals are subject to regulation under two different sections of the law, even though they may be the same substances, given in the same manner, for the same purpose. Currently, FDA and other organizations such as the Association of American Feed Control Officials (AAFCO) "are struggling to reconcile the realities of manufacturers' desire to market products containing novel dietary ingredients having nontraditional functions, and the public's desire to purchase these products with the existing statutory and regulatory framework" (Perron and Lambert, 2000). More complete information about the current regulatory environment for dietary supplements for both humans and animals is provided in Chapter 2.

COMMITTEE CHARGE

To assist in making decisions about the safety of dietary supplements for animals, the Center for Veterinary Medicine (CVM) of the FDA commissioned the Board on Agriculture and Natural Resources of the National Academies to produce a report on the safety of supplements in general and to review three specific supplements (lutein, evening primrose oil, and garlic). A committee of experts, consisting of animal nutritionists, veterinarians, clinical pharmacologists, and toxicologists, was established for this purpose and asked to examine the safety of the three different supplements when given orally. The committee's task was to collect and examine data about these supplements and to review factors that should be considered when evaluating the safety of any dietary supplements for horses, dogs, and cats. The results of this examination are intended to provide FDA with sufficient information to assess whether the addition of lutein, evening primrose oil, and garlic to the diets of horses, dogs, or cats may cause a significant adverse health effect that changes normal function in the animals. The FDA will also be able to incorporate information in the report into a framework for evaluating the safety of dietary supplements for animals more generally. The specific statement of task given to the committee is in Box 1-1.

The Committee's Approach to Its Task

The committee held four in-person meetings and several conference calls while preparing this report. The first meeting included an open session during which federal agencies, other organizations, businesses, and interested individuals were able to provide input. The committee also contacted and received helpful information from other organizations, commercial companies, and individuals. A list of those who contributed data or other information is given in Appendix D. Committee members also performed extensive searches of the published scientific literature. The results of these searches provided the primary basis for the conclusions reached, although personal commu-

BOX 1-1
Statement of Task

A committee will collect and examine data related to the safety of three dietary supplements offered for horses, dogs, and cats, whether in feed or separately. During its review of the data for each of the three supplements, the committee will reflect on whether the compounds raise unique issues for safety and on their implications for general and specific considerations that need to be taken into account in determining supplement safety. In a report to the FDA, the committee will describe its findings and conclusions about the safety of the three supplements and provide recommendations for factors to consider in future analyses. Although not meant to be comprehensive, these considerations will help form the basis of a more general framework for evaluating supplement safety.

nications and an established history of usage were also considered.

Boundaries of the Report

To limit the task and enable the committee to produce a report in a relatively short period, several restrictions were established. First, the study addresses only safety, not utility. Although numerous utility studies were examined while seeking data on safety, no effort was made to assess the nutritional or other value of any dietary supplements or the need to supplement the diet of these animals. Second, the study is limited to only three animal species—horses, dogs, and cats. In the United States these animals are not generally consumed as human food and therefore the question of residues from dietary supplements entering the human food chain was not considered. Third, the primary focus of the study was on three specific supplements selected by the CVM—lutein, evening primrose oil, and garlic. Fourth, although factors to be considered in the evaluation of the safety of dietary supplements for animals are discussed in the report, this should not be considered a "framework" report. Decision trees, specific weightings of evidence, and other factors are not part of this study. Finally, the study did not examine any potential effects on human health, such as effects on persons administering the supplement, residues in animal tissues or products, or environmental pollution.

GENERAL TERMINOLOGY AND DEFINITION OF DIETARY SUPPLEMENT

Several technical and scientific terms are used throughout this report. Most of these are well established and are contained in the list of abbreviations and acronyms and glossary in Appendixes B and C. However, the committee struggled with the term "dietary supplement." When DSHEA was enacted, it contained a legal definition of dietary supplement (Box 1-2). Although there is little in the definition to preclude its application to supplements intended for animals, the FDA decision that DSHEA does not apply to products for animals makes the use of the term problematic. Furthermore, for the purpose of this report, the DSHEA definition does not accurately describe the substances and products of interest to the CVM. The committee initially attempted to avoid the term in this report and considered numerous alternates (e.g., nutraceutical, nutritional supplement, oral supplement, novel ingredient, functional food, phytomedicinal, and dosage form animal health products), but none was considered satisfactory. The committee therefore decided to use the term "animal dietary supplement," as defined in Box 1-3.

BOX 1-2
Legal Definition of a Dietary Supplement as Defined by the Dietary Supplement Health and Education Act of 1994

The term dietary supplement means a product (other than tobacco) intended to supplement the diet that bears or contains one or more of the following dietary ingredients:

(A) a vitamin;
(B) a mineral;
(C) an herb or other botanical;
(D) an amino acid;
(E) a dietary substance for use by man to supplement the diet by increasing the total dietary intake; or
(F) a concentrate, metabolite, constituent, extract, or combination of any ingredient described in clause (A), (B), (C), (D), or (E).

Dietary supplements are further defined as products that are labeled as dietary supplements and are not represented for use as a conventional food or as a sole item of a meal or the diet. Supplements can be marked for ingestion in a variety of dosage forms including capsule, powder, softgel, gelcap, tablet, liquid, or, indeed, any other form so long as they are not represented as conventional foods or as sole items of a meal or of the diet.

SOURCE: IOM-NRC (Institute of Medicine-National Research Council), 2005.

BOX 1-3
Animal Dietary Supplement

A substance for oral consumption by horses, dogs, or cats, whether in/on feed or offered separately, intended for specific benefit to the animal by means other than provision of nutrients recognized as essential or for provision of essential nutrients for intended effect on the animal beyond normal nutritional needs, but not including legally defined drugs (Committee definition).

The committee's definition of "animal dietary supplement" deviates significantly in several respects from the DSHEA definition of "dietary supplement." The DSHEA definition applies only to products in specific form (e.g., pills, powders, liquids, bars, drinks) that are labeled as "dietary supplements" and are not represented as conventional food or as sole items of a meal or diet. Further, they must contain one or more dietary ingredients, which may include dietary essential nutrients such as vitamins, minerals, and amino acids. On the other hand, the committee's definition applies to ingredients of products in any form, including standalone supplements, added to conventional animal feed items, or even as components of a complete ration. Also, the committee's definition expressly excludes recognized dietary essential nutrients unless provided in excess of normal nutritional needs. This was done to encompass more precisely the range of substances of interest as stipulated by CVM in its charge to the committee.

Figure 1-3 shows the various components of an animal's diet. As illustrated in the figure, animal dietary supplements can be provided in feeds, treats, or water or separately. The terms in Figure 1-3 are defined in the Glossary (Appendix C). Thus, for the purpose of this report, "animal dietary supplements" are not only distinct from human dietary supplements but also from primary feed ingredients, feed/food additives, and drugs. They are considered a category by themselves, although from a regulatory standpoint no such category currently exists in the United States.

ORGANIZATION OF THE REPORT

The next chapter of this report reviews the current laws that regulate dietary supplements in the United States. The chapter covers both supplements intended for humans and those for animals. The history of regulation is described and potential modifications to current approaches are discussed.

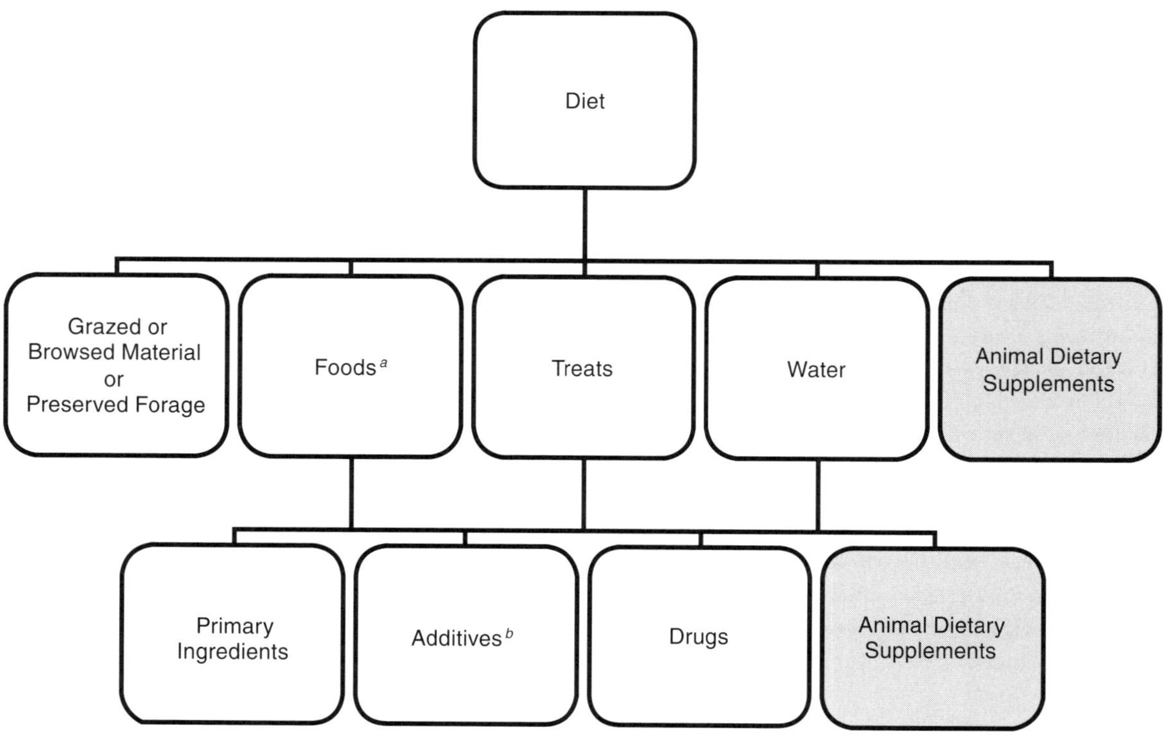

FIGURE 1-3 Components or final products of animal diets.
[a]Also known as feeds or formula feeds.
[b]Additives are generally called feed additives (AAFCO) and food additives (FFDCA)—see Glossary (Appendix C).
NOTE: See Glossary (Appendix C) for additional definitions of terms.

Chapters 3, 4, and 5 provide information that must be considered in the evaluation of safety of dietary supplements for animals. Chapter 3 covers the various elements of safety assessment such as different types of adverse events, Chapter 4 discusses a wide range of safety issues such as the dose and duration of administration, and Chapter 5 reviews the various categories of scientific evidence.

In the following three chapters, the safety of three dietary supplements for the three animal species is reviewed: Chapter 6 covers lutein, Chapter 7 discusses evening primrose oil, and Chapter 8 presents garlic.

Finally, Chapter 9 provides a review of general considerations in determining safety of animal dietary supplements.

REFERENCES

AHC (American Horse Council Foundation). 2005. The Economic Impact of the Horse Industry on the United States. Online at: horsecouncil.org/publications.html. Accessed November 29, 2007.

APPMA (American Pet Products Manufacturers Association). 2007. National Pet Owners Survey. Online at: www.appma.org. Accessed August 23, 2007.

Freeman, L. M., S. K. Abood, A. J. Fascetti, L. M. Fleeman, K. E. Michel, D. P. Laflamme, C. Bauer, B. L. E. Kemp, J. R. Van Doren, and K. N. Willoughby. 2006. Disease prevalence among dogs and cats in the United States and Australia and proportions of dogs and cats that receive therapeutic diets or dietary supplements. J. Am. Vet. Med. Assoc. 229:531–534.

HSUS (Humane Society of the United States). 2007. Pet Overpopulation Estimates. Online at: www.hsus.org. Accessed August 23, 2007.

IOM-NRC (Institute of Medicine-National Research Council). 2005. Dietary Supplements: A Framework for Evaluating Safety. Washington, DC: The National Academies Press.

NAHMS (National Animal Health Monitoring System). 1998. Equine '98, Part II: Baseline Reference of 1998 Equine Health and Management. Online at: http://www.aphis.usda.gov/vs/ceah/ncahs/nahms/equine/equine98/eq98pt2.pdf. Accessed November 8, 2007.

NAHMS. 2007. Equine 2005, Part II: Changes in the U.S. Equine Industry, 1998–2005. Online at: http://www.aphis.usda.gov/vs/ceah/ncahs/nahms/equine/equine05/equine05_report_part2_trends.pdf. Accessed November 8, 2007.

NASC (National Animal Supplement Council). 2007. Situation Analysis. Online at: http://www.nasc.cc/Situation_Analysis.aspx. Accessed September 17, 2007.

National Geographic. 2004. U.S. Faces Growing Feral Cat Problem. Online at: http://news.nationalgeographic.com/news/2004/09/0907_040907_feralcats.html. Accessed January 4, 2008.

Perron, J., and E. I. Lambert. 2000. DSHEA and structure/function claims for animal feed. Food Drug Law J. 55:151–183.

2

Regulation of Dietary Supplements in the United States

The passage of the Dietary Supplement Health and Education Act (DSHEA) in 1994 had a dramatic impact on the dietary supplement market for both human and animal consumption. While DSHEA itself arguably did not affect prevailing law as it applies to regulation of products intended for animal use, the influx of a great number of dietary supplements of all types available for people as a result of the change in law increased consumer expectations as to the availability of similar products for animal consumption. Since that time, the market has been attempting to fill the void, notwithstanding significant regulatory restrictions. To understand how animal dietary supplements are currently regulated in the United States, an overview of the regulation of human dietary supplements is warranted.

REGULATION OF DIETARY SUPPLEMENTS FOR HUMAN CONSUMPTION

In the United States, dietary supplements intended for consumption by humans are regulated under the provisions of the DSHEA. The act amends the Federal Food, Drug, and Cosmetic Act of 1938 (FFDCA) to place dietary supplements under the umbrella of "foods," but in a special category (FDA, 2001). Products in this category are afforded allowances with respect to ingredients and labeling that are not granted to foods in "conventional" form. On the other hand, there are regulatory requirements for dietary supplements that do not apply to conventional foods.

According to DSHEA, a dietary supplement is a product taken by mouth that contains one or more of the following "dietary ingredients": a vitamin; a mineral; an herb or other botanical; an amino acid; a dietary substance for use by man to supplement the diet by increasing the total dietary intake (e.g., enzymes or tissues from organs or glands); or a concentrate, metabolite, constituent, extract or combination of the aforementioned substances (FDA, 1995a). It excludes tobacco and approved drugs, certified antibiotics, and licensed biologics. The DSHEA definition of "dietary supplement" can be found in Chapter 1, Box 1-2.

Dietary supplements are most often available in dosage form (e.g., tablet, capsule, liquid, or powder), but may be in forms such as bars or drinks, as long as the labeling does not represent the product to be a conventional food or intended to be the sole item of a meal or diet. It must be clearly identified as a "supplement" on the label.

Ingredients and Manufacturing of Dietary Supplements for Human Consumption

A major exemption for dietary supplements from the laws pertaining to permissible ingredients in food has resulted from passage of DSHEA. Normally, ingredients that are not "generally recognized as safe" (GRAS) substances, prior sanctioned for use in food (i.e., expressly approved by FDA before passage of the Food Additives Amendment of 1958), or otherwise excluded from the definition (e.g., color additives, allowed pesticides or pesticide residues, approved new animal drugs) are deemed "food additives" [21 USC 321(s)]. The FDA must approve food additives through submission of data adequate to prove safety as well as to establish utility (i.e., the food additive will have the intended physical or technical effect, may reasonably be expected to become a component, or to directly or indirectly affect the characteristics of the food) [21 CFR 571.1(c)C] prior to marketing (see the section on Regulatory Assessment of Safety later in this chapter). Foods containing ingredients that are not approved food additives, GRAS substances, or prior sanctioned are subject to regulatory action as adulterated foods. Possible actions include seizure of the noncompliant product, injunction against the manufacturer or distributor, or, in the most egregious cases, criminal charges.

However, the law as amended by DSHEA expressly notes that dietary ingredients in or intended for use in a dietary supplement are *not* food additives and are exempt from the premarket safety evaluations normally required for new food ingredients (FDA, 1995a). Also, DSHEA does not dictate minimum or maximum amounts of nutrients or other dietary ingredients per serving of dietary supplements. In other words, although it is the responsibility of the manufacturer or distributor to ensure the product is safe when used as recommended, FDA has no authority to review safety data for dietary supplements before they reach the consumer.

There is, however, a premarket notification procedure for a "new dietary ingredient." This is defined as a substance that meets one of the categories of "dietary ingredient" as defined by DSHEA that was not marketed in a dietary supplement prior to passage of DSHEA on October 15, 1994 (FDA, 1995a). Substances in use in dietary supplements prior to the act are exempt from the notification requirement. There is no authoritative list of these "grandfathered" ingredients, however, so it is the burden of the manufacturer or distributor to document pre-DSHEA use.

For a dietary supplement containing a new dietary ingredient, a manufacturer or distributor must notify FDA at least 75 days prior to introducing the product into interstate commerce unless the new dietary ingredient is chemically identical to a substance already in the food supply [21 CFR 190.6]. Accompanying the notification must be the name of the new ingredient, a description of its inclusion rates and conditions of use, and evidence to show why the ingredient may be reasonably expected to be safe when used as directed on the label of the dietary supplement. Suitable evidence may include history of use or citations from the published scientific literature, but FDA has not issued guidelines as to the type and extent of data likely to be deemed sufficient to demonstrate reasonable expectations of safety.

Use of a new dietary ingredient for which there is insufficient evidence of safety when used as recommended on the label of the dietary supplement may render the supplement adulterated and subject to enforcement action. The FDA may also take action if a dietary supplement presents a significant or unreasonable risk of illness or injury under conditions of use recommended in labeling (or if no conditions are specified, under ordinary conditions of use), if it contains a poisonous or deleterious substance that may render it injurious to health under the conditions of use recommended or suggested in the labeling, or if the secretary of health and human services declares it poses an imminent hazard to public health or safety (FDA, 1995a). Under all these provisions, FDA bears the burden of proof to show that a dietary supplement is adulterated prior to action against a marketed product. This is exactly opposite in the case of a conventional food containing an unapproved food additive, where it is the burden of the manufacturer or distributor to demonstrate the ingredient is safe. To date, only one dietary ingredient, ephedrine alkaloids, has been codified in the regulations as presenting an unreasonable risk of illness or injury [21 CFR 119.1].

In 2007, FDA issued its final rule regarding Good Manufacturing Practices (GMPs) for dietary supplements separate and distinct from those already required for foods (FDA, 2007a). Provisions in the rule include minimum requirements for the design and construction of physical plants, sanitation, manufacturing operations, quality control procedures, testing of final product or incoming and inprocess materials, handling of consumer complaints, and maintenance of records. Products not manufactured in accordance with GMPs after they became effective in June 2008 may be considered to be adulterated and subject to enforcement action as such. However, to accommodate small businesses, full compliance by some manufacturers may not be required until June 2010.

Labeling of Dietary Supplements for Human Consumption

Labeling requirements for dietary supplements are similar to foods, in that a label must bear a suitably descriptive name of the product, the name and place of business of the manufacturer or distributor, a complete list of ingredients, nutrition labeling (if the small-business exemption is not applicable), and a net content declaration (FDA, 2001). However, the format in which some of this information is provided may differ. For example, the nutrition labeling takes the form of a "Supplement Facts" panel, similar in presentation to the "Nutrition Facts" panel required on all conventional food labels [21 CFR 101.36]. The Supplement Facts panel must list the serving size (e.g., "two tablets"), each dietary ingredient present in the product (and, if necessary, the source of the dietary ingredient), and the amounts of each of these ingredients per serving. Exceptions are made for "proprietary blends" of dietary ingredients, in which case only the total amount of the blend per serving must be declared. Dietary ingredients for which a Reference Daily Intake (RDI) or Daily Reference Value (DRV) has been established must also declare a "% Daily Value." Ingredients without established values must be indicated as "Daily Value not established."

As with conventional food labeling, all ingredients in the product must be declared on the dietary supplement label. However, unlike conventional food labels, where all ingredients must be declared together in descending order of predominance by weight irrespective of their function, those ingredients in dietary supplements already declared in the Supplement Facts panel do not have to be repeated in the ingredient list. Rather, only those not declared in the Supplement Facts panel (e.g., excipients, fillers, artificial colors, sweeteners, flavors, or binders) are listed under "other ingredients," immediately below the Supplement Facts panel [21 CFR 101.4 (a)(1)].

Since dietary supplements are "foods" by law, they are restricted in the types of claims that can be made on the label or labeling and are strictly prohibited from labeling that would indicate or imply intended use for the treatment, prevention, cure, mitigation, or diagnosis of disease. This is because such a claim would identify the intent to offer the product as a "drug." Further, because that drug was not subject to approval by FDA through submission of sufficient data to prove safety and efficacy for that intended use, it would be subject to enforcement action as an "adulterated drug."

There are exceptions, however. For example, claims of benefit related to a classical nutrient deficiency disease, for example, vitamin C and scurvy (provided it discloses the prevalence of such disease in the United States), may be considered a "food," and not a "disease" claim. Also, dietary supplements and other foods may make "health claims" or "qualified health claims" that relate the level of a nutrient or dietary substance with a disease process (e.g., calcium and osteoporosis, sodium and hypertension), provided that the claim has been expressly approved and codified by FDA (FDA, 2003).

The statutory definition of "drug" also includes articles intended to affect the structure or function of the body, with the caveat "other than food." Foods, through provision of nutrients to the body, do have an effect on normal structure or function. For example, calcium is a dietary essential nutrient necessary for proper bone formation and maintenance. Therefore, claims relating to this property of food (e.g., "with calcium for strong bones") are allowed and precede passage of DSHEA.

However, DSHEA extends the means by which dietary supplements may make certain "structure/function" statements compared to conventional foods. In addition to claims relating to the normal role of dietary essential nutrients as allowed for any food, DSHEA also allows dietary supplement labels to describe the role of any dietary ingredient in the product intended to affect structure or function, even for those ingredients without recognized nutritive value. For example, a herbal dietary supplement containing saw palmetto may claim its presence "to help support a healthy prostate," despite the fact that its function in affecting prostate health is not necessarily related to provision of specific vitamins, minerals, or other known dietary essential nutrients. A similar claim would not be acceptable on a conventional food label. In addition, DSHEA allows dietary supplement labels to characterize the documented mechanism by which a dietary ingredient acts to maintain such structure or function, or to describe general well-being from consumption of a dietary ingredient.

There are still some restrictions. First, structure/function claims must be accompanied by the disclaimer "This statement has not been evaluated by the Food and Drug Administration. This product is not intended to diagnose, treat, cure, or prevent any disease." Also, no later than 30 days after first marketing a dietary supplement whose label bears a structure/function claim, the manufacturer or distributor must notify FDA that it has included such a statement on the label or labeling of its product [21 CFR 101.93]. In addition to the name of the product and text of the claim, the notification must include certification from the responsible party that the information contained in the notice is complete and accurate and that the party has substantiation that the statement is truthful and not misleading. The FDA will review the notification and will require correction of the label or labeling if it finds the statements to be "disease" claims or otherwise objectionable.

REGULATION OF ANIMAL DIETARY SUPPLEMENTS

In a notice published in the Federal Register on April 22, 1996, FDA opined that Congress neither considered nor intended DSHEA to apply to dietary supplement products intended for use in animals (Federal Register, 1996). Evidence to that effect comes from repeated references in DSHEA and its supporting documentation of dietary supplements "for use by man," or for "improving health status of United States citizens," with no hint at contemplated use of supplements in animals. Further, FDA concluded that DSHEA should not apply to animal products for several reasons.

First, a prevailing rationale for passage of DSHEA was the purported long history of use of dietary substances by humans to beneficially affect health without significant risk of illness or injury. However, FDA found a paucity of historical evidence or scientific data to show the same from use in animals. Another reason is that application of DSHEA to animal products would circumvent a key safety consideration of approval of new animal drugs and food additives, namely, review of data to show the absence of unsafe residues in meat, milk, or eggs of animals consuming the substance. Finally, DSHEA would unfairly allow "production claims" (i.e., claims to affect performance, such as weight gain, feed efficiency, or milk yield), while for products that were not covered under DSHEA, the same statements would be considered to be drug claims requiring premarket clearance.

To date, FDA's opinion on the inapplicability of DSHEA, in whole or in part, to animal products has been subject to intellectual discourse, but not challenged by any legal procedure (Perron and Lambert, 2000). Without DSHEA, the provisions in the prevailing law (Federal Food, Drug, and Cosmetic Act) apply to animal products. As such, animal dietary supplements are typically regulated simply as "food" without the special consideration afforded human dietary supplement products. However, there may be plans to regulate some animal dietary supplements as drugs (see the section on Animal Dietary Supplements as Drugs later in this chapter).

Ingredients and Manufacturing of Animal Dietary Supplements

Because DSHEA does not apply to animal dietary supplements, all ingredients in both conventional feed or dosage form products must be GRAS, approved food additives, or otherwise sanctioned for use in animal feed. A product containing an unapproved food additive may be subject to enforcement action by FDA or individual state feed control officials. Many states require registration of products and/or licensure of companies before products may be distributed in that state. In addition to the remedies imposed by FDA, states often have the additional power to simply deny registration/licensure.

The Association of American Feed Control Officials (AAFCO) Feed Ingredient Definition process is another means by which an ingredient may be sanctioned for use in animal feeds (AAFCO, 2007). Although AAFCO is a private organization, its members are all federal, state, or foreign government officials charged with the regulation of animal feeds in their respective jurisdictions. In fulfilling its mission to achieve uniformity in animal feed regulation, AAFCO publishes a Model Bill and Regulations that are subsequently adopted and enforced by a majority of states. While an ingredient that passes the AAFCO feed ingredient definition process is still an unapproved food additive from FDA's perspective, FDA is integrally involved in the process, and the agency most often reviews data to determine safety of the feed ingredient for its intended use prior to acceptance by AAFCO. Therefore, FDA most often chooses to exercise enforcement discretion, and does not initiate or recommend action against a product solely by virtue of it containing an AAFCO-defined, albeit not formally "approved," ingredient. Recently, AAFCO and FDA signed a Memorandum of Understanding wherein FDA will assume more direct responsibility for the AAFCO Definition process, which will allow FDA to formally recognize AAFCO-defined ingredients (FDA, 2007b).

The FDA and state feed control officials may also exercise enforcement discretion when it comes to non-AAFCO-defined ingredients, provided certain conditions are met. The best example of this is glucosamine and chondroitin sulfate. While they do meet the definition of "dietary ingredient" as codified by DSHEA for human dietary supplements, neither ingredient is GRAS, an approved food additive, or AAFCO-defined for use in animal feeds. However, most states do not deny registration of products containing these ingredients as long as the labels otherwise meet the state's requirements (see the section on Labeling of Animal Dietary Supplements later in this chapter). The Office of the Texas State Chemist imposes additional restrictions, however (OTSC, 1999). In Texas, use of glucosamine (hydrochloride form only) and chondroitin sulfate are permitted in dog products intended for adult maintenance only (i.e., not to be used in products for puppies or gestating/lactating bitches or in products for species other than dogs). Also under the Texas policy, maximum inclusion rates are limited to those that would provide no more than 15 mg/kg body weight (BW) per day of glucosamine and 12 mg/kg BW per day of chondroitin sulfate when the product is fed as recommended on the label.

Except for dog and cat food products intended to serve as the sole source of nutrition ("complete and balanced"), AAFCO does not dictate minimum or maximum amounts of nutrients allowed in a product. Thus, there are no explicit restrictions in AAFCO on nutrient content of animal dietary supplements. However, FDA does have a Compliance Policy Guide that stipulates a dog or cat supplement product (for purposes of this policy, defined as products containing vitamins, minerals, protein, fatty acids, or similar nutrients) must contain "nutritionally meaningful" amounts of the nutrients it purports to contain (FDA, 1995b). This has been interpreted as a minimum of 10 percent of the dog's or cat's minimal daily requirement of the nutrient for its given body size and life stage as recommended in the 2006 National Research Council publication *Nutrient Requirements of Dogs and Cats*, when the product is fed as recommended (NRC, 2006; Dzanis, 2007). When no minimal requirement is recommended, the adequate intake value is used (Dzanis, 2007). Presumably, FDA also would act if the supplement delivered a nutrient in excess of any established safe upper limit on a body weight per day basis. Also, since this policy appears to pertain only to nutrients for which dietary recommendations have been established by the NRC, it could not be used to dictate "meaningful" amounts of non-dietary essential substances such as herbs or glucosamine.

Except for feeds containing an approved new animal drug ("medicated feeds") or canned foods, at present there are no GMPs applicable to animal feeds. Both AAFCO and FDA are developing regulations to address this lack of oversight of the manufacturing process.

Labeling of Animal Dietary Supplements

Regardless of form (conventional or supplement), all animal feeds must comply with labeling requirements as stipulated by FDA and each state in which the products are distributed. Because a majority of states follow the AAFCO Model Regulations to some degree, any product in regional or national distribution usually must follow the models. The federal regulations for labeling of animal feeds are not as extensive as those developed for human foods. They cover the basic requirements for a proper statement of identity, net content declaration, ingredient list, and manufacturer's or distributor's name and address [21 CFR 501]. The FDA regulations do not address nutrient content. Rather, these requirements appear in the AAFCO Model Regulations.

Under AAFCO, nutrient content must be declared in terms of a "guaranteed analysis," not a "Nutrition Facts" or "Supplement Facts" panel as required on human product labels (AAFCO, 2007). In most cases, the guaranteed analysis includes a declaration of minimum percentages of crude protein and crude fat, and maximum percentage of crude fiber. There is exception from requirement for any or all of these guarantees when the product is intended for purposes other than to furnish these substances or of minor significance relative to the product's primary purpose (i.e., a vitamin or mineral supplement). Dog and cat food labels, but not horse feed labels, must also declare a maximum percentage moisture content, without exception.

For horse feed products in either conventional or dosage form, labels must make additional guarantees for minimum content of specified minerals and vitamins when added or the product is represented or serves as a principal source of those nutrients. Labels of dog and cat foods in conventional form must bear additional guarantees of minimum content to support claims for nutrient content made in the labeling, but are otherwise voluntary. However, if the dog or cat food is formulated or represented to provide supplemental vitamins or minerals (in either conventional or dosage form), then guarantees of minimum content of every vitamin or mineral in the product (as evidenced by its listing in the ingredient declaration) are required.

Guarantees for minimum content of substances that are not listed in the AAFCO Dog and Cat Food Nutrient Profiles, such as glucosamine and chondroitin sulfate, must be listed after all other required or voluntary guarantees. Each guarantee for a non-AAFCO-recognized substance must be accompanied by an asterisk, leading the reader to a second asterisk and disclaimer immediately below and the same type size as the last guarantee that reads "Not recognized as an essential nutrient by the Dog (or Cat) Food Nutrient Profiles."

With respect to allowable label claims, there are no provisions by FDA or AAFCO to distinguish those made for animal dietary supplements from those made for any other animal feed. As such, no claims that indicate or imply treatment, prevention, or similar effect on a disease or condition may be made. Structure/function claims are limited to those related to a recognized nutritional function of the substance, e.g., "taurine helps maintain a healthy heart in cats" or "methionine is an essential amino acid important for healthy muscle growth." Claims for effects that go beyond classical nutritional principles are generally objectionable as "drug" claims. However, in the case of glucosamine and chondroitin sulfate, statements such as "for healthy joints" are typically tolerated by regulators.

While there is no written policy on the matter, FDA objects to animal product labels bearing the "Not evaluated by FDA/Not intended to treat, prevent disease" disclaimer required under DSHEA for human dietary products bearing structure/function claims. This is because it may falsely imply applicability of DSHEA to animal products. For the same reason, FDA discourages labeling of animal products as "dietary supplements," although similar verbiage, such as "food supplement" or "nutritional supplement," is generally acceptable.

Animal Dietary Supplements as Drugs

While typically regulated as foods, there is interest by both regulators and segments of the industry in regulating some animal dietary supplements as drugs. The FDA does exercise enforcement discretion to allow some drugs on the market without formal approval provided certain conditions are met (FDA, 2007c). Some examples of "unapproved drugs of low regulatory priority" include petrolatum-based cat hairball treatment products, some topical agents, and products equivalent to human over-the-counter drugs.

There is no general guidance as to what may qualify an unapproved drug for low-priority status, and FDA decides the status of a substance on a case-by-case basis. However, from guidance available for drugs intended for use in aquaculture, some insight as to FDA's criteria may be derived (FDA, 2007c). Some of the conditions to allow "low regulatory priority" status of unapproved drugs would appear to include lack of availability of an approved drug for a similar intended purpose; reasonable expectations of safety and effectiveness in the target animal when used as directed; and human food, environmental, and occupational safety. Products granted low-priority status must conform to labeling required for drugs, which may include removal of claims that connote use as food or nutritive value. Products must be drug-listed, and must conform to pharmaceutical GMPs as codified in 21 CFR 211.

Labeling an animal dietary supplement as a drug has some potential advantages for manufacturers and distributors. Since it is no longer "food," the product escapes the authority of most state feed control officials. However, some states enforce "animal remedy" laws as well as feed laws. Although FDA retains authority over whether the product is a food or drug, the restrictions on ingredients and labeling of foods do not apply. While the ingredients and type and extent of claims allowed on low-priority drugs are left to FDA's discretion, in most cases it is more lax than if the product was regulated as a food.

With respect to disadvantages, products containing what would be an unapproved food additive are now and forever drugs under the law. The marketing advantage of dietary supplements as nondrug alternatives to maintenance of health is lost. Also, as unapproved drugs, FDA reserves the right to take enforcement action against these products at any time (but typically chooses not to unless new information raises question as to safety) (FDA, 2007c). Finally, at the present time, the use of dietary ingredients in feeds are regulated the same manner, regardless of whether they are added to a conventional feed or provided in a dosage form product. Because conventional feeds cannot easily meet the labeling and other conditions put on low-priority drugs by FDA, this approach arguably creates an unfair advantage for products in dosage form.

The FDA intends to issue a Compliance Policy Guide for products containing glucosamine and chondroitin sulfate. Although the details have not been released, it is anticipated that the guide will stipulate that products marketed in dosage form containing these ingredients are to be regulated as unapproved drugs of low regulatory priority. It is unclear if and how this affects conventional feeds containing these substances, or whether this guidance will be used as a template for regulation of other animal dietary supplements in dosage form.

REGULATORY ASSESSMENT OF SAFETY

There are several means by which the safety of a new feed ingredient may be established. In this section, regulatory requirements for demonstrating safety of a feed ingredient are compared to that required for drug approval.

Food Additives

Food additives are substances other than those exempted under the Federal Food, Drug, and Cosmetic Act that are intended to result or may be reasonably expected to result in becoming a component or otherwise affecting, directly or indirectly, the characteristics of a food [21 USC 321(s)]. Exempt substances include those determined to be generally recognized as safe (GRAS) for its intended use. Examples of food additives include nutrients, preservatives, and other processing aids, as well as substances that may migrate to the food by contact with packaging. For purposes of regulation, ionizing radiation is a food additive.

Food additives must be approved by FDA prior to marketing. Among other requirements for approval, the petitioner must submit data sufficient to prove reasonable certainty in the minds of competent scientists that the substance is not harmful under the intended conditions of use [21 CFR 570].

The Food Additive Petition must include full reports of all available data regarding safety of the food additive use [21 CFR 571]. These data should address issues of acute, subchronic, and chronic toxicity; mutagenicity; teratogenicity; and carcinogenicity. Each report should clearly describe methods used, as well as detailed findings from appropriate animal and other biological experiments. The petition may not omit any reports of investigations that would bias an evaluation of the safety of the food additive without explanation.

In determining safety, FDA considers the specific biological properties of the compound and the adequacy of the methods employed to demonstrate safety for the proposed use, the probable consumption of the substance and of any substance formed in or on food because of its use, the cumulative effect of the substance in the diet (taking into account any chemically or pharmacologically related substance or substances in such diet), and other safety factors considered appropriate in the opinion of experts [21 CFR 570.3]. The regulations indicate that FDA is guided by the principles and procedures for establishing the safety of food additives stated in current publications of the National Academy of Sciences-National Research Council, although a petition will not be denied simply because procedures other than outlined in those publications were followed [21 CFR 570.20]. In practice, the type and extent of data normally required to prove safety of a New Animal Drug is sufficient.

Generally Recognized as Safe (GRAS) Substances

General recognition of safety requires common knowledge about a substance throughout the scientific community knowledgeable about the safety of substances added to food [21 CFR 570.30]. This common knowledge may be established by documentation of a history of use in feeds or foods or by scientific procedures. This determination must be conducted by experts qualified by scientific training and experience to evaluate the substance's safety.

The FDA has codified a list of substances it considers GRAS for intended use in animal feed in its regulations. For the most part, this list includes substances known to be safely used in food prior to 1958 (the year the Food Additives Amendments were enacted). However, FDA recognizes that because of the large number of substances that may be used in feed, it is impractical to list all substances that may be GRAS [21 CFR 582.1]. Examples by FDA of noncodified GRAS substances are salt, pepper, sugar, vinegar, baking powder, and monosodium glutamate. A feed ingredient will ordinarily be regarded as GRAS without specific inclusion in the regulations if it is of natural biological origin, has been widely consumed for its nutrient properties prior to 1958, is subject only to conventional processing as practiced prior to 1958, and has resulted in no known detrimental effects from consumption of the substance as processed [21 CFR 570.30(d)], although that does not necessarily exclude substances that do not meet these provisions from also becoming GRAS. In other words, most ingredients with long histories of use in feed are GRAS, as are all substances shown to be safe under the intended conditions of use, whether through historical precedent or through scientific procedures.

However, designation as GRAS does not mean that the substance cannot be toxic. Cholecalciferol (vitamin D_3) is GRAS, for example, but excess amounts in the diet may have severe adverse consequences. To be considered GRAS, substances may only be used for their intended purposes, and some GRAS regulations specify conditions or limitations of use, such as maximum amounts that may be added to feed, type of feed to which it can be added, or species for which the feed is intended. All GRAS substances, however, must be used in accordance with good manufacturing or feeding practice. It is the burden of the manufacturer or distributor to ensure that GRAS substances are consumed at safe levels when fed as recommended. Safe practice also requires use of a substance that is of appropriate grade and is prepared and handled as a food ingredient. Further, the quantity of a substance added to animal food should not exceed the amount reasonably required to accomplish its intended physical, nutritional, or other technical effect in food, although the regulations do not specify how that amount should be determined. In the case where a substance becomes a component of animal food as a result of its use in the manufacturing, processing, or packaging of food, and which is not intended to accomplish any physical or other technical effect in the food itself, the quantity should be reduced to the extent reasonably possible. Substances that are not used for their intended purposes, or used contrary to specified or general conditions or limitations, are not GRAS. For example, rosemary extract, which is GRAS as a flavor in animal feed under 21 CFR 582.20, is not GRAS if used as a food preservative. Thus, any indication on the label for preservative function of rosemary extract would identify its intended use beyond that provided for by the regulation, effectively negating its GRAS status in that circumstance. Further, in a 2006 letter to the pet food industry, FDA opined that the typical use levels of rosemary extract in animal feed as a flavoring agent was ≤ 50 ppm (Nancy K. Cook, Pet Food Institute, personal communication). At these levels of inclusion, its function as a preservative is presumed negligible by FDA. Thus, it may be inferred from FDA comments that any use of rosemary extract in excess of 50 ppm in the final feed product would be considered de facto evidence of use for non-GRAS purposes, regardless of any stated intended use.

A manufacturer may conduct its own determination of GRAS status for a substance without submission of data to FDA. The FDA regulations dictate a formal procedure by which a substance may be considered GRAS through the filing of an Affirmation Petition [21 CFR 570]. The FDA would review the data to support safe use, and if it agreed, would codify the substance as such. However, at this time, FDA is moving from this system to a notification process, wherein the manufacturer notifies FDA of the basis by which it determined the substance to be GRAS, including data used in the determination. FDA would then have 90 days upon which to respond if it disagreed with the manufacturer's conclusion. If FDA does not respond, it does not mean the agency has reached an independent conclusion that the substance is GRAS, but only that it chooses not to question the GRAS determination. At this time, GRAS notifications are being accepted for human food ingredients, but not animal feed ingredients (FDA, 2007d). Regardless of the process, the data required for GRAS determination are the same for substances intended for addition to human food or animal feed.

The first means to establish safety is through historical use. Common use in food prior to 1958, ordinarily based upon generally available data and information, and sufficient in the views of experts qualified by scientific training and experience to evaluate the safety of substances directly or indirectly added to food, is adequate to establish GRAS status. The regulations do not specify that the historical use must be in the species for which the new use is anticipated. Data from scientific procedures as required for approval of a food additive are not necessary by this means.

The more common means is through documentation of safety through scientific procedures. To be GRAS, the scientific procedures require the same quantity and quality of scientific evidence as is required to obtain approval of a food additive. The distinction between a GRAS substance and a food additive is that for the former, the scientific procedures ordinarily are based upon studies published in the scientific literature, although the determination may be corroborated by unpublished studies as well as other data and information.

The AAFCO Feed Ingredient Definitions

To facilitate uniform interpretation and enforcement of animal feed regulations, AAFCO publishes definitions for commonly used feed ingredients. The FDA has long considered, albeit informally, the definitions to constitute the "common or usual" names of ingredients for purposes of meeting label declarations (FDA, 1995c). More recently, FDA has signed a Memorandum of Understanding with AAFCO to formalize its recognition of AAFCO-defined feed ingredients (FDA, 2007b).

Not all ingredients used in feeds are defined, but state feed control officials may deny registration of a product containing an ingredient not defined by AAFCO unless it is otherwise sanctioned or is known to be a food in common use (e.g., fruits and vegetables). A procedure to incorporate new or modified ingredient definitions has been established (AAFCO, 2007).

In addition to other required information (name and description of ingredient, purpose, data to support utility, manufacturing methods), petitioners for a new ingredient definition must submit information sufficient to provide reasonable assurances of safety when used as recommended. This information is forwarded to FDA for review prior to acceptance by AAFCO.

Data to support safety may include published literature citations and observations from unpublished studies and feeding trials conducted by the petitioner or third party (Ekelman, 2004). The "No Observed Adverse Effect Level" (NOAEL) as determined by the studies is divided by a suitable safety factor to derive an "Acceptable Daily Intake" (ADI). The ADI is compared to estimates of intake of the ingredient in animals when fed the ingredient as recommended. Generally, the ADI must be greater than the estimated intake to allow for safe use.

The quantity and quality of data required to support safety of a new feed ingredient are similar to those required for a food additive. However, if data suggest that an ingredient or one of its components is a potential carcinogen, FDA is likely to reject the proposal for an AAFCO ingredient definition and require a formal Food Additive Petition be submitted and approved prior to marketing.

Considerations are also given to the expected duration of consumption, although in the case of feed ingredients for dogs, cats, and horses, lifetime feeding is not unusual. Feed ingredients that may constitute a large percent of the diet (> 5 percent) are more difficult to assess by traditional safety studies. This is because test animals cannot be fed the ingredient at high enough levels so that ADIs can be derived without adversely affecting other factors in the normal diet. Thus, these ingredients may require alternative testing procedures (e.g., metabolism studies) to help assess safety.

Drugs

Among other requirements of a New Animal Drug Application is submission of data to demonstrate target animal (i.e., the species in which the drug shall be used) safety. The FDA has published extensive guidance on the quality and quantity of data required (FDA, 1989).

The position of FDA is that animal testing should derive the maximum amount of useful scientific information using the minimum number of animals necessary, so consideration should be given to the use of accepted alternative methods to whole animal testing. The classical LD_{50} test is not required by FDA for determining safety. The FDA allows data collected from nontarget animals to be used to focus studies in target animals. In this way, target animal toxicity studies can concentrate on target tissues and functional changes identified in the nontarget animal studies. However, the nontarget animal studies cannot be used to replace studies in target animals.

Target safety studies may include a drug tolerance test, which is accomplished by inducing toxicity under controlled conditions and recording the clinical sign(s) manifested by the test animals following administration of specific doses. This type of test includes observation of clinical signs, including changes in behavior and appearance, gross lesions in animals that die during the test, and clinical pathologic and histologic data. For drugs intended for long-term, continuous use (15 days or longer), the drug should be administered up to 10X the maximum proposed use level for up to 21 days.

With characterization of the nature of toxicity in the target species through a drug tolerance test, a margin of safety test compares the recommended dose level to multiples of the dose. Generally, it examines the response of the animal to one of at least four levels: zero, the recommended dose, and two or three non-zero multiples of the recommended dose (in most cases three times and five times the recommended dose). For drugs intended for continuous, long-term use, the study generally must run for six months. Physical examinations and observations, clinical pathology tests, and gross pathology and histopathology upon necropsy are to be used to determine the margin of safety between the recommended dose and the highest multiple of the dose where no signs of toxicity are observed.

Reproductive studies are required if the drug is intended for use in breeding animals. Studies are conducted on both sexes. The drug should be administered at a level at least three times the recommended amount, along with a control group. Males are treated during the 90-day period prior to mating and at appropriate times during the breeding period, with semen evaluations conducted just before breeding and at appropriate intervals.

For the study of drug action on female fertility, treatment is conducted through all phases of the estrous cycle. Teratogenic and embryotoxic studies are conducted with repeated administration of the drug in pregnant females throughout the entire period of fetal organogenesis. Finally, the drug is administered to the female from the final one-third of gestation throughout lactation. The duration of gestation, signs of abortion, dystocia, agalactia, or prolonged labor, as well as neonatal viability and growth of the newborn, are noted. Future breeding potential of young animals exposed to a drug in utero or through suckling may be conducted through multiple generation studies using offspring allowed to reach sexual and physical maturity.

REFERENCES

AAFCO (Association of American Feed Control Officials). 2007. Official Publication. Oxford, IN: Association of American Feed Control Officials.

Dzanis, D. A. 2007. U.S. regulatory report. Pp. 65–72 in Proc. Petfood Forum, Chicago, IL.

Ekelman, K. B. 2004. Safety assessment for feed ingredients. Presentation at the AAFCO Mid-year Meeting, Fort Worth, TX.

FDA (Food and Drug Administration). 1989. Target Animal Safety Guidelines for New Animal Drugs. Online at: http://www.fda.gov/cvm/Guidance/Guideline33.htm. Accessed October 8, 2007.

FDA. 1995a. Dietary Supplement Health and Education Act of 1994. Online at: http://www.cfsan.fda.gov/~dms/dietsupp.html. Accessed October 8, 2007.

FDA. 1995b. Nutritional Supplements for Companion Animals (CPG 7126.04). Online at: http://www.fda.gov/ora/compliance_ref/cpg/cpgvet/cpg690-100.html. Accessed October 8, 2007.

FDA. 1995c. Common or Usual Names for Animal Feed Ingredients (CPG 7126.08). Online at: http://www.fda.gov/ora/compliance_ref/cpg/cpgvet/cpg665-100.html. Accessed October 8, 2007.

FDA. 2001. Overview of Dietary Supplements. Online at: http://www.cfsan.fda.gov/~dms/ds-oview.html#what. Accessed October 8, 2007.

FDA. 2003. Claims That Can Be Made for Conventional Foods and Dietary Supplements. Online at: http://www.cfsan.fda.gov/~dms/hclaims.html. Accessed October 8, 2007.

FDA. 2007a. Dietary Supplement Current Good Manufacturing Practices (CGMPs) and Interim Final Rule (IFR) Facts. Online at: http://www.cfsan.fda.gov/~dms/dscgmps6.html#fr. Accessed October 8, 2007.

FDA. 2007b. FDA, AAFCO Sign Agreement on Feed Ingredient Listing. Online at: http://www.fda.gov/cvm/CVM_Updates/AAFCO_MOU.htm. Assessed November 26, 2007.

FDA. 2007c. Enforcement Priorities for Drug Use in Aquaculture. Online at: http://google2.fda.gov/search?q=cache:-zdGgXkP3FkJ:www.fda.gov/cvm/Policy_Procedures/4200.pdf+enforcement+discretion&access=p&output=xml_no_dtd&ie=UTF-8&lr=&client=FDA&site=veterinary&proxystylesheet=FDA&oe=UTF-8. Accessed October 8, 2007.

FDA. 2007d. FDA's Regulation of Pet Foods. Online at: http://www.fda.gov/cvm/petfoodflier.html. Accessed October 8, 2007.

Federal Register. 1996. Inapplicability of the Dietary Supplement Health and Education Act to Animal Products. Vol. 61, No. 78, Pp. 17706–17708.

NRC (National Research Council). 2006. Nutrient Requirements of Dogs and Cats. Washington, DC: The National Academies Press.

OTSC (Office of the Texas State Chemist). 1999. Distributing Products Containing Glucosamine Hydrochloride and/or Chondroitin Sulfate. Online at: http://otscweb.tamu.edu/policy%20memos/Feed%20Industry%20Memoranda/Fd%20Ind%203-17.pdf. Accessed October 8, 2007.

Perron, J., and E. I. Lambert. 2000. DSHEA and structure/function claims for animal feed. Food Drug Law J. 55:151–160.

3

Assessing Safety of Animal Dietary Supplements

The safety of a compound might be assessed through directed (e.g., toxicity) studies, generally occurring prior to market, with the intent of identifying a causal relationship between compound administration and an adverse event, or through surveillance studies, generally occurring post market with the intent of identifying anticipated or unanticipated adverse events that did not emerge during premarket assessment. Although they are not the sole source of safety information, adverse events are particularly important as a category of evidence (addressed in Chapter 5). Because animal dietary supplements share commonalities with both nutrients and drugs (see Chapter 4), their safety assessments accordingly should draw from the safety assessments of both.

ADVERSE EVENTS DEFINED

Adverse events have been variably defined. For the purposes of this document, the definition of adverse events will be that established by the International Harmonization Conference (IHC): any untoward medical occurrence that may present during treatment with a (pharmaceutical) product, but which does not necessarily have a causal relationship with this treatment (as reviewed by Nebeker et al., 2004). In 2006, Congress passed the Dietary Supplement and Non-prescription Drug Consumer Protection Act (2006). In response, the Food and Drug Administration (FDA) has drafted a guidance document for industry in which it defines an adverse event to dietary supplements as any health-related event associated with the use of a dietary supplement that is adverse (FDA, 2007a). A "serious adverse event" involving a dietary supplement is defined in that document as one that "results in death, a life-threatening experience, inpatient hospitalization, a persistent or significant disability or incapacity, or a congenital anomaly or birth defect; or requires, based on reasonable medical judgment, a medical or surgical intervention to prevent an outcome described above" (FDA, 2007a). Neither definition (i.e., IHC or FDA) of adverse event establishes a causal relationship between the adverse event and the product.

Adverse events might be further subdivided into medication errors and adverse drug reactions (Figure 3-1). Medication errors are any preventable event that may cause or lead to inappropriate medication use or patient harm while the medication is in the control of the health care professional, patient, or consumer. Medication errors might result from miscommunication, confusion regarding packaging, improper dose or interval, the wrong product, or any variety of errors made on the judgment of the caregiver (Nebeker et al., 2004) or, in the case of animals, the animal owner. Examples of serious or lethal medication errors associated with animal dietary supplements include treatment with a nonsteroidal anti-inflammatory drug with a trade name very similar to the prescribed animal dietary supplement (D. M. Boothe, personal experience, May 2007) and the accidental overdosage in dogs of a weight loss dietary supplement intended for humans (Ooms, 2001).

In addition to medication errors, adverse events include adverse reactions. The IHC has defined adverse reactions as any noxious and unintended response to a compound when it is administered according to dosing regimens recommended for the intended use (i.e., prophylaxis, diagnosis, or therapy of a disease) (Nebeker et al., 2004). An adverse reaction differs from an adverse event in that a causal relationship between the drug (compound) and adverse event exists, meaning that the reaction is in response to the compound and reflects its inherent (pharmacodynamic) properties. Adverse reactions can be further divided into those that are Type A ("augumented") or those that are Type B ("bizarre"); these reactions are also occasionally referred to as Type I and II, respectively (Figure 3-1). Type A reactions generally are recognized as being related to the concentration of the compound at the site of action (Pirmohamed et al., 1998). Type A reactions may reflect an exaggerated manifestation of the intended response (e.g., bleeding due to excessive antiplatelet effects of garlic) or an undesired, but

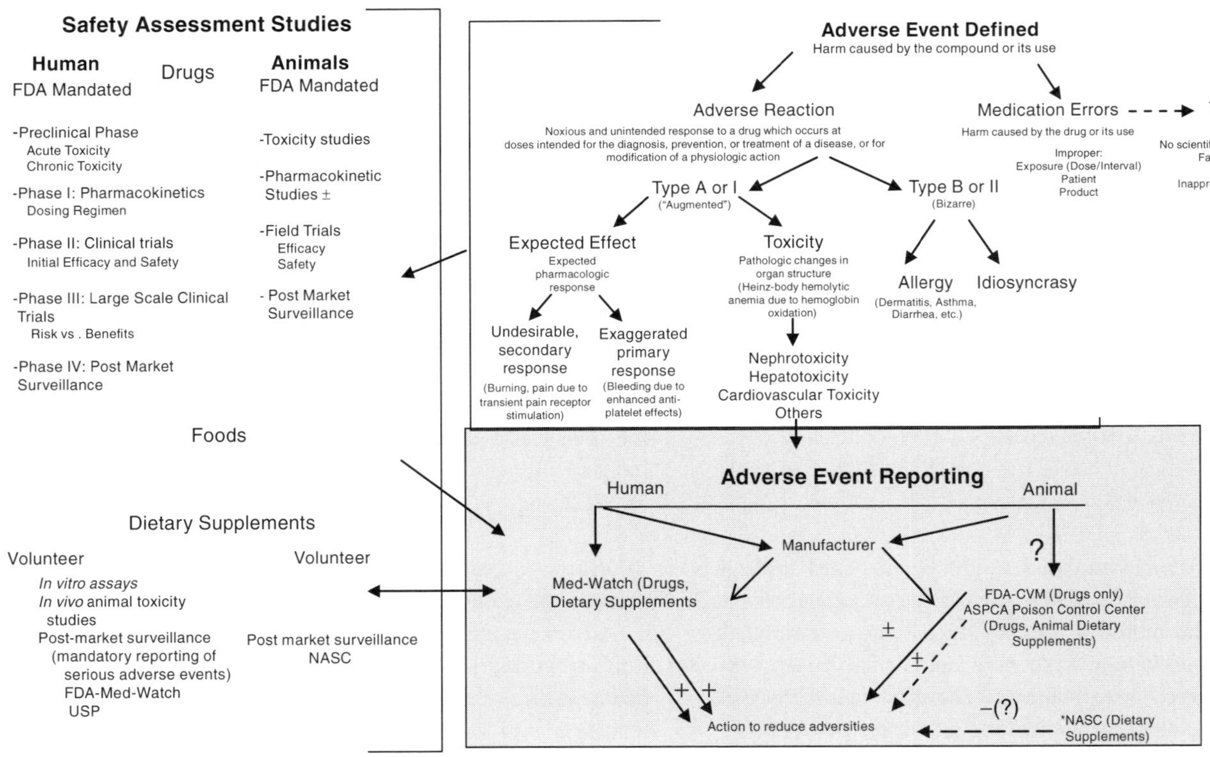

FIGURE 3-1 Flow chart summarizing the definition of adverse events.
NOTE: Safety assessment studies vary with the product. For drugs, studies are mandated by FDA for both human and animal drugs, although the extent varies. Postmarket surveillance is the most likely source of adverse event data. For dietary supplements, all testing and reporting is voluntary, with the exception of reporting of serious adverse events to human dietary supplements, which must be reported to FDA. For the purposes of this document, therapeutic failure has been added as a subset of medication errors in recognition of the greater risk associated with harm when an animal dietary supplement (which undergoes no premarket approval) is used in lieu of accepted therapies. Adverse event reporting programs developed for human dietary supplements may be useful for identifying signals of adverse events in animals. Programs specific for animals would be ideal, but currently only one exists: the NASC Compliance Plus® program, which is limited in both scope and review but holds promise of an effective reporting system.

nonetheless predicted, effect of the drug (e.g., stimulation of pain receptors by garlic). Type A reactions occur in a sufficiently large proportion of the populations if the conditions of risk are met (e.g., physiologic, pharmacologic, and pathologic factors described in Chapter 4). Type A reactions often are avoidable if actions are taken to accommodate for these risk factors. Because type A reactions occur in a large proportion of the at-risk population, their occurrence is more easily detected, particularly during the postmarket period. At-risk populations include those characterized by unique physiology or the presence of disease or because they are receiving multiple interventions that might lead to interactions among drugs, nutrients, and supplements (Chapter 4). For animal dietary supplements, the risk of Type A adverse reactions also is increased by the lack of premarket approval for these products. The absence of toxicity or safety data is self-evident, whereas the impact of the absence of quality assurance data (which might identify contaminants or other mislabeling concerns) or pharmacokinetic data (which might help identify patients at risk for adverse events) is less obvious.

In contrast to Type A reactions, Type B reactions are unrelated to the concentration of the drug, occur in a small population of individuals receiving the compound, and thus may not be evident until very large numbers receive the compound. Idiosyncratic reactions, which may reflect genetic polymorphisms or allergic responses (e.g., dermatitis or asthma associated with garlic), are examples of Type B adverse reaction. Again, garlic serves as an example of an animal dietary supplement to which allergic reactions have been ascribed (see Chapter 8). Because their incidence in the population is very low, they generally are not recognized until a very large number of patients have received the medication.

The term "side effect" is frequently used in association with the assessment of product safety (Nebeker et al., 2004).

A side effect is usually a predictable or dose-dependent effect of a drug that is not the principal effect for which the drug was chosen; the side effect may be desirable, undesirable, or inconsequential. Side effects are considered to be common and unavoidable consequences of medical care. The difference between adverse events (including adverse reactions) and side effects reflects the level of harm sustained in consumption of a product (Nebeker et al., 2004). Although they occur quite commonly, most side effects are not associated with serious outcomes. However, serious side effects are not considered rare, thus the term side effect increasingly is being avoided in lieu of adverse drug reaction (Nebeker et al., 2004). Accordingly, for the purposes of this study, safety assessment of animal dietary supplements will focus on adverse events, which will include side effects that cause serious harm. One additional adverse event might be considered for animal dietary supplements. An animal dietary supplement may harm an animal if it is chosen in lieu of recognized medical therapies. This is particularly likely to occur if an animal dietary supplement is heavily promoted without scientific evidence of efficacy. Therapeutic failure may also occur if a product is mislabeled such that it does not contain the labeled contents. Both causes of therapeutic failure are more likely with animal dietary supplements than with drugs because the approval process for drugs is intended to prevent these types of failure. The harm to an animal due to therapeutic failure when receiving an animal dietary supplement inappropriately is likely to be subtle and, thus, difficult to detect; furthermore, it may be impossible to discriminate from therapeutic failure due to failed response. It is not within the committee's purview to address the risk of harm associated with therapeutic failure of animal dietary supplements. However, the committee recognizes that the lack of evidence of quality assurance or efficacy for animal dietary supplements may contribute to harm to the animal and suggests that this concern be given consideration in the future safety assessment of these products.

SIGNALS OF ADVERSE EVENTS TO ANIMAL DIETARY SUPPLEMENTS

Signals indicative of an adverse event will vary with the test assay. In humans, premarket assessment based on in vitro assays has been suggested as sufficient to preclude the need for whole animals studies (IOM, 2005). However, the ability of in vitro assays to address adequately the safety of any compound should be considered limited, in part because applicability to target animal species varies with the assay. For example, studies involving transporter or metabolic enzymes may be more likely to be species specific than assays dependent on ion channel activity and electrophysiology. In vivo toxicity studies involving whole animals should reveal adverse reactions in organs particularly susceptible to Type A adverse events, but as with in vitro tests, results may not be relevant to the target species (see Chapter 4). Organs particularly at risk generally are those subjected to the greatest exposure, which includes concentration (dose) and duration. Thus, organs with the greatest blood flow and organs capable of concentrating compounds, such as the liver and kidney, are at the greatest risk for toxicity. Highly metabolically active organs are also more likely to manifest toxic effects for two reasons. First, such organs depend on the presence of energy; anything that impairs acquisition of energy (including blood flow) can lead to malfunction. Second, if the metabolic activity includes metabolism of compounds, the production of potentially reactive metabolites can increase the likelihood of cytotoxicity if these metabolites interact with cellular structures. The organs most susceptible to damage by Type B reactions tend to be the organs that contain tissues that act as haptens for drug-induced allergy (e.g., skin and blood-forming units) or tissues that filter and trap immune complexes (e.g., glomerulus and joints). Signals of adverse events will include clinical signs and data indicative of organ damage or altered organ function (e.g., clinical, gross, and histopathology).

OTHER RELEVANT SAFETY ASSESSMENT TERMS

General Terms

As a general rule, compounds used to supplement the diet with the intent to support or enhance normal structure or function, or to treat or prevent a disease, should be subjected to toxicity studies that attempt to establish a potential dose-toxic response relationship. Several terms are used to describe this relationship.

Intake of excessive amounts of nutrients, even dietary essential nutrients, can have toxic consequences, although the risk is likely to be greater for xenobiotics (i.e., foreign compounds). Toxicity describes the quantitative amount or dose of a poison that produces a toxic response or effect. A poison is any substance that is injurious to animals; the term is synonymous with toxic substance, toxic chemical, and toxicant. The word "poison" is often used interchangeably with "toxin"; however, toxins are poisons that originate from biological sources, also referred to as biotoxins. Presumably, any compound can become a poison ("the dose makes the poison"), and the toxic response to the poison tends to correlate with the dose (or duration) (Osweiler, 2006). A toxic response refers to the effects manifested by an organism in response to a toxic dose of the substance. Acute toxicity generally occurs from a single dose or exposure or from multiple doses within a 24-hour period. Most acute toxicants rapidly interfere with critical cellular processes. Subacute and subchronic toxicity occurs after 1 week and 1 month of exposure, respectively. Chronic toxicity occurs after ≥ 3 months of exposure (Osweiler, 2006). Toxic chemicals, including their metabolites, can act directly by injuring the cells with which they come in contact or indirectly by injuring a group of cells that subsequently precipitate injury to others. Toxic effects of nutrients also can be direct (e.g., vitamin A toxicity) or secondary due to interaction with another nutrient (e.g., zinc deficiency secondary to excess calcium intake in dogs). Alternatively, toxins can act indirectly by interfering with a physiologic process on which a group of cells are vitally dependent (e.g., xylitol interference with glucose metabolism in dogs). Most toxins act systemically, whereas others (such as acids and bases) act locally. Some toxic effects reflect a combination of local and systemic effects.

A common indicator of toxicity of a compound is the LD_{50}, or the dose per unit weight of a chemical that kills 50 percent of animals receiving it (the median lethal dose). Dosage refers to the amount of toxicant per unit of body weight (BW) administered; however, dose is the more commonly used term. The therapeutic index offers a measure of the relative safety of a compound by comparing the LD_{50} to the ED_{50} (IOM, 2005), which is the median effective dose (ED) necessary to induce a desired dynamic response in a targeted percent of the sample population. The companion index EC_{50} describes the concentration at which 50 percent of individuals respond. Establishing ED_{50} or EC_{50} may not be achievable for many animal dietary supplements because discreet outcome criteria for the response may be neither available nor measurable. Like the LD_{50}, both indices of efficacy are generally based on single dosing and do not take into account duration of exposure and so by themselves are insufficient measures of safety. Further, because directed toxicity studies often involve only a small number of study subjects, adverse events that emerge only when a large sample population is receiving the compound are likely to be missed. For example, an adverse event that occurs in 1:1,000 subjects might be considered to occur at a high incidence, yet detection of that adverse event in a toxicity study might require 3,000 or more subjects. Hazard or risk assessment should be more clinically relevant because each expresses the probability of harm under conditions expected with use of or exposure to the compound. Hazard is the potential to cause harm; risk is the likelihood of harm. Thus, risk takes into account both hazard (the inherently toxic nature of the compound) and exposure (the amount of the toxin ingested) (IOM, 2005).

Risk-benefit analysis is the comparison of the risk of a situation (e.g., intake of a compound) to its potential benefits (Colbert and Biron, 2002). The risk/benefit ratio is a measure of the acceptability of an adverse reaction and is based on importance, frequency, and duration of both the therapeutic benefit and the adverse reaction. However, these measures generally are not quantifiable. Thus, the term "assessment" might be more relevant than ratio as a descriptor. Regardless of the descriptor, risk-benefit should be based on postmarket use of a product. This presumes first that the benefits of a product have been well established and second that a postmarket surveillance program is in place to detect and assess adverse events to a product (Hughes et al., 2007). For animal dietary supplements, benefits are not likely to have been established, potentially precluding a favorable risk-analysis. However, a model that assesses hazard and exposure has been proposed for toxicity of human nutrients (IOM, 2007). The proposal characterizes risk by estimating a tolerable upper level (UL) in the context of an estimated range or distribution of intake. This model may be more relevant to animal dietary supplements, because it does not take into account estimates of benefits (or lack thereof). However, relevance to supplements might be lessened by the lack of obvious nutritive value of some supplements.

ASSESSMENT OF NUTRIENT SAFETY

Assessment of drug safety was discussed in Chapter 2. Unfortunately, data to support accurate estimations of maximum safe levels of nutrient intake are often lacking. Particularly when compared to studies designed to determine minimum nutrient requirements, relatively few studies are conducted for the purpose of determining the upper range of appropriate nutrient intake. Thus, estimating maximum safe intake levels often requires evaluation of studies not designed to address the issue of safety or extrapolation of findings from studies in other species. Several terms have been used to describe the maximum safe intake of nutrients. The National Research Council's publication *Mineral Tolerance of Animals* uses the term "Maximum Tolerable Level" to mean "the dietary level that, when fed for a defined period of time, will not impair animal health or performance" (NRC, 2005). The older NRC publication *Vitamin Tolerance of Animals* makes its recommendations in terms of "Presumed Upper Safe Levels," which are defined in part as those that "will not impair any aspect of animal health or production efficiency" (NRC, 1987). It considers these values to be necessarily lower than maximum tolerable levels, but does not clearly define the distinction between the terms.

The NRC's *Nutrient Requirements of Dogs and Cats* defines "Safe Upper Limits," or SUL, as the "maximal concentration or amount of a nutrient that has not been associated with adverse effects" (NRC, 2006). For human nutrition, "tolerable upper intake levels," are established for vitamins and minerals that, "if consumed below the specified level on a continuing basis, should not cause specific identified adverse effects of overconsumption" (IOM, 2005). The NRC's *Nutrient Requirements of Horses* does not define a preferred term, but refers to a variety of similar terminology, such as "upper safe diet concentration," and "maximum tolerable concentration," when discussing the aspect of excess intake of specific nutrients (NRC, 2007). Through its yearly publication, the Association of American Feed Control Officials (AAFCO) reports values in its Dog and Cat Food Nutrient Profiles simply as "maximums" (AAFCO, 2007). Dog or cat foods that exceed the maximum value for a nutrient can still be marketed, but they cannot claim nutritional adequacy (i.e., "complete and balanced") by reference to meeting the nutrient profiles.

This varying terminology may be responsible, at least in part, for misperceptions as to the meaning and application of this value. A critic of the *Nutrient Requirements of Dogs and Cats* (NRC, 2006) opined that the SUL were not determined in a manner consistent with the definition (Cook, 2006). Also, it was argued that the term implied that intake of a nutrient in excess of the SUL was necessarily harmful, when commercial products that exceeded one or more SUL with no apparent adverse effects suggest that premise to be false (Cook, 2006). Specific, explicit examples were not provided. Regardless, it reflects a misunderstanding of how SUL are derived from available data.

Means of Assessing Nutrient Safety

Micronutrients, such as trace minerals and vitamins, are in the diet at relatively low concentrations, so levels in the test diet can be experimentally adjusted to provide a wide range of intake most often without affecting the nature, form, taste, or other attributes of the diet. In that way, they may be studied similarly to drugs, i.e., multiples of the "1X" amount (in this case, that required for nutritional adequacy, or better, typical levels of intake already known to be safe) can be administered to the animal, with the amount titrated until the level at which adverse effect occurs was observed. The difference in the study of a nutrient versus a drug would be that a "0X" control group, where the diet is devoid of the nutrient of study, would likely be very difficult to formulate, at least without use of extremely purified or elemental ingredients. Also, in the case of a dietary essential nutrient, a diet in which the nutrient of study was completely absent or even nutritionally deficient could result in observed adverse effects of its own.

Evaluation of dose and response to varying levels of a nutrient can eventually yield a "no observed adverse effect level" (NOAEL) and/or "lowest observed adverse effect level" (LOAEL). The LOAEL is helpful in identifying initial clinical or pathologic signs associated with toxicity, which can be used to verify absence of these signs in the NOAEL. Comparing the NOAEL to an estimated typical intake level would provide a margin of safety determination. However, depending on how close in dose the treatment groups are, there may be a significant gap between the NOAEL and the true maximum safe intake level. For example, a study may look at a nutrient fed at 1X, 10X, 100X, and 1,000X the minimum dietary requirement. If clinical or pathologic signs of adverse effect are observed at 1,000X but not 100X, the LOAEL is 1,000X and the NOAEL is 100X. In reality, 500X may still be totally safe, but without further study that cannot be assumed. Determining the LOAEL and/or NOAEL for an animal dietary supplement requires experimental studies designed specifically for this purpose. As will be seen in the committee's review of lutein, evening primrose oil, and garlic, these data often are not available for animal dietary supplements.

While the nature of micronutrients make them amenable to study by means of classical toxicologic methods, studies on safety of nutrients in the species of interest in this report (dogs, cats, and horses) may be difficult to obtain at this time. Most pet food companies are reluctant to conduct, fund, or otherwise support studies that are designed to reveal potential harm to the experimental subjects. The costs and limits on equine studies also make them largely infeasible in this application.

Adverse reactions to macronutrients, such as protein, fat, and major minerals, are particularly difficult to assess by classical toxicologic methods. This is because multiples of the typical intake levels may be hard to duplicate without adversely affecting the diet itself. For example, potassium salts are bitter to the taste, so an animal may eat less of, if not outright refuse, a diet that contains much higher than typical levels. This confounds any reasonable comparison between groups and there may not be enough of a range in the nutrient intake levels to establish an NOAEL. Anything more than minor changes in levels of nutrients that may normally constitute a large portion of the diet and/or affect caloric density, such as fat or insoluble fiber, may overtly change the nature of the food itself, wherein the consistency in intake of other nutrients cannot be maintained. For example, a macronutrient that is normally 25 percent of the diet cannot be tested at 2X without disrupting the normal intake of other macronutrients. Effects due to different diet compositions may obscure any observed effect due to the nutrient of interest.

For dog and cat foods, but not horse feeds, an assessment of the safety of a food containing an animal dietary supplement might include feeding trials that follow AAFCO protocols (AAFCO, 2007). Protocols have been designed to evaluate nutritional adequacy for adult maintenance, growth, and gestation/lactation. Successful passage of a growth or gestation/lactation trial is considered substantiation of nutritional adequacy for adult maintenance as well. An "all life stages" designation requires a gestation/lactation trial, followed by a growth trial using the offspring of the gestation/lactation trial with continual use of the same food between the trials.

Animals on an AAFCO feeding trial are fed the diet as the sole source of nutrition except for water. Depending on the species and life stage being tested, specified physical, hematologic, and biochemical measurements are taken (see Table 3-1). These findings are compared to stated average and individual minimum values and/or to the values measured in a suitable historic or concurrent control group of animals that were fed diets that passed that feeding trial. Veterinary examinations for signs of nutritional deficiency or excess are also performed.

Such AAFCO feeding trials lack specificity (i.e., they can detect a potential problem with the nutritional adequacy of a food, but not necessarily the cause). However, in the case

TABLE 3-1 AAFCO Feeding Trial Protocols

Item	Dog (maintenance)	Dog (growth)	Dog (gestation/lactation)	Cat (maintenance)	Cat (growth)	Cat (gestation/lactation)
Minimum number of animals	8	8	Enough to confirm 8 pregnant	8	8	Enough to confirm 8 pregnant
Age of animals	≥ 1 year	≤ 8 weeks	≥ 1 year	≥ 1 year	≤ 9 weeks	≥ 1 year
Other animal specifications	Start at optimal body weight	Must be weaned, from ≥ 3 different bitches	At least in second estrus	Start at optimal body condition	Must be weaned, from ≥ 3 different queens	At least in second estrus
Minimum duration of test	26 weeks	10 weeks	Estrus through 4 weeks of lactation	26 weeks	10 weeks	Estrus through 6 weeks of lactation
Measurements	1. Body weight 2. Whole blood hemoglobin 3. Packed cell volume 4. Serum albumin 5. Serum alkaline phosphatase	1. Body weight gain 2. Whole blood hemoglobin 3. Packed cell volume 4. Serum albumin	**Bitches** 1. Body weight 2. Whole blood hemoglobin 3. Packed cell volume 4. Serum albumin **Puppies** 1. Litter size 2. Body weight	1. Body weight 2. Whole blood hemoglobin 3. Packed cell volume 4. Serum albumin 5. Serum alkaline phosphatase 6. Whole blood taurine	1. Body weight gain 2. Whole blood hemoglobin 3. Packed cell volume 4. Serum albumin 5. Whole blood taurine	**Queens** 1. Body weight 2. Whole blood hemoglobin 3. Packed cell volume 4. Serum albumin 5. Whole blood taurine **Kittens** 1. Litter size 2. Body weight

of assessment of an animal dietary supplement, a food that successfully passed the feeding trial can be reexamined with inclusion of the supplement at levels both at and multiples above intended use levels until adverse effect (compared to performance of the unsupplemented food) is noted. If necessary (especially for macronutrients), the supplement can replace in whole or in part another ingredient so that overall nutrient balance is preserved. Observation of adverse effect can be used to establish a LOAEL or NOAEL. However, lack of observed adverse effect does not necessarily prove safety at the level of inclusion, since the AAFCO trials are not designed to look at all possible adverse effects. For example, an AAFCO trial may detect measurable loss of packed red blood cell volume, but would not routinely detect subtler signs of toxicity such as Heinz body formation. To improve the likelihood of detecting an adverse effect if it exists, additional measurements (e.g., blood smears or serum liver enzymes), including any suspected of being affected by the supplement, are desirable.

Setting Safe Levels of Intake

Where definitive data are sufficient to establish an NOAEL in the intended species, establishment of the SUL may be relatively straightforward. Additional safety factors may be added on to account for the potential variety of ages, body weights, and other physical attributes of the intended population compared to those used in the study. For example, an NOAEL of 1,000 mg of a nutrient per kg of diet as tested in a group of nonbreeding adult dogs does not account for increased consumption of food by growing puppies or pregnant/lactating bitches. A rule of thumb for calorie intake for newly weaned puppies is twice the requirement for adult maintenance, while a bitch with a large litter in heavy lactation may consume up to three times maintenance. Thus, barring available data specifically in dogs in other life stages, a three-fold decrease in the NOAEL to account for potential increased consumption may be used to establish the SUL at 333 mg/kg of diet for all life stages.

In other cases, though, safety factors may be added that are not based on any specific formula or rule, but rather reflect the consensus of opinion of the expert panel reviewing the data. Where there is a large margin of safety between the NOAEL and typical use levels, a dramatic reduction in the SUL compared to the NOAEL is most often considered prudent and does not cause issues. In some cases, though, the margin of safety does not allow for such conservatism. For example, several studies conducted in the 1980s supported safe inclusion of total fat in the diet of dogs at levels up to 82.5 g per 1,000 kcal metabolizable energy (ME), while an older study found adverse effect in dogs at 92 g/1,000 kcal ME (NRC, 2006). Thus, the NRC Nutrient Requirements of Dogs and Cats committee set the SUL for total fat at the level deemed safe by the 1980s studies, even though it was only 10 percent lower than shown to be potentially harmful to dogs. Most commercial dog foods do not contain near the SUL for fat, although there may be exceptions in the marketplace. Still, establishment of any SUL for total fat has been criticized because it implies some commercial products to be unsafe (Cook, 2006).

In many cases where safety studies are lacking, SUL may be derived from looking at utility studies (e.g., technical functionality studies, clinical trials to assess animal benefit or performance, or other studies not designed to directly assess safety). Failure to report adverse effect of a nutrient at a level specified in a study may be evidence of safety, especially when corroborated by other similar studies. The SUL for various carbohydrates in dog and cat foods were established based on maximum reported use levels in the literature (NRC, 2006). Because the levels of use of a nutrient in a utility study may not be in great excess of typical inclusion rates, basing SUL on these data may result in values much lower than if determined by traditional toxicologic methods. However, while there may be no data to suggest adverse effects from higher inclusion rates, the available data on carbohydrate levels in pet foods did not provide sufficient evidence for that committee to make an assumption of safety at higher levels.

Occasionally, data from other species are used to support an SUL where there is concern for toxicity but no species-specific data are available. Lacking such data, AAFCO established a maximum for zinc and copper in dog food at 3,000 and 250 mg/kg of diet dry matter, respectively, based on NRC recommendations for swine available at that time (AAFCO, 2007). The SUL for vitamin D in dog food conforms to a previous "rule-of-thumb" recommended by NRC for all mammals (4 to 10 times the minimum requirement for that species), although data specific in cats allow for higher inclusion rates than would be predicted by the same rule (NRC, 1987, 2006).

An SUL may not be established where there is no practical need. For example, while sodium or potassium toxicity in dogs or cats is possible, the likelihood in a healthy animal is negligible, since excess levels in a pet food will negatively affect palatability to a degree where adverse effects due to excess consumption will not be observed (assuming available access to plain water and alternative food sources). However, failure to set an SUL should not be inferred as evidence of lack of safety concern, but rather a lack of available data sufficient to estimate safe intake. For example, AAFCO set a maximum for selenium in dog foods consistent with that recommended for other species (2 mg/kg of diet dry matter; DM) (AAFCO, 2007). Considering the typical selenium content of commonly used ingredients, that level did not represent a burden to dog food manufacturers. However, although practical experience showed that cats had a long history of consumption of fish-based diets that contained significantly higher amounts of selenium without any evidence of adverse effect, it is not clear if a similar intake level would have been safe in a non-fish diet. Therefore, in the opinion of AAFCO, an SUL the same as for other species would be unreasonably burdensome, but without other available data to confirm safe intake, an SUL that was set arbitrarily high would falsely imply safety where none was confirmed.

From all descriptions used to assess nutrient safety (e.g., safe upper limit, maximum tolerable concentration), it should be clear that the terminology intends to define a level of a nutrient that is known to be safe, not what is considered to be unsafe, and there can be considerable gaps between the two. Admittedly, use of the terms "maximum," "tolerable," or "upper" could be inferred as a firmly defined limit, where anything in excess was imminently dangerous. Perhaps a term that does not imply such definitiveness would better characterize the intended meaning of the value (Fahey, 2007).

To this end, the committee chose the term "Presumed Safe Intake (PSI)" as a means to convey a level of exposure that it felt is safe yet has not been determined with the rigor of an NOAEL or SUL because of lack of appropriate data.

ADVERSE EVENT DETECTION AND REPORTING FOR ANIMAL DIETARY SUPPLEMENTS

Limitations of Adverse Event Reporting for Animal Dietary Supplements

Reporting of adverse events is dependent, in part, on an expectation that they will occur. Reports will be facilitated if actively sought. As such, the absence of reported adverse events to a dietary supplement should not be taken as evidence of safety unless data show that adverse events were sought through scientific, controlled studies or reporting mechanisms. Because dietary supplements, including those for animals, are perceived to be safer than drugs, even if an adverse event is recognized, the causal relationship between the supplement and the adverse event is often lost. Education of consumers regarding the potential for an adverse event to occur is indicated to facilitate adverse event reporting. However, the most profound limitation to an effective means of assessing the risks and benefits of adverse events to dietary supplements is the lack of an effective identification, reporting, and reacting system. Issues that limit identification of and reaction to adverse events to animal dietary supplements were recognized to exist in the current reporting system for dietary supplements in humans (OEI, 2001).

Adverse Event Reporting for Drugs

The drug approval process in humans is designed to identify adverse reactions. Collection of data begins with the preclinical phase (short- and long-term animal testing) (Figure 3-1). It continues through first (pharmacokinetics and dynamics in healthy volunteers), second (effects in patients with the targeted disease), and third (expanded clinical trials to evaluate safety and efficacy in diseased patients) clinical phases during which risk benefit associations are identified (FDA, 1998). For some drugs, a fourth clinical phase of postmarket surveillance is mandated. The approval process for animals is much less regimented, with the actual requirements often based on the individual drug undergoing consideration (FDA, 2007b). Although adverse drug events in animals that are reported to manufacturers must be reported to FDA, data generally are not actively sought but reflect voluntary reporting on the part of the health care provider. The veterinary profession, probably more than the human medical community, is less likely to report adverse events. Further, the mechanism by which the information is forwarded to the veterinary health care provider is limited in scope. If mechanisms of adverse drug event reporting in veterinary medicine are lacking, deficiencies in reporting of adverse events to dietary supplements are likely to be worse.

Adverse Event Reporting for Human Dietary Supplements

Mechanisms for the reporting, processing, and reacting to adverse events to dietary supplements is markedly scaled down compared to that for drugs. This probably reflects, in part, the misguided assumption that adverse events to dietary supplements are unlikely to cause morbidity and mortality. Dietary supplements were not mentioned in the workshop summary titled *Adverse Drug Event Reporting: The Roles of Consumers and Health-Care Professionals* (IOM, 2005). Yet, the Office of Evaluations and Inspections has indicated that the current method of detecting, reporting, and assessing human adverse events to dietary supplements is insufficient to allow actions necessary to assure consumer safety (OEI, 2001). The information regarding an adverse event caused by a supplement becomes useful only when reported back to health care professionals after a fair and unbiased assessment that indicates a reasonable-cause and effect. A mechanism for reporting the incidence and clinical manifestations of adverse events and the probability of a cause and effect relationship does not currently exist for dietary supplements (Figure 3-1).

The absence of an approval process for dietary supplements precludes collection of information that might otherwise be generated during the preclinical and clinical phases of drug approval (Figure 3-1). Postmarket assessment of adverse events associated with animal dietary supplements will be limited by the lack of an obvious mechanism by which adverse events might be reported (Figure 3-1). Although the FDA is mandated by the Dietary Supplement Health and Education Act (DSHEA) to monitor adverse events to dietary supplements, it cannot mandate postmarket surveillance of dietary supplements. Furthermore, manufacturers of dietary supplements are compelled to report only serious adverse events to the FDA. Because DSHEA does not apply to animals, FDA is not mandated to monitor animal dietary supplements and its role in the detection of adverse events to animal dietary supplements is not clear.

Adverse Event Reporting for Animal Dietary Supplements.

Although several potential programs exist in which adverse events to animal dietary supplements might be assessed, each is characterized by limitations that vary in impact. The FDA's Medwatch program accepts volunteer reports for human, but not animal, dietary supplements. The FDA-CVM adverse event reporting program addresses adverse events in animals, but does not address animal adverse events to animal or human dietary supplements. The American Society for the Prevention of Cruelty to Animals (ASPCA) collects information on adverse events related to any compound ingested by an animal in the context of a fee-for-service (counseling regarding treatment of the adverse event) basis. The information collected is that which is necessary to guide the diagnosis and treatment of the adverse event in the animal patient. The database is cumulative, and intermittently reviewed for patterns of adverse events that might be attributed to a compound, with reports of clinically relevant findings in scientific journals. However, the data are generally biased toward those adverse events that are life-threatening. Currently, the data are not generally accessible for systematic review, although collaboration with the ASPCA might be pursued. An alternative source of adverse event data for animal dietary supplements may be the manufacturers of animal dietary supplements. They have implemented a voluntary adverse event reporting program known as the "Compliance Plus Program," which is promoted by the National Animal Supplement Council (http://nasc.cc/). Members (manufacturers) that register with NASC must report adverse events to the program. The NASC has defined an adverse event as "a type of complaint where a patient has suffered any negative physical effect or health problem that may be connected to or associated with use of the product," whereas a serious adverse event is defined as an "adverse event with a transient incapacitating effect (i.e., rendering the animal unable to function normally for even a short period of time, such as with a seizure) or nontransient (i.e., permanent) health effect. Transient vomiting or diarrhea do not constitute serious adverse events. A purported serious adverse event requires follow-up with a veterinarian. A layperson diagnosis does not constitute a serious adverse event."

One of the attributes of the NASC adverse event reporting program is the inclusion of units sold, thus allowing correction for presumed intake. Although the NASC and similar programs are important first steps toward adverse event reporting for animal dietary supplements, several criteria are paramount to the effectiveness of any program. These include the need for active, rather than passive, solicitation of adverse events (i.e., promotion of the program and assuring easy access to user-friendly reporting forms); assurance that data collection and analysis are able to detect adverse events, including the discrimination of serious adverse events; a sufficient level of oversight by an independent regulatory agency; and public access to the data (currently NASC data are available to FDA and, upon request, to state feed regulators). Furthermore, a mechanism for reporting the specific product may be particularly important because of the variability that characterizes the contents and formulations of animal dietary supplements. A disadvantage to the collection of adverse event reporting through voluntary registration programs is the limited scope; only products that have been registered will be included. Manufacturers of products that present the greatest risk may not participate in such programs.

AN ALGORITHM OF SAFETY ASSESSMENT FOR ANIMAL DIETARY SUPPLEMENTS

The assessment of the safety of an animal dietary supplement might be based on three sources of information: (1) quality assurance data, reflecting all aspects of manufacturing, storage, and distribution that might lead to adverse events; (2) safety data generated during the evaluation of biologic response, including efficacy when the animal supplement is used as a drug; and (3) data collected with the specific intent to assess safety (Figure 3-2) (Boothe, 2004).

Quality Assurance

The DSHEA, including its discussion of Good Manufacturing Practices (GMP), does not apply to animal dietary supplements. Further, the Verified Program for Dietary Supplements is extended to manufacturers of dietary supplements recognized under DSHEA, which does not apply to animal dietary supplements. Accordingly, extra care should be taken to ensure the quality of animal dietary supplements. A path to assessment of product quality has been reviewed (Groot and Van der Roest, 2006). Assessment should include the product itself, but also the facilities, including the site of manufacture and its surrounding grounds, sanitation, equipment, quality control, production and process controls, warehouse, and postdistribution practices. Accuracy of the label can not be overemphasized. Evaluation should assure that the labeled ingredients are present in an active form at the indicated strength, that the label contains an expiration date, and that the product is not adulterated. Adulteration can be defined as "the addition of an impure or inferior component not ordinarily part of that substance; or removal of a crucial entity; usually used to imply that a substance is debased (desecrated) as a result" (Cole and Fetrow, 2003). Contamination is a type of adulteration with the "presence of foreign material that renders impure a material whose composition is degraded" (Cole and Fetrow, 2003). Contaminants include, but are not limited to, materials

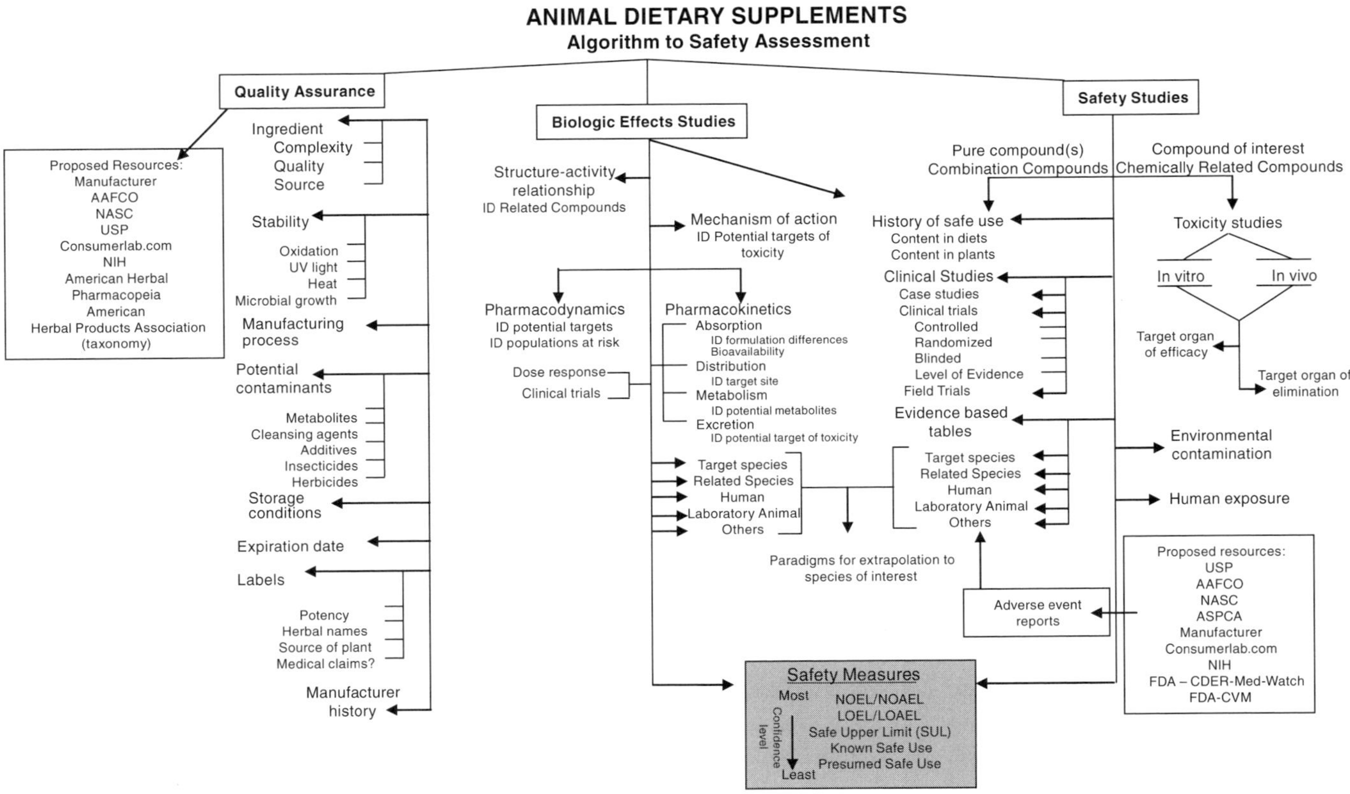

FIGURE 3-2 A proposed algorithm for assessing safety of animal dietary supplements.
NOTE: Each of the three major categories of assessment provides information that supports the safety of a supplement. Although safety assessment is most directly relevant, information regarding biologic effects gathered and reported scientifically can be useful if it helps to identify target organs and signals of adversity or populations at risk. The ideal measure of safety would be a no observed adverse event level (NOAEL). However, lack of scientific information may limit assessment to determination of a presumed safe use level.

present in the pure or active "pharmaceutical/nutrient" ingredients or in excipients, that are either intentionally added or inadvertently acquired during manufacturing (i.e., degradation of materials, environmental contamination, or intentional "spiking" with drugs). Residual environmental contaminants (e.g., herbicides, insecticides, heavy metals, or microbes) are particularly relevant to herbs or biologicals (Priyadarshini et al., 2004). These contaminants are discussed in more depth in Chapter 4. Although more difficult to identify, contaminants also include those intentionally included to enhance therapeutic effects or to reach quality standards (e.g., melamine supplementation of pet foods; Anonymous, 2007). Standards for herbs have been discussed by Fennell et al. (2004). These standards include the need to state the part of the plant and the use of both herbal and medically recognized names, when relevant.

Potential sources of quality assurance data for animal dietary supplements include the manufacturer of the product, the Association of American Feed Control Officials (http://www.AAFCO.org), the National Animal Supplement Council (http://nasc.cc), and laboratories such as ConsumerLab (http://www.consumerlab.com). ConsumerLab is an independent publishing company that provides information about the quality of dietary supplements (Abourjaily, 2001; Glassman, 2004). Although it offers a voluntary certification program, the majority of its analytical investigations are not sponsored by manufacturers. Selected information regarding its testing procedures and results is accessible at its website. ConsumerLab reports that animal dietary supplements consistently perform more poorly than human supplements in their tests, with the most common reasons for failure being the lack of the labeled ingredient at the labeled strength and the presence of contaminants (Tod Cooperman, President, ConsumerLab, personal communication, May 2008). The committee did not have an opportunity to review relevant data and independently validate this observation.

Two other programs evaluate dietary supplements on a volunteer basis. The United States Pharmacopeia offers a dietary supplement verification program for human dietary supplements (http://www.usp.org/USPVerified/dietarySupplements). Supplements are evaluated to ensure they contain the ingredients stated on the label in the stated amounts and that contaminants such as heavy metals, pesticides, dioxins, furans, polychlorinated biphenyls, and microbes do not surpass acceptable limits. The program ensures that the products are manufactured using safe, sanitary, and well-controlled procedures. The National Sanitation Foundation, International (NSF International) also sponsors a certification program (http://www.nsf.org/certified/consumer/listings_main.asp) for both animal and human supplements, although information about performance of supplements apparently is not available to the public.

For herbs, additional resources include the American Herbal Pharmacopeia (http://www.herbal-ahp.org). The American Herbal Products Association offers the *Botanical Safety Handbook* and *Herbs of Commerce*, which provide information about proper taxonomy and common names of herbs (http://www.ahpa.org/Default.aspx?tabid=68). Several other interactive, web-based sources of information about dietary supplements are available (Larkin, 2004).

Evidence of Biologic Effects

Data offered in the context of evidence of a desired biologic response, including efficacy in the prevention or treatment of a disease, may facilitate safety assessment of an animal dietary supplement for several reasons. First, efficacy studies may provide evidence of safety, particularly if an adverse event emerges or if an adverse event does not emerge but was actively sought by the investigators. Second, if safety assessment includes an assessment of risk-benefits, failure to promote evidence of efficacy may inappropriately lean the balance of the risk-benefit assessment toward risk. Data demonstrating tolerance or lack of adverse event when the compound is administered at therapeutic doses for pharmacodynamic or pharmacokinetic studies should support risk-benefit assessment. Third, documented mechanisms of biologic action or pathways of disposition (i.e., absorption, distribution, metabolism, or excretion) may identify a signal that will direct safety assessment toward target organs to be reviewed more in depth for evidence of an adverse event. Demonstration of safe use of the compound through pharmacokinetic or pharmacodynamic studies may support determination of a presumed safe level (or dose) in the absence of specific toxicity or safety studies. Finally, pharmacokinetic or pharmacodynamic modeling involving compartments is particularly well suited for nutritional compounds and may be useful for extrapolating information across species (Novotny, 2005).

The complexity of the disposition of the compound might be assessed as a greater risk compared to a compound whose absorption, distribution, and elimination are straightforward, in part because of the risk that compound disposition might be altered in susceptible populations. Demonstration of oral bioavailability (that is, the degree to which or rate at which the compound is absorbed or becomes available in the plasma) of the labeled compound (including the specific salt), either as the intact molecule or as its component "building blocks," will facilitate comparison of studies with different forms of the compound. Efficacy studies in the target or related species (e.g., cats and ferrets, dogs and wolves, horses and donkeys) should be ranked highest in regards to applicability to risk assessment, whereas data collected from distant species should be given the least consideration. Sources of data might include manufacturers, academicians with known expertise, and literature searches that reveal clinical trials or kinetic/dynamic studies in related or unrelated species.

Evidence of Safety

Sources of safety data include studies involving both the pure compound or combination products and might also include data generated for a related compound. Relatedness has been described in terms of chemical relatedness, in which the chemical structure is similar to known toxic chemicals or contains constituents that are similar in structure to known toxicants; taxonomical relatedness, in which the source of the herb is taxonomically related to a known toxic plant; or functional relatedness, referring to a shared common biologic effect or mechanism of action (IOM, 2005). However, care must be taken in defining chemical relatedness. For herbs, information about the species and variety must be included. For example, while *Salvia officinalis* is a condiment, *Salvia divinorum* is associated with psychogenic effects. For chemicals, some that seem to vary little chemically have profoundly different physiological effects, as is exemplified by enantiomers (see Chapter 5).

The highest level of confidence in the safety of an animal dietary supplement would be provided by availability of an NOAEL or LOAEL. In their absence, a recommended maximum safe dose might be determined for the animal dietary supplement. Although the applicability of in vitro toxicity studies to in vivo use may be unclear, such data should not be ignored if limited information is otherwise available. Ideally, in vivo toxicity studies implemented following multiple dosing at several-fold higher doses compared to that recommended on the label will be available in the target species. Such studies should focus on organs of elimination and the target organ of efficacy, but should not be limited only to these body systems. Data collected from distant species may also be useful, but it is also essential to assess the data according to relevance to the target species. A number of types of clinical studies might be evaluated for evidence of safe use. This might include a history of safe use if sufficiently long and used in a large population; case reports including series and retrospective studies, particularly if cohort controlled; and clinical trials, with randomized, controlled clinical trials providing the best evidence. Generation of evidence-based tables might allow most effective assessment. Postmarket surveillance studies or data merit high consideration. In-depth systemic reviews may be accepted as part of the assessment package. As with toxicity data, clinical trial data supporting safe use are most relevant if generated in the target species. Resources of data directly supporting the safety of an animal dietary supplement include previously cited resources, with the addition of data generated through volunteer adverse event reporting programs (human) and the ASPCA Poison Control Center.

A final aspect of safety of animal dietary supplements that prudently might be assessed is public health considerations resulting from consumption and subsequent elimination of the supplement or its active components into the environment. Such contamination might eventually present a potential harm to either humans or animals. This aspect of supplement safety was not considered by the committee.

REFERENCES

AAFCO (Association of American Feed Control Officials). 2007. Official Publication. Oxford, IN: Association of American Feed Control Officials.

Abourjaily, P. 2001. Nutrition in Clinical Care. 4:118–120.

Anonymous. 2007. Chemical combination poisons pets and enters human food chain. Ethical Insights 64, May 03, 2007. Online at: http://www.ethical-insight.com/issue64/analysis_28.html. Accessed January 2008.

Colbert, B. L., and P. Biron. 2002. Pharmaco-vigilance from A to Z: Adverse Drug Event Surveillance. Malden, MS: Blackwell Science.

Boothe, D. M. 2004. Balancing fact and fiction of novel ingredients: definitions, regulations and evaluation. Vet. Clin. N. Am. Small Anim. Pract. 34:7–38.

Cole, M. R., and C. W. Fetrow. 2003. Adulteration of dietary supplements. Am. J. Health Syst. Pharm. 60:1576–1580.

Cook, N. K. 2006. Deficiencies and difficulties: New NRC guide fails to make the grade for PFI. Petfood Industry 48(8):26–27.

Fahey, G. C. 2007. The 2006 NRC publication on the nutritional requirements of dogs and cats: Response to critics. Proc. Petfood Forum 2007, Chicago, IL.

FDA (Food and Drug Administration). 1998. The CDER Handbook. Online at: http://www.fda.gov/cder/handbook/. Accessed March 13, 2008.

FDA 2007a. Questions and answers regarding adverse event reporting and record keeping for dietary supplements as required by the Dietary Supplement and onprescription Drug Consumer Protection Act. Guidance for Industry. Online at: http://www.cfsan.fda.gov/~dms/dsaergui.html. Accessed May 15, 2008.

FDA. 2007b. Information and Requirements for Review and Approval of New Animal Drug Applications (NADAs). Online at http://www.fda.gov/cvm/nadaappr.htm. Accessed March 13, 2008.

Fennell, C. W., M. E. Light, S. G. Sparg, G. I. Stafford, and J. van Staden. 2004. Assessing African medicinal plants for efficacy and safety: Agricultural and storage practices. J. Ethnopharmacol. 95:113–121.

Glassman, N. R. 2004. ConsumerLab.com. J. Med. Libr. Assoc. 92:509–510.

Groot, M. J., and J. Van der Roest. 2006. Quality control in the production chain of herbal products. Pp. 253–260 (Chapter 18) in Medicinal and Aromatic Plants, J. Bogers, L. E. Craker, and D. Lange, eds. Dordrecht, Netherlands: Springer.

Hughes, D. A., A. M. Bayoumi, and M. Pirmohamed. 2007. Current assessment of risk-benefit by regulators: Is it time to introduce decision analyses? Clin. Pharmacol. Ther. 82:123–127.

IOM (Institute of Medicine). 2005. Dietary Supplements: A Framework for Evaluating Safety. Washington, DC: The National Academies Press.

IOM. 2007. Nutritional Risk Assessment: Perspectives, Methods, and Data Challenges, Workshop Summary. Washington, DC: The National Academies Press.

Larkin, M. 2004. Complementary and alternative medicine. Lancet-Oncology. 5(1):66.

Nebeker, J. R., P. Barach, and M. H. Samore. 2004. Clarifying adverse drug events: A clinician's guide to terminology, documentation, and reporting. Ann. Intern. Med. 140:795–801.

Novotny, J. A. 2005. What can pharmacokinetic models tell us about the disposition of lycopene and the potential role of lycopene in cancer prevention? J. Nutr. 135:2048S–2049S.

NRC (National Research Council). 1987. Vitamin Tolerance of Animals. Washington, DC: National Academy Press.

NRC. 2005. Mineral Tolerance of Animals, 2nd Revised Edition. Washington, DC: The National Academies Press.

NRC. 2006. Nutrient Requirements of Dogs and Cats. Washington, DC: The National Academies Press.

NRC. 2007. Nutrient Requirements of Horses, 6th Revised Edition. Washington, DC: The National Academies Press.

OEI (Office of Evaluations and Inspections). 2001. Adverse event reporting for dietary supplements. An inadequate safety valve. OEI-01-00-00180. Boston: Department of Health and Human Services.

Ooms, T. G., S. A. Khan, and C. Means. 2001. Suspected caffeine and ephedrine toxicosis resulting from ingestion of an herbal supplement containing guarana and ma huang in dogs: 47 cases (1997-1999). J. Am. Vet. Med. Assoc. 218:225–229.

Osweiler, G. D. 2006. General toxicological principles. Pp. 2–17 in Small Animal Toxicology, M. E. Peterson, and P. A. Talcott, eds. St. Louis, MO: Elsevier Saunders.

Pirmohamed, M., A. M. Breckenridge, N. R. Kitteringham, and B. K. Park.1998. Adverse drug reactions. BMJ 25(316):1295–1298.

Priyadarshini, R., L. C. Patino, and M. G. Nair. 2004. Evaluation of metal and microbial contamination in botanical supplements. J. Agric. Food Chem. 52:7822–7827.

4

Factors Affecting Animal Dietary Supplement Safety

Many factors, both intrinsic and extrinsic, can influence the safety of an animal dietary supplement. Proper evaluation of these factors is vital for safety assessment, particularly when little traditional safety data are available. This knowledge can improve comfort level about the safety of an animal dietary supplement or can raise red flags that otherwise would not have been obvious. This chapter provides an overview of a number of these important factors.

EXTRINSIC AND INTRINSIC FACTORS AFFECTING ANIMAL DIETARY SUPPLEMENT SAFETY

Supplement Source

Animal dietary supplements are typically of plant, bacterial, algal, fungal, mineral, or animal origin; they may also be synthetic. Plant source supplements can come from bulbs, roots, leaves, stems, fruit, seeds, or other parts of the plant. Supplements of animal origin can be isolated from muscle, organs, blood, or parts of the body that are not typically considered food sources (e.g., shark cartilage). The putative active component(s) can be purified or consumed as part of a complex matrix or an intact part of the plant. The source will determine potential for contamination and presence of other beneficial or toxic substances, as well as metabolism by the animal. Therefore, the risk of an adverse reaction to an animal dietary supplement and the level of safety assessment will depend on its source.

For the purposes of this discussion, animal dietary supplements will be further divided into those that are native to the body (e.g., nutrients) and those that are foreign to the body. Foreign substances are also known as xenobiotics and are defined as "any substance, harmful or not, that is foreign to the animal's biological system" (Blood et al., 2007). The risks associated with foreign compounds are likely to be greater than for nutrients. The distinction between nutrient and foreign may not be clear for some compounds, such as lipids, but is clear for others. For example, several herbal constituents are considered to be associated with high risk (IOM, 2005) and are clearly foreign. However, some lipids of plant origin contain high levels of essential fatty acids and are, therefore, natural to the animal, inherently safe, and treated as native substances by the body. The risk of harm for foreign compounds reflects not only their intrinsic toxicity, but also their tendency to require the body to develop new transport or metabolic pathways or to induce normally quiescent transport or metabolic pathways for processing. As such, foreign compounds are more likely than nutrients to be involved in drug interactions. These interactions will be discussed later in this chapter.

Contaminants

Figure 4-1 illustrates examples of potential sources of contamination and other extrinsic factors that could affect the safety of animal dietary supplements. Likely contaminants should be determined and then monitored for animal dietary supplements. Good Manufacturing Practices (GMP) should be followed to minimize safety hazards resulting from contamination. The GMP will vary according to the type of animal dietary supplement. Examples of GMP are outlined in Codex Code of Practice on Good Animal Feeding (http://www.codexalimentarius.net) and in 21 CFR 110 and 111.

Contaminants Obtained During Supplement Production

The animal dietary supplement may unintentionally contain contaminants resulting from the use of fertilizers, herbicides, and pesticides as well as from exposure to pollutants (e.g., heavy metals) during production and harvesting. Most botanicals evaluated in recent surveys (Huggett et al., 2001; Raman et al., 2004) were contaminated with bacteria and/or fungi, organochlorine pesticides, and metals. In addition, the growth of bacteria, fungi, or yeasts may result in the formation of a variety of unwanted chemical compounds such as aflatoxin, lipopolysaccharide, and fumonisins, which may

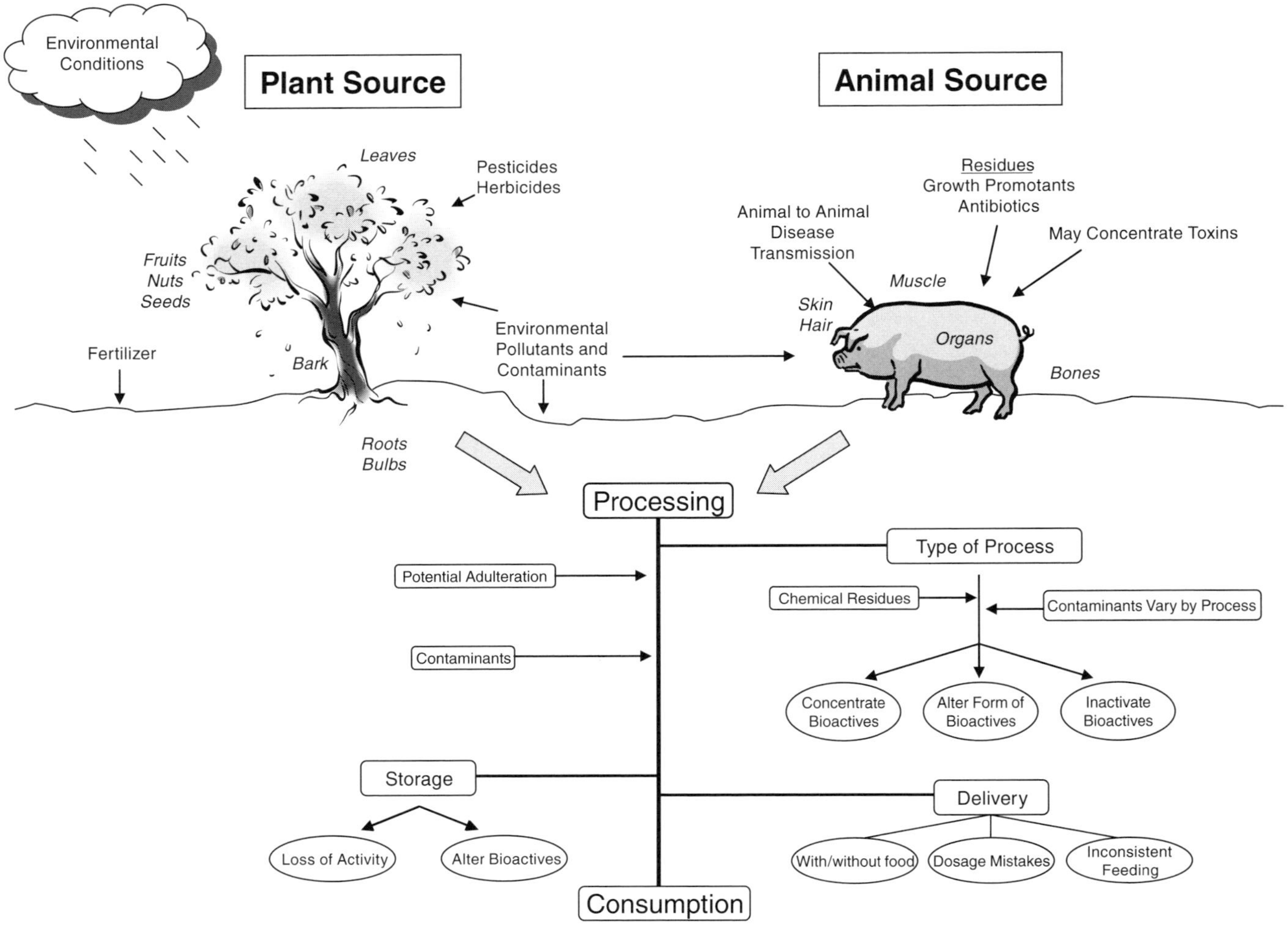

FIGURE 4-1 Examples of extrinsic factors affecting animal dietary supplement safety.

have potent physiological and toxic effects. In the case of supplements of animal origin, the formation of chemical components because of fermentation or decay needs to be considered. Examples include the formation of histamine and tyramine (from histidine and tyrosine, respectively) in supplements of animal origin that have been pickled, aged, smoked, fermented, or marinated. Both substances have potent physiological effects, ranging from mediating arousal and attention to hypertension and modulation of the immune response.

Contaminants Obtained During Supplement Processing

While some supplements are consumed in their natural form, others are processed before incorporation into the diet. Common forms of processing include solvent or mechanical extraction, heating, drying, enzymatic or chemical treatment, fermentation, and encapsulation. Contamination due to processing must be taken into consideration as a potential source of introducing unwanted substances into animal dietary supplements. For example, natural vitamin E supplements have recently been found to contain high concentrations of two highly toxic substances, dioxin and furan (Halbert and Archer, 2007). The researchers indicated that the contamination originated from the extraction process of the deodorizer distillate, a byproduct of the refinement of vegetable oil and the source for natural vitamin E.

Production and Harvesting

Harvesting, growing, and storage conditions can influence the concentration and form of the bioactives of interest. For example, grasses grown in humid tropical conditions contain more lutein than the same grasses grown in dry conditions (Reynoso et al., 2004). Lutein is particularly sensitive to destruction by heat and solar radiation (Bailey and Chen, 1988). The chapters in this report on garlic, evening primrose oil, and lutein include a full discussion of production and harvesting factors affecting bioactive content for these animal dietary supplements.

Processing

The type of processing used during production of an animal dietary supplement, and during production of animal feed it may be incorporated into, can influence the potency of the bioactive ingredients, the formation of secondary compounds that are potentially more toxic, and the type and concentration of potential contaminants and antinutrients. Therefore, understanding the complete process involved in producing the animal dietary supplement is necessary for identification of safety concerns. Specific effects of processing are discussed in more detail in the chapters evaluating the safety of lutein, evening primrose oil, and garlic.

Raw Ingredient Processing

Ingredients are often processed to improve storage stability, increase concentration and/or bioavailability of bioactive components, destroy antinutrients and other toxins, and kill bacteria, fungi, and molds. Common processing methods include milling, grinding, drying, roasting, extruding, saponification, cooking, micronizing, flaking, crushing, cracking, rolling, crimping, pelleting, and enzyme treatment. An excellent overview of these processes is provided in the book *Feed Manufacturing Technology* (Schofield, 2005). Lipids are typically extracted by mechanical or solvent extraction. Solvent extraction will not only increase the concentration of essential fatty acids, but also the concentration of other lipid-soluble compounds. Hence, processing may increase the concentration of compounds that are much more toxic than the bioactive component.

Diet Processing

A detailed description of feed processing methods is provided by the American Feed Industry Association (Schofield, 2005); only a brief overview is provided in this text. Processed horse feeds are typically pelleted or extruded, or some combination of the two. Horses may also be fed textured or sweet feeds where the cereal grains usually have been processed via rolling, crimping, or steam-flaking prior to incorporation into the feed, which may also contain pelleted or extruded components as well as molasses or vegetable oils. In addition, some horse feeds that contain significant quantities of forage (e.g., an equine "complete" feed) may contain chopped forage or chaff. Processing conditions for dog and cat foods depend on the product type (e.g., dry, wet, semi-moist, biscuit). Wet pet foods are produced by cooking a mixture of ingredients by a process called retorting. One of the main functions of retorting is to sterilize the product. Retort temperatures and times will vary based on the ingredients, form of the product (e.g., loaf vs. chunk-in-gravy), packaging type, and package size. Typically, retort temperatures are approximately 120–130°C for up to 120 minutes. In contrast, most dry pet foods undergo extrusion processing. Typically, a blend of ingredients is exposed for 20 to 240 seconds to steam and/or hot water in a preconditioner before being forced through the extruder. Depending on the type of extruder and the processing conditions, the product may be exposed to low or high shear. After extrusion, the product is cooled and then dried in an oven. An additional coating of fat and/or palatability enhancers is typically applied at some point after extrusion. Because extruded products are exposed to thermal and mechanical energy for a brief but intense time, extrusion can alter the structure of dietary components. For example, starch granules are gelatinized during extrusion, making them more available for digestion. Steam flow rate, retention time, extruder configuration, and macronutrient levels all affect the degree of expansion and starch gelatinization in an extruded product. Processing conditions can also induce interactions between ingredients and/or nutrients (Tran et al., 2007). An example is the formation of Maillard compounds during retorting/extrusion if free amino groups are available in the presence of reducing sugars. As a result, the bioactive component may be destroyed or altered in a way to make it less effective or more toxic. Understanding the potential effects of processing on animal dietary supplements and the active ingredient is necessary for adequate safety assessment.

Intrinsic Factors

Intrinsic factors such as antinutrients, other nutrients, and other biologically active compounds can affect the safety of an animal dietary supplement. Examples of antinutritive factors include tannins and trypsin inhibitors in soybean meal and other oil seeds (including evening primrose seeds). These factors may be concentrated or eliminated during processing of the animal dietary supplement. For example, if both the bioactive and the antinutrient components of the animal dietary supplement are lipid soluble, lipid extraction of the ingredient will concentrate both components. A full understanding of potentially harmful intrinsic factors and how these factors are affected by the harvesting, processing, and storage conditions specific to an animal dietary supplement is vital for evaluating the safety of an animal dietary supplement.

BIOLOGICAL FACTORS AFFECTING ANIMAL DIETARY SUPPLEMENT SAFETY

Natural Diet

Evaluation of the natural diet of an animal species can help predict whether a dietary component will be well tolerated. Items that are commonly consumed by an animal species in the wild are likely to be safe components of that species' domestic diet. Aversion to consumption of an ingredient that is abundantly present in the natural environment of the animal raises a red flag about safety of that ingredient (e.g., *Senecio jacobaea* tends to be avoided by horses in good pastures). Thus, knowledge of the natural diet is an important component of assessing potential safety of animal dietary supplements.

Horses

The generally recognized ancestor of the earliest equids existed in the Eocene epoch 65 million years ago. At their maximum diversity in the fossil record, there were some 13 Equid genera, of which *Equus* is the only surviving genus today. The genus is thought to have included approximately 30 separate species. Today, there are just eight to ten *Equus* species remaining (depending on interpretation), including the horse, donkey, ass, onager, kiang, and the various zebras (MacFadden, 2005).

The evolutionary adaptation of the horse from a browsing animal to a predominantly grazing animal is believed to have taken place in the later Miocene between 20 and 15 million years ago (MacFadden, 2005). Diversification in tooth morphology included high-crowned cheek teeth adapted for grazing on the extensive grasslands of more open-country biomes, which spread during the Miocene. In addition, these equids became increasingly adapted to select and contend with the highest-fiber, lowest-protein diet in the grazing community by perfecting hindgut fermentive digestion (i.e., cecal and colonic fermentation) in conjunction with increased rate of intake and passage (Janis, 1976).

Until the mid-1900s, there were two subspecies of wild horse in Europe and Asia: the Tarpan (*Equus ferus ferus*) in Central Europe and the Przewalski or Mongolian wild horse (*Equus ferus przewalskii*). Both are now extinct in the wild, but an attempt to reconstruct the Tarpan from domestic hybrids has been made in Poland. In addition, the Przewalski is maintained as a captive population, some of which have been released into semi-natural reserves in Mongolia (Goodwin, 2002). In contrast to wild horses, there are numerous populations of feral horses in existence worldwide. Feral horses are descendents of horses that were once domesticated but have escaped captivity and are essentially self-sufficient. The success of these many feral populations provides evidence that the behavior of the horse has changed very little during 6,000 years of domestication (Goodwin, 2002). Thus, the feeding preferences and behavior of feral and free-ranging horse populations probably provide a reasonable estimation of the domestic horse.

Time budget experiments have shown that free-ranging feral and domestic horses, and horses housed at pasture, generally graze for 10–17 hours daily (Martin-Rosset et al., 1978; Salter and Hudson, 1979; Crowell-Davis et al., 1985; Duncan, 1985; Mayes and Duncan, 1986; Crane et al., 1997; Boyd and Bandi, 2002). Nocturnal intakes may account for between 20–50 percent of the total time spent grazing (Doreau et al., 1980; Crane et al., 1997). Feral horses in Alberta spent nearly 75 percent of the day in foraging activities (Salter and Hudson, 1979), while Camargue mares spent 71 percent of daylight hours and 49–56 percent of nighttime hours grazing during winter and spring (Duncan, 1985). Meal length on pasture by feral horses ranged from a few minutes to 13.5 hours (Mayes and Duncan, 1986).

Although horses are herbivores, they do not possess the capacity for extensive foregut fermentation, as seen in ruminants, and they do not ruminate. Horses have been observed to spend more time grazing (47 percent of daylight hours) than cattle (32 percent) or sheep (37.5 percent) grazing the same pasture (Arnold, 1984). Consequently, dry matter intake by horses on pasture is higher than cattle when examined relative to metabolic body weight (Menard et al., 2002). The consumption of small amounts of forage with each bite, coupled with the lengthy time spent grazing, has earned horses the descriptor of, "trickle feeder."

Although graminoids (e.g., grasses, sedges, and rushes) are the main component of feral horse diets (75–98 percent), microhistological analysis of plant cuticular fragments in feces have also demonstrated significant consumption of shrubs and minor amounts of forbs (see Table 4-1) (Hubbard and Hansen, 1976; Hansen et al., 1977; Salter and Hudson, 1979, 1980; Krysyl et al., 1984; McInnis and Vavra, 1987). Similar preference for forage variety has been shown by domesticated horses (Goodwin et al., 2002). On a year-round basis, feral horses seem to select more mesic communities (e.g., bogs, meadows, and riparian areas) in their foraging behavior when available (Hubbard and Hansen, 1976; Salter and Hudson, 1979; Crane et al., 1997). These wetter areas contain more succulent forage and are often used in greater proportion to their availability compared to other habitats. The diet of feral and free-ranging horses often shows changes through the year with seasonal abundance and primary productivity of forage species (Table 4-1). For example, analysis of plant fragments in feces collected from New Forest ponies showed that graminoids constituted > 90 percent of the diet in the summer, but only 48 percent in the winter (Putnam et al., 1987). In the winter, New Forest ponies shifted to a more sheltered habitat in evergreen and deciduous woodland, where forbs and shrubs made up the majority of their diet. Similarly, analysis of fecal material deposited by feral horses has demonstrated a greater consumption of graminoids in the summer and spring, which mirrors a greater availability of these feed sources during these times of year (Salter and Hudson, 1979, 1980; Krysyl et al., 1984; McInnis and Vavra, 1987).

Studies on forage species preference by domestic, pasture-housed horses have yielded inconsistent results, which is likely due to differences in maturity of the herbage at the time of study. Despite the difficulties in interpreting such data, it has generally been found that pastures of mixed species were preferred to monocultures (Archer, 1973) and grasses were preferred to legumes and herbs (Archer, 1973, 1978; Odberg and Francis-Smith, 1976; Krysyl et al., 1984).

TABLE 4-1 Feeding Ecology of Feral and Free-ranging Horses (*Equus caballus*)

Location	Horse Population	Season/Habitat	Component (% of diet)[a]			
			Graminoids[b]	Forbs	Shrubs	Other
Alberta[c]	Feral	Annual Average	93	< 1	4	2
Alberta[d]	Feral	Winter	85	< 1	6	8
		Summer	94	< 1	1	4
Colorado[e]	Feral	Mountain shrub	85	5	10	—
		Ecotone	98	< 2	< 1	—
		Pinyon-juniper	89	8	3	—
Colorado[f]	Feral	Summer	94	3	3	—
Oregon[g]	Feral	Summer #1	91	7	2	—
		Fall #1	89	7	4	—
		Winter #1	90	7	3	—
		Spring #1	98	2	< 1	—
		Summer #2	87	6	7	—
		Fall #2	79	14	7	—
		Winter #2	86	12	2	—
Wyoming[h]	Feral	Summer	75	3	22	—
		Winter	63	1	36	—
New Forest, England[i]	Domestic, free-range	Spring	69	< 1	20	10
		Summer	92	4	1	3
		Fall	79	6	10	5
		Winter	46	2	39	11

[a]In all cases, botanical compositions of diets were identified and quantified by microhistological analyses of plant fragments in fresh or undecomposed fecal material.
[b]Includes grasses, sedges, and rushes.
[c]Salter and Hudson (1979).
[d]Salter and Hudson (1980).
[e]Hubbard and Hansen (1976).
[f]Hansen et al. (1977).
[g]McInnis and Vavra (1987).
[h]Krysyl et al. (1984).
[i]Putnam et al. (1987).

Dogs

The domestic dog (*Canis familiaris*) is believed to have evolved from the gray wolf (*Canis lupus*) and is one of the oldest domesticated animal species. Archaeological evidence suggests that domestication occurred some 15,000 years ago but new mitochondrial DNA sequence analysis suggests that domestication may have occurred much earlier because early dogs may have been phenotypically indistinguishable from gray wolves (Ostrander and Wayne, 2005). Domestic dogs are believed to have originated in East Asia, according to the multiple and diverse origin model, where a number of populations and hundreds of individuals made multiple contributions to the gene pool (Vila et al., 2005). The subsequent limited interbreeding has resulted in a vast number of breeds that represent distinct genetic pools that can be divided into at least four genetic groupings: Asian/Ancient, Herding, Hunting, and Mastiff breeds (Ostrander and Wayne, 2005).

As dogs have no direct wild ancestors, nutritional information on the evolutionary diet of this species can best be investigated through the natural diet of the closest related free-living ancestor alive today, the gray wolf (*Canis lupus*). However, it must be taken into account that directed interbreeding since its domestication might have affected the nutrient metabolism of modern-day dogs. These studies show that the gray wolf can be classified as a dedicated carnivore with a certain capability for opportunism. A number of studies (Gade-Jørgensen and Stagegaard, 2000; Jedrzejewski et al., 2000; Sidorovich et al., 2003; Andersone and Ozolins, 2004; Chavez and Gese, 2005; Ansorge et al., 2006) across various geographical locations have investigated quantitative aspects of the dietary habits of gray wolves. A variety of methods were used to estimate diet composition, relying mainly on analysis of scat and/or stomach contents. Accordingly, some researchers have questioned the accuracy of the methods. These studies show (Table 4-2) that in Poland, Finland, and Germany, almost 100 percent of their diet consists of wild ungulates. In these studies, the major proportion of these wild ungulates consists of cervids such as red deer (*Cervus elaphus*), roe deer (*Capreolus capreolus*), and moose (*Alces alces*). In Belarus, however, Sidorovich et al. (2003) found that about two-thirds of the wild ungulates' biomass was represented by

TABLE 4-2 Diet Composition of Gray Wolves (*Canis lupus*) in Different Countries (Percent of Total Diet)

Source:	1		2	3		4	5	6
Country:	Poland		USA	Finland		Belarus	Latvia	Germany
Methodology:	Scat Analysis		Scat Analysis	Scats		Scat Analysis and Direct Observations	Scat and Stomach Content Analysis	Scat Analysis
Component	May–Sept	Oct–Apr	Mar–Nov	May–Sept	Oct–Apr	—	Apr–Sept	—
Wild ungulates	96.6	98.1	52.8	87.0	96.0	32.1	81.8	97.4
Domestic ungulates	–[a]	1.2	14.7	5.0	3.0	26.7	2.3	–
Rodents	+[b]	+	3.3	1.0	–	5.1	12.6	–
Small rodents	+	0.1	18.1	+	+	0.3	2.0	+
Hares	0.9	0.1	–	6.0	1.0	17.2	0.1	2.6
Rabbits	–	–	3.6	–	–	–	–	–
Raccoon dogs	–	0.2	–	–	–	5.9	–	–
Other mammals	2.3	0.2	2.4	1.0	0.1	10.0	–	–
Birds	0.1	+	1.8	+	+	1.0	0.2	+
Reptiles	+	+	–	–	–	–	+	–
Amphibians	+	+	–	–	–	–	–	–
Fish	–	–	–	+	+	–	–	+
Invertebrates	–	–	–	+	+	–	–	–
Insects	–	–	1.0	–	–	–	+	–
Plant material	+	0.1	0.8	+	+	0.6	0.2	–
Other	–	–	1.5	+	+	0.1	0.2	–

[a]Food item not consumed.
[b]Food item was present but not clearly quantifiable.
SOURCES: 1, Jedrzejewski et al. (2000); 2, Chavez and Gese (2005); 3, Gade-Jørgensen and Stagegaard (2000); 4, Sidorovich et al. (2003); 5, Andersone and Ozolins (2004); 6, Ansorge et al. (2006).

wild boar (*Sus scrofa*). The contribution of domestic ungulates to the diet of the wolf is relatively small in comparison to wild ungulates. Only in the study in Belarus (Sidorovich et al., 2003) was the difference small, with 32.1 percent of the diet coming from wild ungulates and 26.7 percent from domestic ungulates.

The content of medium-sized and small mammals in the natural diet of wolves is relatively low. The highest levels were found by Chavez and Gese (2005), who reported 18.1 percent of the diet of gray wolves consisted of small rodents, predominantly muskrats (16.6 percent). Also in the study in Belarus (Sidorovich et al., 2003), the content of medium-sized and small mammals was relatively high. Intake of beaver (*Castor fiber*), hare (*Lepus europaeus*), raccoon dog (*Nyctereutes procyonoides*), and domestic dog (*Canis familiaris*) accounted for almost 40 percent of the total diet and exceeded the intake of wild and domestic ungulates.

The contribution of plant material to the diet of gray wolves seems to be very low (Table 4-2). Gade-Jørgensen and Stagegaard (2000) and Sidorovich et al. (2003) reported the plant component consumed by gray wolves consists of grass, leafs, fruit (apples, pears, plums, figs, grapes, berries), seeds, and grains (corn, wheat). Other components like reptiles, birds, fish, and insects are frequently found in the diet, but similar to the plant material, contribution to the overall diet is small.

Cats

A recent genetic assessment of domestic cats and their wild progenitors—the European wild cat (*Felis silvestris silvestris*), near Eastern wild cat (*F. s. lybica*), central Asian wild cat (*F. s. ornata*), southern African wild cat (*F. s. cafra*), and Chinese desert cat (*F. s. bieti*)—shows that all house cats are descendants from a group of Eastern wild cats (*F. s. lybica*) around 9,000 years ago coinciding with agricultural village development in the Near East (Driscoll et al., 2007).

A number of studies (Coman and Brunner, 1972; Fitzgerald and Karl, 1979; Jones and Coman, 1981; Tidemann et al., 1994; Medina and García, 2007) have investigated quantitative aspects of the dietary habits of feral cats introduced into previously cat-free ecosystems in New Zealand, Australia, Canary Islands, and Christmas Island. These studies indicate that domesticated cats once introduced (deliberately or accidentally) into the ecosystem quickly become the most dominant predator. Their diet is highly versatile exploiting a wide variety of prey depending on local availability. The most common prey size for cats is about 1 percent of their body weight, which is much less than most previously reported values for carnivores (Pearre and Maass, 1998). When available in sufficient quantities, mammals (rabbits, rats, and mice) are the predominant prey item consumed (Table 4-3).

TABLE 4-3 Diet Composition of Feral Cats (*Felis catus*) in Different Countries

Source:	1	2	3	4			5	
Country:	New Zealand	Christmas Island	Canary Islands	Australia			Australia	
Methodology:	Scat Analysis	Gut Content Analysis	Scat Analysis	Stomach Content Analysis			Stomach Content Analysis	
Component	—	—	—	Site 1	Site 2	Site 3	Site 1	Site 2
Mammals	93.0	54	88.3	85	68	85	85.7	91.5
Birds	4.5	30	4.6	9	18	13	5.8	–[a]
Fish	–	–	–	1	9	–	–	–
Reptiles	–	3	7.1	< 1	2	< 1	1.1	–
Arthropods	2.5	12	< 0.1	1	1	< 1	0.8	–
Amphibians	–	–	–	< 1	–	< 1	0.0	1.0
Plant material	0	–	–	–	–	–	2.5	–
Other	–	1	–	> 2	2	0	3.5	6.0

[a]Food item not consumed.

SOURCES: 1, Fitzgerald and Karl (1979); 2, Tidemann et al. (1994); 3, Medina and García (2007); 4, Jones and Coman (1981); 5, Coman and Bruner (1972).

Jones and Coman (1981) reported that the occurrence of prey, rather than preference, seems to explain differences in food items consumed. Quantitatively less important food items include reptiles, amphibians, fish, and arthropods. Plant material, although often present in the feces, does not seem to contribute to the daily nutrient intake of feral cats, a result consistently observed across studies. Whether specific components in the plant material consumed by feral cats have a hitherto unidentified physiological or metabolic function remains to be established.

> Guiding Principle: The composition of the evolutionary diet can provide information on the "foreignness" or "nativeness" of a compound to the body raising concern about the safety of use in the target animal species.

Eating Behavior

Eating behavior can influence the ability of a species to tolerate an animal dietary supplement (Table 4-4). Understanding the natural eating pattern of a species of animal is also one component in determining whether safety data obtained with one animal species can be extrapolated to another. For example, when compared to an animal that nibbles, an animal that consumes its entire daily intake in one or two meals may have larger fluctuations in blood concentration of a xenobiotic or nutrient. Plasma concentration of xenobiotics is correlated with both efficacy and toxicity (Figure 4-2). As a result, the same daily intake could result in different outcomes depending on the intake pattern. In other situations, a nutrient or xenobiotic may be less efficiently absorbed when ingested as a large bolus than when ingested in small steady doses. In this case, the maximum tolerable level may be lower in the animal that nibbles.

In the domestic environment, the animal owner can have a large influence on the dog, cat, or horse's feeding behavior and pattern of supplement intake. Cats are often provided dry food ad libitum and/or canned food once or twice per day. However, some owners choose to feed their cats dry food only once or twice per day. Adult dogs at maintenance are often fed one or two meals per day. However, puppies and lactating bitches may be fed much more frequently. One bag of commercial dog or cat food may take one or more months to consume ensuring consistent day-to-day consumption of an animal dietary supplement if it is incorporated into the commercial food. Thus, compliance typically is better than if the supplement is manually added to the food by the pet owner.

The feeding behavior of domestic horses has been reviewed by others (Houpt, 2006; NRC, 2007). Feral and free-ranging horses spend a considerable amount of time feeding (10–17 hours per day); they rarely fast voluntarily for more than 2–4 hours at a time. In general, the grazing horse will take a few bites of forage, with each bite consisting of only a small amount (≈ 100 g), walk a step or two forward, and repeat the process (Houpt, 2006). Unless they are grazing a monoculture pasture, grazing horses will select from a variety of grass species and may also consume smaller amounts of forbs and shrubs. In contrast, many of today's horses are housed in confinement in stalls or small pens for all or most of the day, with little opportunity to graze and select their own diet. These horses are often fed preserved forages in the form of hay, haylage, or silage that is often, but not always, made up of a monoculture of grass species. Many horses (particularly growing horses, pregnant and lactating mares, and working horses) are also fed nutrient-dense concentrates, including cereal grains, oilseed meals, oils, and mineral and vitamin supplements. These

TABLE 4-4 Species Differences in Digestive Physiology and Eating Behavior

Species	Rat	Human	Dog	Cat	Horse
Digestive Physiology	Nonruminant omnivore; large cecum	Nonruminant omnivore	Nonruminant opportunistic carnivore	Nonruminant, obligate carnivore	Nonruminant herbivore; predominantly a hind gut fermenter (with some fermentation occurring in the stomach and SI)
Consumption Pattern (domestic)	Nibbles; coprophagizes	Eats 3 meals per day	Eats 1–3 large meals per day; in the wild, may go days without eating. Tends to gorge when presented with palatable food. Consumes decomposing carcasses, buries bones for later consumption.	Nibbles; eats 10–15 meals per day; in the wild most food is consumed during twilight	Nibbles; forages for the majority of the day in the wild
Implications	Potentially toxic substances are consumed in small, steady increments. Stomach rarely empty. Coprophagy results in consumption of microbial sources of vitamins and microbial metabolites.	—	Intake of potentially toxic dietary substances occurs in large boluses rather than small increments throughout the day	Potentially toxic substances are consumed in small, steady increments. Stomach rarely empty in the wild.	Potentially toxic substances are consumed in small, steady increments. Stomach rarely empty.
Primary Diet	—	Muscle meat; plants including fruits and vegetables	In the wild, opportunistic carnivore. Domesticated dogs tend to consume a more omnivorous diet with a mix of plant and animal protein sources.	Small prey—mice, birds, rabbits; occasionally insects; consumes the entire carcass	In the wild, eats a variety of plants; domestic horses typical consume a more limited selection of plant species
Implications	Readily adapts to a variety of diet types	Readily adapts to a variety of diet types	Readily adapts to a variety of diet types	Well-adapted to carnivorous diet (see Table 4-8)	In the wild, not likely to over-consume a plant containing a toxin

concentrates are usually offered as one or two meals per day, to accommodate the owners' schedule and to avoid the risk of digestive upset that would be associated with allowing ad libitum access to these types of ingredients. Some horses may be managed by a combination of pasture turnout for grazing combined with periods of stall confinement, where they are offered concentrates in meal form.

If incorporated into the food, the intake pattern of the animal dietary supplement will mimic that of the food. However, animal dietary supplements may also be administered as a bolus, with or without food. The total intake of the animal dietary supplement may vary with the food intake if incorporated into the food, or may be constant from day to day if administered separately. The presence of food and the frequency of administration can potentially affect the absorption, and hence tolerance, of the animal dietary supplement.

Digestive Physiology

The digestive physiologies of the dog and cat were recently reviewed by the National Research Council (NRC, 2006) and, therefore, will not be reviewed in depth in this text. Gastric emptying, transit time, enzyme and hormone concentrations, microbiota populations, and pH influence absorption and metabolism in the intestinal tract. Dogs and cats are nonruminant carnivores/omnivores, whereas horses are nonruminant herbivores. These species typically have limited fermentation capacity in the upper intestinal tract when compared to their lower intestinal tract or to the upper gastrointestinal tract of ruminants. As a result, nutrients and xenobiotics that are bound in a indigestible matrix will be poorly absorbed in the small intestines of dogs, cats, and horses. Rats are often used as models for other species when evaluating the safety of xenobiotics. Rats are nonruminants, but have a large cecum relative to body size when compared to that of other nonruminant species. In addition, rats practice coprophagy. The combination of a large cecum and coprophagy allows rats to have access to compounds that are bound in indigestible matrices. Because of this difference in digestive physiology between rats and dogs or cats, care must be taken when extrapolating rat data on fiber sources or xenobiotics that are bound in non-digestible matrices.

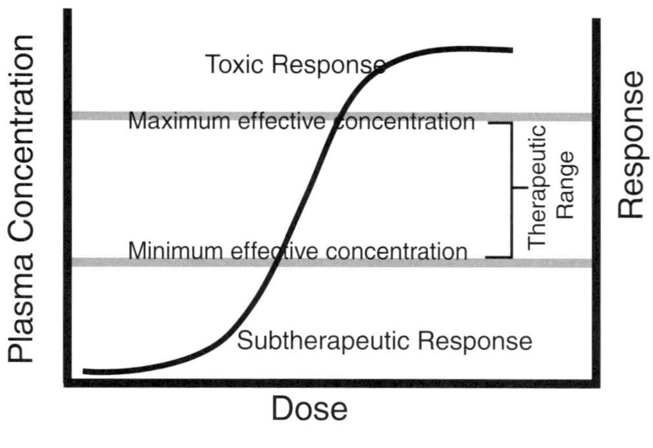

FIGURE 4-2 Relationship between dose and plasma concentration and response to a xenobiotic.
NOTE: The relationship between dose and plasma concentration and response to a xenobiotic such as a drug most commonly can be represented by a sigmoidal curve. The magnitude of response increases very little despite marked changes in dose at very low and high doses, but is essentially linear within the range considered therapeutic. The risk of therapeutic failure is increased at low doses, whereas the risk of toxicity is greatest at high doses. However, for some compounds in some animals, adverse events may occur within the therapeutic range.

Due to the horse's capacity for hind-gut fermentation, the extent of nutrient and xenobiotic release from these indigestible matrices and their subsequent absorption in the lower intestinal tract potentially would be higher in the horse than in the dog or cat. In contrast, nutrients and xenobiotics that are synthetic, processed, or otherwise in a highly available form could be absorbed in the small intestine of any of these species. Therefore, the source of supplement can have a large influence on extent and site of absorption; these effects will be dependent upon the digestive physiology of the animal consuming the supplement.

Metabolic Response to Nutrients and Xenobiotics

Xenobiotics are compounds that are foreign to the body. The most obvious example is drugs, but other compounds, including some animal dietary supplements, are also foreign. Because the goal of the body is to remove the foreign compounds, animals have developed specialized systems for their metabolism and excretion. Figure 4-3 contrasts the response of an animal to varying concentrations of a xenobiotic and the classical response to nutrients. Xenobiotics such as drugs produce optimal performance at low intake levels followed by a decrease in health and performance at higher levels. No response is apparent at intakes below the effective dose. In contrast, deficient intake of nutrients results in suboptimal health and performance, deficiency signs, and potentially death; increasing nutrient consumption improves health and performance. This response gradually tapers off until the minimal nutrient requirement is met as measured by a specific response criterion or criteria. A wide range of optimal intake follows until, eventually, performance and health gradually decline and nutrient toxicity becomes apparent. While many nutrients have wide ranges of optimal intake, others have much narrower safety limits. These ranges often vary between species of animals. For example, when compared to dogs, cats are much more tolerant to excess dietary calcium. The tolerable range can even vary within species. For example, Japanese canine breeds are thought to be at a greater risk to react adversely to garlic and onion compared to other breeds due to altered sodium-potassium pumps in red blood cell membranes (Yamoto and Maede, 1992). Some nutrients have such broad ranges of optimal intake that negative effects of excess consumption are not observed under practical situations.

Xenobiotic and Nutrient Metabolism

Avoidance of adverse events is best accomplished with an understanding of those factors that alter dynamic response to an animal dietary supplement. Response to a nutrient or xenobiotic supplement reflects physiologic considerations such as receptor numbers and affinities, but also those factors that alter the concentration of the compound at the site of action (e.g., kinetics).

At any point in time, plasma and tissue concentrations of a xenobiotic or nutrient reflect several movements that act in concert (Figure 4-4). These movements include absorption (A) from the site of administration to systemic circulation, defined as the major vessels and well-perfused organs; distribution (D) of the xenobiotic or nutrient from systemic circulation to tissues (target and nontarget) and back again; and elimination of the xenobiotic or nutrient from the body by metabolism (M) and excretion (E). Absorption, distribution, metabolism, and excretion are often referred to collectively as ADME. These movements are dynamic, occurring simultaneously, and their net effects determine plasma or tissue concentrations at any time following consumption of the nutrient or xenobiotic (Box 4-1).

> Guiding Principle: Factors that influence any facet of ADME (absorption, distribution, metabolism, excretion) can affect animal dietary supplement safety.

Each movement is accomplished largely by passive diffusion, with facilitated and active transport as secondary mechanisms. Determinants of passive diffusion largely reflect the chemical characteristic of the compound, and include lipophilicity, frequently described as an (octanyl-water) partition coefficient, molecular size, and pKa. The

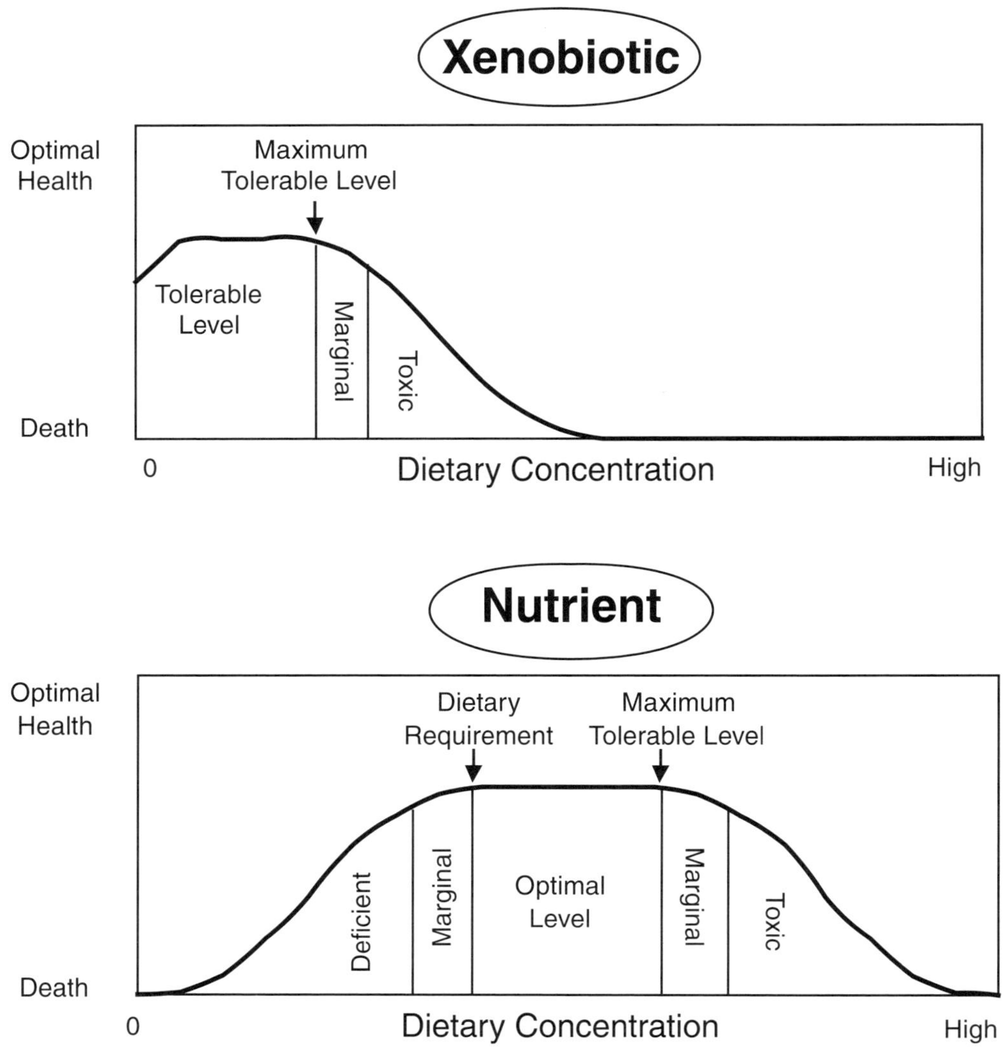

FIGURE 4-3 Effect of various concentrations of xenobiotics and essential nutrients on animal health.
SOURCE: Adapted from *Mineral Tolerance of Animals* (NRC, 2005).

pKa, in the context of the external environment, determines the degree to which a molecule is ionized and thus lipid soluble. In addition to chemical characteristics, each xenobiotic movement is simultaneously affected by multiple host factors, each reflecting host physiology (Figure 4-4). Although some of these host factors influence all compound movements (e.g., blood flow), most are unique to each movement. Each of these factors, in turn, is subject to changes or differences among special populations, increasing the risk of adversity to an animal dietary supplement. Factors that reflect differences in normal physiologic states, including but not limited to age, gender, pregnancy, lactation, or physiologic activity, may alter the risk of adversity to an animal dietary supplement in any species. However, for products intended for use in (nonhuman) animals, the risk for adversity can be profound if evolutionary differences in species physiology are not taken into account. The risk is magnified if the animal shifts from a state of normalcy to one of pathology due to disease, or due to the presence of other therapeutic agents with which an animal dietary supplement might interact. The impact of physiologic changes, species differences, pathology, and compound interactions can be profound and warrant a discussion on the most relevant to the safety of animal dietary supplements.

Relevant Kinetic Terms

Assessment of compound disposition includes a description of the disposition of the compound in kinetic terms. These terms are summarized in this section and discussed in more detail by Riviere (2003). Relevance of these terms and their predictability from one species to another will facilitate

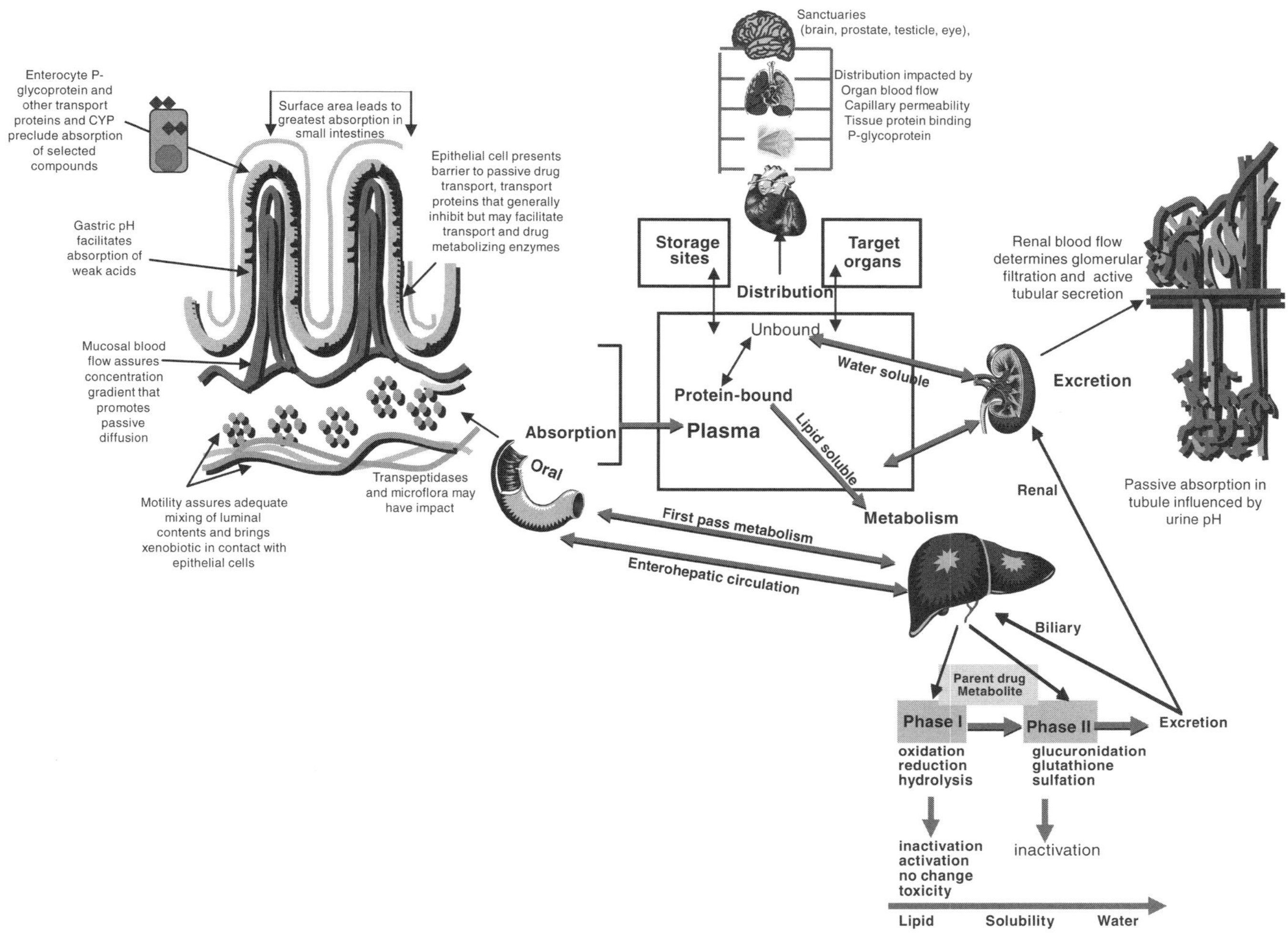

FIGURE 4-4 Factors determining plasma and tissue xenobiotic concentrations.

NOTE: Concentrations at any point in time reflect the dynamic interactions of four movements: absorption, distribution, metabolism, and excretion. Each of these four movements is largely dependent on passive diffusion of dissolved and unbound molecules. Each movement is, in turn, determined by a number of physiologic (animal) and xenobiotic factors, the latter including molecular weight, lipid vs. water solubility, and pKa. For an animal dietary supplement, the first movement is oral *absorption* of the dissolved compound. Influencing factors include local pH, surface area (greatest in the small intestine), epithelial permeability, mucosal blood flow, smooth muscle motility, and epithelial transport proteins, particularly those that efflux (e.g., P-glycoprotein) compounds (including nutrients) into the lumen. Once absorbed, selected compounds in the portal circulation may be almost completely removed during the first passage through the liver (first-pass metabolism). Once in circulation, the unbound (free) xenobiotic is distributed into tissues, where it may be bound to tissues, cleared, or distributed back into circulation. Host factors influencing *distribution*, the second movement, include extent of protein binding, regional (organ) blood flow, vascular permeability (e.g., extent of sanctuaries), body compartment size (i.e., extracellular vs. total body water), and transport proteins. After distribution, the intent of disposition of xenobiotics diverges from that of nutrients in that movements are intended to eliminate the former, but incorporate the latter. Elimination of the (generally unbound) lipid soluble xenobiotic reflects *metabolism* that occurs primarily, but not exclusively, in the liver. Phase I metabolism chemically changes the compound. The changes are accomplished predominantly by cytochrome P450 (CYP) enzymes that are subject to induction or inhibition by other compounds. The xenobiotic becomes more water soluble and amenable to phase II conjugation. Phase I metabolites may be inactive, active, or toxic. Phase II metabolism is a synthetic process that adds a large water-soluble molecule, inactivating the parent compound or metabolite and facilitating renal excretion. Depletion of phase II enzymes may increase toxicity of phase I metabolites. The last movement, *excretion*, is largely accomplished by the kidney but requires water solubility and is affected by glomerular filtration, which is passive and limited by protein binding; active tubular secretion, which occurs in the proximal tubules and is rapid and is not influenced by protein binding; and passive absorption, which can occur throughout the renal tubules and is influenced by urinary pH. Both active tubular secretion and glomerular filtration depend on renal blood flow. Biliary excretion of conjugated larger (> 600 MW) lipid-soluble molecules is less common, but may increase exposure of the body to a compound if the molecule is freed by intestinal microbes such that it can be resorbed (enterohepatic circulation).

BOX 4-1
Nutrients and Xenobiotics Are Managed Differently by the Body

The disposition (absorption, distribution, metabolism, and excretion, or ADME) of a compound that enters the body differs with the state of "foreignness" or "nativeness" to the body. Compounds perceived by the body as nutrients are incorporated into the body, becoming part of the body structure or contributing to its function and support. In general, mechanisms by which these compounds are "handled" have developed over evolution in response to the animal's physiologic needs and typical dietary intake. In contrast, specific pathways have evolved for compounds that are perceived by the body as foreign. These pathways target the elimination of xenobiotics to protect the body from toxicity. As such, xenobiotics are associated with a greater inherent risk, with the magnitude of risk dependent upon the existence and efficiency of pathways for metabolism and/or excretion of these materials. Consequently, it is often easier to predict the safety of compounds that are incorporated into normal physiology as compared to compounds that require development of specialized metabolism and elimination pathways.

accurate extrapolation of disposition data for animal dietary supplements when supplementation regimens are based on an alternative species.

Bioavailability

For the purpose of this report, the committee has defined bioavailability as the degree to which, or rate at which, a compound is absorbed or becomes available at the site of physiologic activity after administration. For the purposes of this discussion, the site of physiologic action is generally the plasma. Absolute bioavailability of a compound, particularly xenobiotics, is often determined by comparing the area under the plasma concentration curve (AUC) of the compound of interest after intravenous administration (thus assuring 100 percent of the compound enters the blood stream) to the AUC after administration via the route of interest. For animal dietary supplements, the route is generally oral.

Apparent Volume of Distribution (Vd)

The volume to which the compound is distributed reflects the chemistry of the xenobiotic and its ability to penetrate and accumulate within tissues. The volume of distribution is in reality a proportionality factor relating administered quantity to concentration achieved in the body. The volume proportionately and inversely impacts the concentration of that compound in plasma. Because it is a theoretical factor, calculated from the ratio of dose and plasma xenobiotic concentration after intravenous administration (Vd = Dose/concentration), the site and true volume to which the compound is distributed cannot be determined, and the term "apparent" is used. In general, the distribution of compounds that are water-soluble will be limited to interstitial fluids and thus is characterized by a volume of approximately 30 percent (0.3 L/kg) or less. In contrast, a volume of 60 percent (0.6 L/kg) or more may characterize a lipid-soluble xenobiotic, which is able to penetrate cell (lipid) membranes. Because protein binding might influence the distribution of a compound, volume of distribution is ideally referring to the unbound compound. Because the amount of a compound in plasma also influences how much of the compound will be cleared, volume of distribution also proportionately and directly influences the rate of elimination of the compound from the body.

Clearance (Cl)

Clearance describes the volume (generally of blood or plasma) that is irreversibly cleared of the compound of interest per unit time.

Half-Life ($t_{1/2}$)

Elimination half-life is among the more clinically relevant pharmacokinetic parameters. It determines the time that must elapse before steady-state concentrations are reached or before a compound is eliminated from the body. Elimination half-life is a proportionality of the rate of elimination (k_{el}): $t_{1/2} = 0.693/k_{el}$. Along with the dosing interval and effective range, half-life determines the amount of fluctuation in xenobiotic or nutrient concentrations during a recommended dosing interval. Half-life assumes that first-order kinetics describe compound movement, and thus is relevant only if a compound follows first-order kinetics. First-order kinetics protect the animal, in part, by ensuring a constant proportion (e.g., 10 percent per unit time and $k_{el} = 0.1\ min^{-1}$) of compound is eliminated per unit time. Saturation of enzymes (e.g., metabolic) may result in conversion to zero order kinetics, in which a constant amount (e.g., 15 mg) of compound is eliminated per unit time (Dayton et al., 1967). In such instances, concentrations of the compound may dramatically and rapidly increase and the concept of half-life becomes irrelevant until concentrations decrease below the point of saturation. Compounds that follow first-order elimination also might accumulate if the dosing interval is frequent enough that the compound remains in the body from the previous dose. The magnitude of accumulation can be predicted by the relationship to dosing interval and half-life. As such, half-life of the active ingredients (parent or metabolite) is a reasonable "must know" characteristic of a compound if extrapolation of dosing regimens is to be attempted. Elimination half-life is a function of both volume of distribution and clearance ($t_{1/2}$ = 0.693 Vd/Cl), with changes proportional to changes in volume of distribution (directly) or clearance (inversely). For example, if the volume of distribution of a compound decreases, more remains in the plasma. Because plasma concentrations increase, more is in the blood that is cleared per unit time, causing the compound to be eliminated more rapidly.

Mean Residence Time (MRT)

A parameter related to $t_{1/2}$ is mean residence time. However, it is more biologically relevant than half-life in that it describes the average length of time a molecule remains in the body. Half-life and mean residence time are equally affected by factors that influence xenobiotic movement because, like $t_{1/2}$, MRT is determined by both clearance (directly proportional) and volume of distribution (inversely proportional).

Physiologic Factors that Influence Xenobiotic Movement

Transport Proteins

Disposition of xenobiotics and nutrients often involve efflux and influx transport proteins. Knowledge of their impact can facilitate assessment of potential safety risk associated with an animal dietary supplement. As technology leads to more sophisticated investigative tools, cell membrane transport proteins will be increasingly linked with factors influencing movement of nutrients or xenobiotics, including physiologic differences (e.g., age, gender, and species), changes induced by disease, and interactions among compounds (nutrients or xenobiotics) administered simultaneously.

Transportation of compounds into or out of cells is mediated via transport proteins located at portals of entry (e.g., enterocyte of the gastrointestinal tract or sinusoidal hepatic cells), precluding entry into systemic circulation, or in "sanctuary" tissues (e.g., brain, cerebral spinal fluid, placenta, prostate, eyes, or testicles). As such, transport proteins influence each drug movement (absorption, distribution, metabolism, and excretion) of compounds that serve as substrates for the proteins. Intestinal transport proteins have been particularly well reviewed (Kunta and Sinko, 2004). Three major families move compounds from the lumen into the enterocyte, thus facilitating absorption, and from the body into the enterocyte, thus facilitating secretion. Transport proteins important to the uptake of nutrients include peptide export transport proteins, proteins located in the brush border of enterocytes where they transport peptides and small amino acid conjugates. Perhaps the most well known of the transport proteins is the ATP-binding cassette (ABC) superfamily of efflux transporters, which includes P-glycoprotein, the multidrug resistance protein (MDRP1), and a multispecific organic anion transporter (CMOAT/MRP2). The impact of the ABC transporters is profound, influencing movement of exogenous compounds, including nutrients and xenobiotics, and endogenous compounds such as steroids. Substrates for P-glycoprotein include both xenobiotics and dietary components that often are not structurally similar (Kunta and Sinko, 2004). Competition for transport increases oral absorption or distribution of one of the competing molecules. Among the better-described interactions between nutrients and drugs involving transport proteins is that of the flavonoids of grapefruit juice that inhibit P-glycoprotein (Zhang and Morris, 2003; Huang and Lesko, 2004; Kunta and Sinko, 2004; Hu et al., 2005). The role of P-glycoprotein in particular is being investigated for its impact on oral bioavailability of nutrients or xenobiotics. Because P-glycoprotein is commonly located in close proximity to, and shares substrates with, cytochrome-P450 enzymes (particularly CYP3A), it may have an additional influence on metabolism (Kunta and Sinko, 2004; Tyden et al., 2004). Polymorphism of P-glycoprotein is a recognized cause of differential response to xenobiotics among human populations.

It cannot be assumed that transport is the same across species. Recent work from Germany (Breves et al., 2007), for example, has suggested that the epithelial mechanism for intestinal chloride secretion in horses is likely to be very different from many other species. In addition, peptide transport is either not mediated by a pH gradient, as shown for pigs and other species, or the surface pH is not affected by luminal pH.

Xenobiotic Metabolizing Enzymes

The role of metabolism in the disposition of xenobiotics is complex and can be an important factor in assessing the potential safety risk associated with an animal dietary supplement. Although metabolism is generally considered a detoxification process for xenobiotics, in fact the compound may not change its activity, may become more active, or may become more toxic through the formation of secondary metabolites. Metabolites of variable activity, including toxicity produced by phase I metabolism and the importance of phase I and II metabolism in removing potentially toxic compounds, warrant special address in this review.

Most xenobiotics are eliminated by hepatic metabolism, renal excretion, or both. Lipid-soluble xenobiotics require enzymatic conversion to a water-soluble form to avoid passive resorption when excreted by the kidney (Figure 4-4). Those xenobiotic metabolizing enzymes located in the smooth endoplasmic reticulum (SER) of the hepatocyte are responsible for the majority of compound metabolism.

These enzymes are comprised predominantly of cytochrome P450 enzymes (CYP 450), referred to as such in recognition of the heme moiety, which mediates their enzymatic activity. This enzyme system is genetically recognized as a superfamily with nomenclature based on sequence similarity. Its role in compound metabolism, with an emphasis on toxicity, recently has been reviewed (Guengerich, 2008). The most important CYP enzymes in humans and the proportion of xenobiotics metabolized by the respective enzyme are 1A2 (13 percent), 2A6 (4 percent), 2B6 (1 percent), 2C (18 percent), 2D6 (1.5 percent), 2E1 (7 percent) and 3A4 (30 percent) (Bogaards et al., 2000). The presence and classification of CYP450 isoenzymes in dogs (Trepanier, 2006), cats (Trepanier, 2006; Shah et al., 2007), and horses (Tyden et al., 2004) were recently published (Table 4-5).

The sequelae of phase I metabolism on substrates includes xenobiotic inactivation, but this may be accompanied by production of metabolites of equal, more, or less activity, as well as reactive (e.g., oxygen radicals) or otherwise toxic metabolites. Among the important roles of phase II metabolism is removal of phase I metabolites whose accumulation may contribute to toxicity of the liver or other tissues. Phase II metabolism is accomplished with the chemical conjugation or addition of a large water-soluble molecule to the parent compound or its metabolite.

Glucuronidation is the most common phase II reaction, with -OH and -COOH functional group common substrates. Glucuronide conjugates are eliminated in the urine and bile; degradation by gastrointestinal microbiota, or less commonly by renal glucuronidases, may release the compound from the conjugate, allowing reabsorption and recirculation of the compound. Therefore, factors that influence composition of the intestinal microbial population could potentially affect toxicity of xenobiotics.

The glutathione transferase system targets electrophiles (compounds seeking electrons) and, as such, has several different roles in the body, including detoxification of radical metabolites. However, the enzyme can be rapidly depleted, which increases the risk of liver disease; N-acetylcysteine is a precursor for glutathione that can be use to replete the system.

With rare exceptions, phase II metabolites are inactive. Both phase I and phase II xenobiotic metabolizing enzymes are active at sites other than the liver, including the skin, lung, and kidney. Their impact on drug movement can be profound. For example, CYP P450 3A4 is the most predominate xenobiotic metabolizing enzyme in the enterocyte (Sagir et al., 2003).

Enantiomers

A second aspect of metabolism that might influence the risk of adversity in susceptible populations is the existence of many compounds (synthetic and natural) as enantiomers. Enantiomers are mirror-image stereoisomers. They are similar in molecular weight but differ in the orientation of four different functional groups that are bonded to a central, or "chiral," carbon. Enantiomers are designated as either D or L (or sometimes as S, sinister or R, rectus) (Landoni et al., 1997). Enantiomers are often interconverted by the body. Although seemingly chemically similar in structure, the different orientation of the side chain can result in profound differences in physiology, absorption, and disposition. Further, enantiomers may interact differentially with receptors, enzymes, or other targets, resulting in marked pharmacodynamic differences. For example, D enantiomers of amino acids are often not as bioavailable as L enantiomers and bioavailability can vary among species (Baker, 2006) so that toxicity may also differ. Compounds that exist as enantiomers are often marketed as racemic mixtures (generally 50:50), thus potentially physiologically representing two different compounds (Landoni et al., 1997). The pro-

TABLE 4-5 Cytochrome P450 Families and Their Importance to Drug Metabolism in Humans and Orthologs in Other Species

Human	% of Drugs	Dog	Cat	Horse
CYP1A1	13	CYP1A1	CYP1A	CYP1A
CYP1A2	—	CYP1A2 (o)	—	—
CYP2B6	—	CYP2B11	—	CYP2A6/2B6
CYP2E1	7	CYP2E2	CYP2E[a]	—
CYP2C9	18	CYP2C1[b]	CYP2C[c]	CYP2B,2C[d]
CYP2D6	1.5	CYP2D15[e]	CYP2D	CYP2D[d]
CYP3A4	30	CYP3A12	CYP3A	CYP3A
—	—	CYP3A26	—	—

[a]Three variants (Tanaka et al., 2005).
[b]Polymorphism (Blaisdell et al., 1998).
[c]Very low (Shah et al., 2007).
[d]Very low.
[e]Three variants (Paulson et al., 1999).

portion of enantiomers in natural compounds might be very different from that in synthetic preparations and may differ with source, processing, storage, and other factors. For such compounds, data should be presented in the context of each enantiomer rather than total compound. Yet, analysis of each enantiomer of a compound (e.g., kinetic or dynamic studies) may be difficult, often requiring expensive methods that force separation despite physical and chemical similarities.

Physiological Factors that Influence Disposition and Response: Populations Potentially at Risk

A number of factors might affect the response to an animal dietary supplement by either altering its disposition such that plasma or tissue concentrations are affected, or altering response at the physiologic level. Among the most important are physiologic differences, interaction with other compounds, and pathologic changes induced by diseases. The more complicated the disposition of a compound, or the more foreign, the greater the likelihood that adversities will occur in selected populations. The impact of kinetic and dynamic differences among populations at risk has received little attention in the past several decades in animals or humans, reflecting, in part, the difficulties encountered in study methods. By their nature, such studies either are based on in vitro models or are invasive. Methods of quantitation often are expensive particularly when attempting to separate exogenous materials that are the same as or similar to endogenous counterparts. Recent investigations in humans have included methods based on tissue dosimetry that can characterize interindividual variability in physiologic and pharmacokinetic indices characterizing xenobiotics (toxins in particular), due to differences in age, gender, and species (Clewell et al., 2002). Although much of this information may be applicable to animals, care must be taken with overextrapolation in the face of uncharacterized species differences.

A number of physiologic factors can influence individual response to an animal dietary supplement. These include, but are not limited to, species or breed differences, age, and gender, as well as altered body states, such as obesity or pregnancy. The information regarding the impact of these factors in animals is limited but has been reviewed and is summarized below. As with much information regarding the disposition of compounds in animals, the information often reflects extrapolation among species, with few specific references to scientific studies in target animals. Those physiological factors that are most likely to affect the disposition and reaction to animal dietary supplements are addressed.

Age

The impact of age on the disposition of compounds can be profound, with differences generally compared to the young adult (Table 4-6). Although limited data are available for target species, most veterinary clinical pharmacologists generally apply disposition patterns described for humans to animals and find this application to be clinical relevant (Dowling, 2005). Changes in disposition have been described in both age extremes in humans (Nouws, 1992; Vestal, 2000) with geriatric people being at a greater risk, not only because of "normal" aging changes in physiology, but also because the likelihood of polypharmacy and disease may increase the risk of adverse events.

Differences in disposition in geriatric and neonatal or pediatric animals compared to young adult animals affects each of the four compound movements; those impacting xenobiotics in particular are delineated in Table 4-6. The most profound differences impact distribution and clearance. Distribution differences reflect different body compartment sizes and differences in the composition and integrity of sanctuary barriers. Clearance differences primarily reflect differences in both the size and function of organs of clearance. Further, in addition to changes in disposition, very young and aged animals tend to be characterized by differences in tissue responsiveness to compounds (Ginsberg et al., 2005; Hurria and Lichtman, 2007).

In general, oral absorption and clearance is slower in both pediatric and geriatric animals. Differences exist for both nutrients and xenobiotics. For example, young kittens have decreased energy, carbohydrate, and organic matter digestibility when compared to kittens over 19 weeks of age (Harper and Turner, 2000). However, when compared to adult animals of the same species, young animals also consume more food per unit body weight resulting in higher intake (per unit body weight) of an animal dietary supplement incorporated into the food.

Digestibility of key nutrients, such as fat, tends to decrease in elderly cats (Taylor et al., 1995; Harper, 1998; Peachey et al., 1999; Perez-Camargo, 2004); therefore, oral absorption of animal dietary supplements may also be impaired. Perez-Camargo (2004) reported that 30 percent of cats over 12 years of age had low fat digestibility (< 80 percent fat digestibility, compared to 90–95 percent fat digestibility for younger adult cats). Peachey et al. (1999) reported lower digestibility of all fatty acid groups in elderly cats when compared to young adult cats. Consequently, absorption of lipid-soluble animal dietary supplements such as evening primrose oil would be expected to be lower in elderly cats. Decreased absorption of an animal dietary supplement implies that the intake of the supplement would need to be higher before adverse effects (other than effects on the gastrointestinal tract) would be observed. Other changes in digestive physiology may also help explain impaired absorption in elderly humans and animals. For example, there is a shift in the intestinal microbiota population of elderly dogs and humans, with lactobacilli decreasing and clostridia increasing (Benno et al., 1992). Elderly cats have lower fecal bifidobacteria concentrations when compared to young adult cats (Patil et al., 2000). Changes in the

TABLE 4-6 The Impact of Age-related Differences in Physiology on Xenobiotic Disposition in Humans

Age	Absorption	Distribution	Metabolism	Excretion
Pediatric ≤ 12 weeks	Increased absorption for 1st 24 hr (during colostrum absorption)	Increased volume of distribution reduced plasma concentrations	Decreased phase I metabolism, being absent for first weeks and reaching adult levels at 3 to 4 months	Decreased renal clearance until 2 to 3 months
	Decreased acidity leads to decreased absorption of weak acids.	Greater proportion of extracellular fluid reduces plasma concentrations of water soluble compounds.	Increased bioavailability of drugs that normally undergo first pass metabolism	Prolonged half-life
	Decreased rate (not extent) of absorption of most drugs	Longer half-life for most drugs unless cleared more rapidly than adults	Decreased response to compounds which must be metabolized to active state	—
	Milk may bind to luminal contents	Decreased distribution of compounds that accumulate in fat	Decreased peripheral metabolism of compounds	—
	Reduced absorption of fat soluble drugs	Decreased protein binding may increase distribution.	—	—
	—	Increased blood flow to brain and heart	—	—
	—	Increased permeability of blood brain barrier	—	—
Geriatric	Decreased motility prolongs absorption time.	Decreased total body water and greater proportion of extracellular fluid	Decreased hepatic mass and drug metabolizing enzymes (phases I and II)	Decreased glomerular filtration rate (GFR)
	Increased risk of bacterial overgrowth	Increased body fat increases distribution of lipid soluble drugs.	Decreased hepatic blood flow	Decreased renal clearance
	Generally decreased absorption	Decreased protein binding compensated for by clearance of free compound	Decreased hepatic clearance and prolonged half-life	Decreased renal protection
	Decreased gastroprotection	Increased distribution to heart and brain as cardiac function declines	Decreased hepatoprotection	—

microbial population can influence enterohepatic circulation of bile acids (Hickman et al., 1992), which are essential for excretion of some xenobiotics.

Differences in distribution reflect differences in body compartments. Pediatric humans generally have larger volumes of distribution for water-soluble compounds whereas geriatric humans generally have a contracted muscle mass but greater body fat. The disposition of several antimicrobials in neonatal animals has been reviewed by Baggott (2000), with differences in disposition generally found to be similar to that described for humans. Studies of the disposition of ampicillin, a water-soluble drug, in kittens and puppies (Goldstein et al., 1995; Lavy et al., 1995) support a larger volume of distribution in this age group. Volumes were 3- to 4-fold higher in kittens compared to that expected in adults, resulting in clinically significant lower drug concentrations. Sequin et al. (2004) also demonstrated marked, yet somewhat unpredicted differences in the disposition of enrofloxacin, a lipid-soluble drug, in kittens. An age-dependent effect of volume was manifested, being smaller at 2–4 weeks but greater at 4–6 weeks. Clearance was more rapid at 6 weeks, resulting in a short half-life compared to adults. Therapeutic concentrations were not achieved with oral administration of an adult dose.

Differences also have been demonstrated in other species, including pediatric horses. For example, differences have been demonstrated for gentamicin, a water-soluble drug (Abo El-Sooud, 2003) in three juvenile species (foal, lamb, calf). Of the three species, the volume of distribution was largest in the foal, being approximately 3-fold that in lambs, 70 percent higher than that in calves, and approximately twice that expected in adult animals.

Like humans, dogs may lose lean body mass and accumulate more body fat as they age (Lawler et al., 2005). This change will increase distribution of fat-soluble components. The impact differs with the chemistry of the compound.

For lipid-soluble compounds, dosing on a mg/kg BW basis should minimize the impact on plasma concentrations, but not elimination rates. For water-soluble compounds, unless dosed on a lean body mass basis, the volume of the water compartment will represent a smaller proportion of total body compartments. Plasma concentrations are likely to be higher whereas elimination will be more rapid (assuming clearance does not change). The effect of aging on body composition is somewhat breed-dependent in dogs. Speakman et al. (2003) reported increased body fat with age in Great Danes, but not Labrador Retrievers or Papillons, although Lawler et al. (2005) reported decreased lean body mass and increased fat mass within one year of death in elderly Labrador Retrievers.

While middle-aged cats tend to be overweight, geriatric cats often become thin (Perez-Camargo, 2004). Accordingly, distribution of both water- and fat-soluble supplements may be more variable in cats as they age, compared to dogs. For the lean geriatric cat, plasma concentrations of lipid-soluble compounds might be expected to be higher compared to the young adult, even if dosing on a mg/kg BW basis. Elimination thus is more likely to increase. For water-soluble drugs, dosing on a mg/kg BW basis might compensate for potential changes in plasma concentrations. However, as with lipid-soluble compounds, the loss in body mass is likely to increase plasma concentrations and thus the rate of elimination, although these changes might be offset by changes in clearance.

Energy requirements of dogs decrease as they age (see NRC, 2006, for a review of the studies), so food intake will be lower in elderly dogs if they are maintaining body weight. Decreased food intake will result in decreased consumption of animal dietary supplements that are incorporated into the food.

Other differences in disposition among ages affecting distribution reflect the integrity of blood-tissue barriers. The blood brain barrier is not well developed in the pediatric human whereas changes in mental activity, motility, cytoprotection, and other factors predispose the geriatric person or animal to greater risks (Ginsberg et al., 2005; Hurria and Lichtman, 2007). Morita et al. (2005) reported alterations in the blood brain barrier in elderly dogs.

Differences in age extremes also will influence metabolism and excretion. Compared to distribution, their impact is seemingly less complex and thus more predictable (Table 4-6). Yet, as scientific studies emerge in target species, complexities might also be anticipated. For example, Ecobichon et al. (1988) found that glucuronidation was the most predominant phase II reaction in Beagle pups, and that sulfonation decreased as puppies got older. Appearance of phase I metabolites for selected drugs also decreased with age. For renal excretion, development of the renal cortex may influence clearance as well as predisposition to toxicity. For example, the risk of nephrotoxicity of the antimicrobial gentamicin seems to be less in neonatal compared to older pediatric dogs (Cowan et al., 1980) because renal cortices are not fully developed. The same is not true, however, for horses, for which differences in disposition seem to increase the risk of nephrotoxicity in foals (Riviere et al., 1983).

Gender

The impact of gender on xenobiotic disposition is not as well characterized as the impact of other factors. In general, female humans, compared to males, are characterized by reduced smooth muscle motility, greater body fat, and greater content and fluctuation in plasma volume, as well as increased organ blood flow, xenobiotic metabolism (increase CYP3A4, others not clear), and transporter protein activity (Tanaka, 1999; Gandhi et al., 2004). Gender differences, when elucidated scientifically, are likely to be complex, as has been demonstrated for CYP enzymes in cats (Shah et al., 2007). Female cats were characterized by greater CYP2D and lower CYP3A compared to males. To the committee's knowledge, the effect of neutering on xenobiotic disposition has not been evaluated. Among gender differences are also those that influence reproduction.

Pregnancy

Selected changes described in pregnant humans are likely to occur in other species, including dogs, cats, and horses. The impact of pregnancy on anticancer drugs in pregnant animals has been reviewed by Autio et al. (2007), although little information was available for target species. In general, pregnancy is associated with physiologic differences that decrease concentrations of xenobiotics. Each compartment—maternal, placental, and fetal—is characterized by its own rate of absorption, distribution, metabolism, and excretion (Welsch, 1982; Krauer and Krauer, 1991). Furthermore, pregnancy is a dynamic state characterized by dramatic changes in placental and fetal growth and in the physiology of the pregnant animal. All pharmacokinetic processes change in the mother, in concert with the progression of pregnancy. Gastrointestinal motility and gastric acid secretion decrease and may lead to decreased xenobiotic absorption. Decreased albumin concentration results in decreased binding of highly protein-bound xenobiotics. Increased volume of distribution of unbound compounds may result in lower concentrations and more rapid clearance. Increases in cardiac output, renal blood flow, and glomerular filtration rate can further decrease xenobiotic concentrations, particularly of antibiotics. High progesterone concentrations may induce hepatic microsomal enzymes and increase xenobiotic metabolism (Papich and Davis, 1986). Variability has been demonstrated among investigators studying drugs that share similar characteristics, as has been demonstrated in pregnant horses. For example, whereas Sanstchi and Papich (2000) failed to detect significant changes in the disposition of a water-soluble drug (gentamicin) in pregnant mares,

Traver and Riviere (1982) found that ampicillin, also a water-soluble drug, achieved lower concentrations in pregnant mares. These studies serve to underscore the complexity that characterizes pregnancy, thus rendering response to chemical compounds largely unpredictable.

Species variability in response to pregnancy should be anticipated. Some differences have been demonstrated, such as differences in increased volume of distribution (increasing less in ruminants compared to up to 50 percent in rats and humans, as reviewed by Autio et al., 2007).

The pharmacologic principles that address risk of fetal exposure to potential teratrogens have been reviewed (Farrar and Blume, 1991; Syme et al., 2004). The drug approval process generally precludes availability of those compounds with a demonstrated risk but premarket assessment does not occur for all animal dietary supplements. The period during which the fetus is most sensitive to adverse effects (greatest in the first trimester) is likely correlated with duration of pregnancy, with the period representing a longer proportion of the pregnancy in animals with a shorter pregnancy (e.g., dogs and cats) compared to those with a longer pregnancy (e.g., horses) (Autio et al., 2007).

The placenta presents a barrier to xenobiotic distribution from maternal blood into the fetus. Transporter proteins on both the maternal and fetal side influence xenobiotic movement. Placental phase I and II xenobiotic-metabolizing enzymes also have been identified throughout gestation in human placenta. As a sanctuary, the barrier to compound distribution presented by the placenta reflects transporter proteins (e.g., P-pg) on both the maternal and fetal side, and both phase I and II xenobiotic-metabolizing enzymes also have been identified throughout gestation in human placenta. Yet, as has been demonstrated in humans, nearly all xenobiotics administered during pregnancy are assumed to enter to some degree the fetal circulation (Syme et al., 2004). Further, a "depot phenomena" has been described in human placenta and reflects the accumulation of selected lipid-soluble xenobiotics in the placenta, with the placenta possibly serving as a storage site (Syme et al., 2004). Extrapolation of data among species regarding maternal to fetal transfer of compounds is complicated by the unique placentation of the human fetus compared to other animals (Carter, 2007). Autio et al. (2007) indicated that placentation in horses, cows, goats, and pigs consists of six layers, compared to five layers found in the dog and cat. Humans and rats have the least number of layers, with maternal blood bathing the fetal trophoblast. The endotheliochorial placentation of carnivores differs from hemochorial placentation of humans only by the presence of maternal endothelium, and it is likely that this single fenestrated layer does not present a significantly greater barrier (Renfree, 1982). In contrast to endotheliochorial placenta in carnivores, the horse has an epitheliochorial placenta, whereby the chorion is in contact with the endometrium everywhere and there is no loss of maternal tissue (Arthur, 1996). As a result, there is an additional tissue barrier (i.e., the endometrial epithelium) separating the maternal blood flow from the fetal blood flow in the horse compared to the dog and cat. Not surprisingly, gentamicin (a water-soluble drug) administered to a pregnant mare was not detectable in foals, whereas trimethoprim (lipid soluble) was detectable (as reviewed by Autio et al., 2007). This is consistent with the differences in gentamicin and ampicillin seen in pregnant horses discussed earlier. The equine placenta further differs from canine and feline placentas in that villi are uniformly dispersed on the fetal chorion in the mare (i.e., diffuse), whereas the villi are disposed in the form of a broad encircling belt in the bitch and queen (i.e., zonary) (Arthur, 1996).

The fetus also is capable of metabolism of nutrients or xenobiotics, although contribution to xenobiotic metabolizing enzymes in near-term animals is negligible (Welsch, 1982). Species differences among fetal metabolism might also increase the risk of adverse events in the dam. For example, compared to other species, the fetal foal depends more on transplacental glucose for energy, rather than amino acids or lactate, due to a limited ability to deaminate amino acids (Fowden, 1997). The foal's high glucose requirement is met through redirection of glucose from maternal tissues. Prolonged hypoglycemia in the mare may result in adverse events, including initiation of early labor.

Lactation

Like the fetus, the nursing animal potentially is an inadvertent recipient of xenobiotics administered to the mother. Most of the pertinent information in the veterinary literature is concerned with excretion of xenobiotics in the milk of food animals; there seems to be no information regarding small animals or horses. Studies of humans indicate that low molecular weight (< 200), unionized, highly lipid-soluble xenobiotics that are minimally protein bound diffuse into the lactating mammary gland rapidly, whereas water-soluble xenobiotics diffuse more slowly (Berlin, 1981). Similar criteria should be reasonably expected in other species. Depending on milk pH and compound pKa, "ion trapping" can concentrate xenobiotics in milk. Generally, the amount of xenobiotics excreted in human milk is less than 2 percent of the maternal dose (Berlin, 1981).

Even if compounds are excreted in milk, they may not be associated with negative sequelae. For example, a xenobiotic that has been excreted into, and subsequently ingested with, milk during nursing may not be absorbed from the gastrointestinal tract of the nursing animal. Milk may decrease the absorption of some compounds (e.g., chelation with calcium), whereas the pharmacokinetic properties of other xenobiotics (i.e., aminoglycosides) preclude their absorption. An exception may be the very young for which the gastrointestinal tract is characterized by marked permeability such that colostrum absorption is facilitated. Compounds that might not be absorbed in older pediatric animals may be absorbed in the neonate that is less than 24 hours of age.

The disposition of compounds may be influenced by changes in energy need in the reproducing animal. Depending on litter size, food intake increases 3- to 4-fold in lactating dogs and cats. As a result, both daily animal dietary supplement intake and animal dietary supplement intake per kg body weight are much higher than in nonreproducing adult cats and dogs. In addition, during their animals' pregnancy and lactation, owners might be more inclined to provide additional supplements. In the lactating mare, voluntary dry matter intake increases over that observed during gestation, but the magnitude of the increase is not as dramatic as that seen in the litter-bearing bitch and queen. Daily dry matter intake of gestating mares is generally 1.75–2.5 percent body weight, whereas it typically does not exceed 3 percent body weight in the lactating mare (NRC, 2007). The upper limit in dry matter intake in the horse can be attributed to, in part, the relatively bulky, high-fiber nature of the feedstuffs consumed. In the domestic horse, the increased nutritional needs of the lactating mare are usually accommodated by providing more nutrient-dense ingredients, such as the addition of greater amounts of cereal grains and oilseed meals.

Exercise

The effect of exercise on nutrient metabolism and energy requirements of dogs and cats was recently reviewed (NRC, 2006) and, therefore, will not be reviewed in depth in this text. Exercise has been shown to cause oxidative stress (Hinchcliff et al., 2000), decrease gastric acid secretion, delay gastric emptying (Kondo et al., 1994), and decrease mucosal blood flow in dogs (Tasler et al., 1974). Little research has been conducted on exercise in cats; however, it is apparent that activity level of indoor pet cats is similar to that of laboratory cats (NRC, 2006). In contrast, kennel dogs typically exercise more and have higher energy requirements than sedentary house pets (Patil and Bisby, 2002). Heavily exercising dogs consume much more food than sedentary dogs. This is particularly true for animals involved in endurance sports such as sled dog racing; these dogs not only run long distances, but also are exposed to extremely low environmental temperatures. Small breed dogs tend to be very active and have higher energy requirements (Kienzle and Rainbird, 1991), and therefore higher food intake, per kilogram body weight than larger breed dogs. Consequently, food intake and breed must be accounted for when extrapolating animal dietary supplement intake from published studies to sedentary house pets, working dogs, or different breeds.

Horses are used for a variety of athletic activities. The intensity, duration, and frequency of training and competition have the biggest effect on the digestible energy needs of the horse. For example, the digestible energy requirement of horses in "light" work (e.g., pleasure riding) may be just slightly greater than that needed to meet maintenance needs. In contrast, horses participating in "very heavy" work, which could be of fast speed (e.g., Thoroughbred racing) or long duration (e.g., endurance racing), may have twice the energy requirement of a sedentary horse (NRC, 2007). If given the opportunity, horses will voluntarily increase dry matter intake to meet the increased energy demands of exercise. However, similar to that mentioned above for the lactating mare, the bulky nature of the horse's diet often limits dry matter intake to 3 percent of body weight. As a result, more energy-dense feedstuffs (e.g., cereal grains and oils) are often added to the diets of exercising horses. Exercise itself has been shown to affect the absorption, distribution, metabolism, and excretion of some nutrients in the horse (see review in NRC, 2007). For example, nitrogen retention is increased in the exercising horse compared to the sedentary horse (see review in NRC, 2007).

Pathologic Factors

The diseased animal is more likely to react adversely to a xenobiotic or excess intake of a nutrient due to changes in the disposition of the compound induced by disease. Selected examples of the more likely sequelae are listed in Table 4-7. Although such reactions occasionally reflect disease-induced differences in receptor number or sensitivity, most often they reflect differences in xenobiotic or nutrient disposition. Pathophysiologic changes in most body systems can alter all phases of disposition, predisposing the animal to adverse xenobiotic reactions. The sequelae of disease on xenobiotic disposition reflect disease-induced changes in volumes of distribution and clearance. The impact on compound disposition can be complex, with the most problematic being those that lead to increased concentrations (e.g., smaller volume of distribution as may occur with dehydration) and longer half-lives (e.g., decreased renal clearance associated with renal disease). As such, supplementation levels generally need to be decreased for those compounds characterized by an increased risk of adversity. Disease may also increase the risk of adverse reactions due to the need for polypharmacy and thus drug-xenobiotic or drug-nutrient interactions. Finally, diseased organs are less able to cytoprotect, increasing the risk for xenobiotic or nutrient-induced diseases, particularly in organs that accumulate the compound or its metabolite (e.g., organs of clearance). Organs whose disease is most likely to increase the risk of adverse events are those exposed to the greatest concentrations, including the gastrointestinal tract and organs of excretion and metabolism, the kidney and liver. The heart and brain may also be predisposed to adverse reactions if disease has resulted in vascular responses that increase their blood flow (e.g., hypotension). Changes in vascular responses (e.g., induced by cardiac, renal, or liver disease) may also affect absorption, distribution, metabolism, and excretion.

TABLE 4-7 Examples of the Potential Impact of Disease on Disposition of Xenobiotics

Pharmacokinetic Changes	Impact	Sequelae
Renal disease	Decreased cytoprotection	Increased risk of xenobiotic-induced nephrotoxicity
	Decreased autoregulation	Increased risk of xenobiotic-induced nephrotoxicity
	Decreased body mass (dehydration)	Decreased volume of distribution (higher xenobiotic concentration, shorter half-life)
	Decreased renal blood flow	Decreased renal clearance (longer half-life)
	Glomerular disease	Increased risk of xenobiotic-induced nephrotoxicity
		Deceased protein-binding (increased fraction of unbound xenobiotic)
		Increased clearance of unbound fraction of highly protein-bound xenobiotics
Liver disease	Decreased hepatic blood flow	Increased oral bioavailability, decreased clearance of highly extracted compounds
Cardiac disease	Decreased phase I enzymes	Decreased hepatic clearance (longer half-life)
	Decreased phase II enzymes	Decreased hepatic clearance (longer half-life)
		Decreased hepatoprotection (increased risk of hepatoxocity
	Decreased albumin	Increased concentration of free xenobiotic
	Decreased renal blood flow	See renal disease
	Decreased hepatic blood flow	See liver disease
	Decreased regional blood flow	Decreased organ delivery (higher concentrations delivered to brain and heart)
Gastrointestinal disease	Decreased cytoprotection	Increased risk of gastrointestinal toxicity
	Altered permeability	Altered absorption
	Altered gastrointestinal motility	Decreased rate of absorption
Pharmacodynamic Changes	Altered receptor number or affinity	Altered response

The impact of renal disease on disposition is relatively straightforward (Table 4-7) (Churchwell and Mueller, 2007). For xenobiotics and nutrients whose elimination depends on renal function and whose clearance is known to be decreased in renal disease, the incidence of adverse events might be reduced by altering the dose of the supplement based on serum creatinine. Xenobiotics and nutrients that are not excreted through or metabolized by the kidney are not expected to be affected by renal disease. The effects of liver disease on xenobiotic disposition are much more complex (Table 4-7) (Delco et al., 2005), reflecting changes in hepatic blood flow, hepatic metabolism, and protein binding. The impact depends in part on the fraction of the xenobiotic extracted from blood with each passage through the liver. Highly extracted compounds are more impacted by changes in hepatic blood flow whereas compounds characterized by low extraction are impacted by protein binding as well as the metabolic capacity of the liver.

While animal dietary supplement tolerance data obtained from healthy animals cannot necessarily be extrapolated to diseased animals, if an animal dietary supplement is shown to be safe in diseased animals, it will most likely be safe in healthy animals of the same physiologic state at the same intake.

Species Differences

Differences among species in the kinetics and response to compounds are profound but not well reviewed. Studies that methodically compare disposition characteristics among species are few, and often oriented toward identifying the (laboratory) animal most predictive of human disposition. For example, Jolivette and Ward (2005) attempted to identify a system whereby the species could be identified that would most accurately predict human pharmacokinetics of specific compounds. They compared selected intravenous pharmacokinetic data (volume of distribution, clearance, and mean residence time) of over 100 molecules (including drugs) reported in the literature for humans, monkeys, dogs, and rats and related differences to detailed chemical descriptors of each molecule. For each pharmacokinetic parameter, the authors attempted to describe "rules" that would increase the predictability of data in each species to human data. For example, for molecules characterized by moderate or high clearance, qualitative and quantitative rules could be described that would allow accurate human predictions based on data collected from dogs, rats, and monkeys. Likewise, molecules could be characterized for which extrapolations among the species would be incorrect. The authors concluded that the combination of computation analysis of the molecular characteristics of each compound with in vivo pharmacokinetic data might be helpful to identify the most appropriate species for predicting pharmacokinetic behavior of a particular molecule in another species.

Absorption

Lin (1995) suggested that drug absorption is simply a process of interaction between drug and biomembrane and might be similar among the species. Predicting adversity resulting from absorption of compounds would be facilitated by such a simplistic mechanism. Yet, profound differences in anatomy, physiology, and biochemistry have been described among species and are likely to differentially impact xenobiotics and nutrients (Kararli, 1995). Differences among species impact xenobiotics and nutrients, although different pathways are likely to be involved with xenobiotics versus nutrients. Evidence for other xenobiotics suggested that marked differences in disposition preclude simplistic extrapolation of data among species, but that extrapolations are more likely to be relevant if species are closely, rather than distantly, related.

Differences in absorption have been demonstrated among species. For example, in dogs, absorption of some hydrophilic compounds is more similar to that in rats whereas others are more similar to that found in humans (He et al., 1998). Different affinities for P-glycoproteins have been demonstrated between humans, nonhuman primates, and Beagle dogs (Xia et al., 2005). Differences in gastrointestinal CYP 450 among species are further complicated by regional tissue differences. For example, Tyden et al. (2004) demonstrated CYP3A4 activity in the duodenum to be 4-fold higher than in the liver, with a gradual decrease distally. The impact of these and other differences has contributed to surprisingly different absorptive patterns for xenobiotics between species. The limited number of oral bioavailability studies of xenobiotics in dogs, cats, or horses demonstrates the lack of predictability. For example, ciprofloxacin is characterized by excellent oral bioavailability in humans but poor to no oral bioavailability in horses (ponies; Langston et al., 1996) and cats (Albarellos et al., 2004) and fair to poor in dogs (Abadia et al., 1995). Accordingly, data regarding absorption of animal dietary supplements may not always be accurately extrapolated among species.

Lipid Absorption

Because two nutrients reviewed in this report are lipids (lutein and evening primrose oil), and because lipid absorption is different from absorption of most drugs, a focus on species differences in lipid absorption from the gastrointestinal tract is warranted.

Understanding of lipid absorption is especially relevant for lipid-soluble nutrients and supplements. Hydrolysis of triglycerides begins with gastric lipase, which, along with churning by the stomach, forms lipid droplets. As the acidic fat emulsion enters the duodenum, it is neutralized and modified by mixing with bile and pancreatic juice. Bile is secreted from the gallbladder of dogs and cats; because horses do not have a gallbladder, bile is secreted continuously from the liver. Biliary secretion and pancreatic fluid are enhanced by cholecystokinin, which is secreted from the duodenal mucosa in response to the entry of acidic chyme from the stomach. In addition to supplying bicarbonate to neutralize the acidic chime, pancreatic fluid contains enzymes that catalyze the hydrolysis of fatty acids from triglycerides, phospholipids, and cholesterol esters. Before pancreatic lipase can continue what gastric lipase started, bile salts must first accumulate on the surface of lipid droplets. This interaction between bile salts and lipid droplets attracts colipase (also secreted from the pancreas). Colipase is essential for the activity of pancreatic lipase, which is otherwise strongly inhibited by bile salts. Pancreatic lipase catalyzes the hydrolysis of fatty acids from positions 1 and 3 of triglycerides, yielding two non-esterified fatty acids (NEFA) and one 2-monoglyceride. As these products are formed, they disperse and form multimolecular aggregates called mixed micelles. Mixed micelles are made up of a monolayer of bile salts, monoglycerides and lysophospholipids, which surround a core of NEFA, cholesterol, and fat-soluble vitamins.

The intraluminal phase of fat absorption involves passage of monoglycerides and NEFA into the absorptive cells of the small intestine. Lipid absorption generally begins in the distal duodenum and is completed in the jejunum. Because of their small size, mixed micelles pass readily into the unstirred water layer at the surface of the microvillus membrane. Monoglycerides and NEFA are then released from the mixed micelle and passively diffuse (or are potentially transported via fatty acid binding proteins) through the brush border membrane.

The intracellular phase of fat absorption involves recombination of monoglycerides and NEFA in the enterocyte and packaging for export into the circulation. Nonesterified fatty acids entering the enterocyte bind to cytosolic fatty acid binding proteins and are taken to the endoplasmic reticulum where they are re-esterified to form triglycerides. Re-esterification is an ATP-dependent process, with acyl-CoA synthase needed to "activate" fatty acids to their acyl-CoA thioesters. The major acceptors for esterification of acyl-CoA are the 2-monoglycerides; therefore, resynthesis of triglycerides occurs mainly via the monoglyceride pathway. Fatty acids can also be re-esterified to the 1 position of lysophospholipids by an acyl transferase located in the villus tips of the intestinal brush border. These phospholipids, along with an apolipoprotein skeleton, are packaged to form the outer monolayer of a chylomicron, with a core of triglycerides, cholesterol, and some carbohydrates.

The final phase of absorption involves the fusion of the triglyceride-rich chylomicron with the basolateral membrane of the enterocyte and secretion into the extracellular space by exocytosis. Animal dietary supplements formulated with nanoparticle delivery systems may potentially also be absorbed via the chylomicron pathway. Chylomicrons do not enter the plasma directly, but instead they are excreted into the tiny lymph vessels (lacteals). From there, chylomicrons transverse the lymphatic system and pass via the thoracic duct into circulation. Compared to the other products of absorption, dietary lipids are unique in that they do not enter the hepatic portal vein and transverse the liver before entering system circulation. The exceptions are short- and medium-chained fatty acids (2 to 12 carbons), which are rapidly absorbed via the portal vein. After digestion, triglyceride-rich chylomicrons transport lipids of dietary origin and deliver them to tissues in need of fatty acids. The enzyme lipoprotein lipase—anchored to the luminal aspect of endothelial cells lining the capillaries of adipose tissue, skeletal and cardiac muscle, mammary glands, and other tissues—binds to chylomicrons passing through the capillaries and rapidly hydrolyzes triglycerides in the core of the chylomicron. Hydrolysis of triglycerides releases NEFA, which can diffuse across the cell membrane (either by simple diffusion or by facilitated diffusion using fatty acid transport proteins). Once inside the cell of a tissue, the NEFA can be oxidized for energy, re-esterified to triglycerides and stored (in adipose tissue and muscle), or re-esterified to phospholipids where they may become a part of the cell membrane. The half-life of a chylomicron-triglyceride once it is released from the enterocyte and enters the circulation has been estimated at about 5 minutes, whereas the half-life of a whole chylomicron particle has been estimated to be about 13–14 minutes (Gurr et al., 2002).

In contrast to that described above, it is not clear whether adult horses transport dietary triacylglycerols in the form of chylomicrons. A chylomicron-like lipoprotein fraction has been identified in the nonfasting plasma of suckling foals, but not in mature horses or ponies maintained on forage and grain diets (see review by Watson et al., 1993). The absence of a chylomicron lipoprotein fraction in mature equids may be related to the relatively low fat content of their normal diet (< 3 percent crude fat), whereas suckling foals are likely consuming more fat from mare milk. However, the fat content of the diet may not be the only factor influencing chylomicron synthesis, as attempts to isolate chylomicrons from adult ponies following an oral fat load were unsuccessful as the animals showed no evidence of postprandial lipemia (Watson, 1991, as cited in Watson et al., 1993). Others have reported very small concentrations of chylomicrons in the plasma of horses fed diets with or without added fat (e.g., van Dijk and Wensing, 1989; Marchello et al., 2000). However, the physical and chemical composition of the lipoprotein fractions retrieved in these studies have not been well described and may not fit the true definition of a chylomicron. The lack of a chylomicron fraction in horses may reflect a mechanistic adaptation to relatively low fat, forage-based diets. Ruminants, which consume diets similar to horses, have been shown to transport dietary triacylglycerols via very low-density lipoproteins (VLDL) when fed normal diets (e.g., hay, silage, or cereal grains) and via chylomicrons when large amounts of polyunsaturated fatty acids are infused into the small intestine (Byers and Schelling, 1988). Even when present, ruminant chylomicrons are typically much smaller, lower in triacylglycerols and higher in phospholipids, and are less prevalent than those generally described for humans (Byers and Schelling, 1988). Certainly, the horse seems to have little difficulty absorbing fat, as crude fat digestibility approaches 100 percent even at levels of fat inclusion up to 23 percent of diet dry matter (Kronfeld et al., 2004). However, more study is needed to elucidate the mechanism(s) of triacylglycerol transport from the equine small intestine.

Distribution

Because most determinants of xenobiotic distribution are largely impacted by cardiac output, regional blood flow, and xenobiotic chemistry, differences among species might be predictable through allometric scaling (Riviere et al., 1997). Exceptions are more likely for xenobiotics or nutrients that might compartmentalize in the large gastrointestinal compartments such as the colon of the horse, or highly lipid-soluble compounds that might be characterized by a large volume of distribution. Differences of xenobiotic or nutrient distribution might also be expected among species based on differences in transport protein type, content, or substrate affinity (Xia et al., 2005).

Metabolism

Xenobiotic Metabolism

In an attempt to identify the best species to predict compound metabolism in humans, multiple investigators have addressed conservation of metabolizing isoenzymes and substrate specificities among species. Not surprisingly, extrapolation is complicated by overlap in isoenzyme substrates specificity, differences in catalytic rates, and differential response to inducers and inhibitors among species. Indeed, even within species, variability exists in breeds. Further, the impact of physiologic states, interactions, and tissue site should not be assumed to reflect the same isoenzyme content among species. A number of studies have attempted to identify a species that is most predictive of human CYP isoenzyme. Yet, a study of nine CYP 450 enzymes in seven species, including the dog, found that no one species best predicted human activity (Bogaards et al., 2000). Guengerich (2008) proposed a general predictability of human CYP, based on extrapolation from other species, to be greatest for CYP2E1 (reasonably predictable); less for 1A1, 1A2, and 4A (cautiously predictable) and 2D and 3A (even more cautiously predictable); and least for 2A, 2B, and 2C (major caution with extrapolation). Bogaards et al. (2000) found that large differences among species were not detected among rodents, rabbits, and dogs for CYP2E1, 3A2, and 4A1. For dogs, only 2D6 was reasonably predictable for humans. These studies indicate that general extrapolation between dogs and humans is not prudent (Ingelman-Sundberg, 2002). Extrapolation between dogs and cats also is not reasonable. The cat has long been described as a species deficient in its xenobiotic metabolizing capabilities when comparisons are made between the dog and cat. Deficiencies in phase I demethylation and hydroxylation as well as phase II glucuronidation lead to much slower elimination of phenols, aromatic acids, and amines in the cat compared to other species (Welch et al., 1966; Baggott, 1977). A recent review of CYP 450 activity-based substrate metabolism in cats suggests that cats have very low activity of CYP2C, but activity of CYP2D and CYP3A approximates that of dogs or humans, depending on gender (Shah et al., 2007). Recent studies have demonstrated a number of CYP 450 enzymes in the horse (Table 4-4) (Tyden et al., 2004). Several studies have been based on substrate specificity rather than immunoreactivity. Marked activity of CYP3A4 in the gastrointestinal tract is proposed to markedly influence first pass metabolism in horses.

Differences in phase II enzymes and their xenobiotic substrates have been better identified and account for many of the differences in xenobiotic disposition between the dog and cat (Baggott, 1977). Most of these differences result from a deficiency of glucuronide conjugation in the cat. The deficiency reflects extremely low concentrations of some glucuronyl transferases. Thus, many xenobiotics excreted as glucuronide conjugates in other species are characterized by a prolonged clearance rate and half-life in the cat. Toxic levels may accumulate much faster in the cat, and exaggerated pharmacologic responses or toxicities occur more easily. Dosing regimens must be modified for such xenobiotics by either decreasing the dose (especially for xenobiotics whose dosing interval is shorter than the elimination half-life) or prolonging the dosing interval. Toxic metabolites might overwhelm the glutathione system. In cats, the scavenging system of feline erythrocytes and hepatocytes may be overwhelmed, resulting in life-threatening methemoglobinemia and (potentially) hepatic necrosis (Savides et al., 1985).

Not all glucuronide conjugates are characterized by deficient metabolism in cats. Some are conjugated efficiently, whereas others are metabolized by alternative pathways, although these pathways may result in the production of toxic metabolites. Faster metabolism of specific xenobiotics to toxic metabolites is a likely cause for high-level toxicity of some xenobiotics, particularly those whose elimination is shunted to alternate (toxic) pathways (e.g., acetaminophen) (Cullison, 1984). Some sulfate conjugation enzymes may be particularly well developed in the cat (Baggott, 1977), and many xenobiotics that are excreted as glucuronide-conjugates by the dog may be excreted as sulfated compounds by the cat. Other sulfate-conjugating systems, however, seem to be easily saturated in the cat.

Deficiencies in both glucuronide and (potentially) glutathione transferase may also predispose the cat to poor scavenging systems in erythrocytes and hepatocytes, leading to toxicity in these or other organs. Other differences in phase II enzymes have been described between the dog and cat. Although acetylation is not a common route of elimination for xenobiotics, it is an enzyme system whose deficiency in the dog is clinically relevant (e.g., procainamide). Sulfonamides are detoxified by n-acetylation in humans. Shunting of the xenobiotic to an alternative pathway in dogs, with the production of the cytotoxic metabolite hydroxylamine may be one mechanism of sulfonamide toxicity in dogs, although alternative mechanism(s) are likely to be responsible (Trepanier, 2006).

Species differences have been documented in the handling of racemic isomers of selected xenobiotics. Inversion (from one isomer to the other) patterns differ and are likely to result in different pharmacologic or toxic effects of the xenobiotics (Landoni et al., 1997).

> Guiding Principle: Marked species differences exist in the ADME of xenobiotics and nutrients.

Nutrient Metabolism

Species differences in nutrient requirements and nutrient metabolism are important considerations when evaluating the safety of an animal dietary supplement and particularly when deciding whether to extrapolate safety data between species. The NRC (2006) summarized these differences for dogs and cats, and they will only be highlighted here. As an example, a number of nutritional adaptations of the cat are summarized in Table 4-8. Many of these adaptations can be related to the fact that the cat has evolved as a strict carnivore. For instance, whole carcasses are rich sources of vitamin A; therefore, the cat would not need to convert β-carotene to vitamin A to meet its vitamin A requirement. Cats are also very tolerant to high intakes of vitamin D, a nutrient likely to be present in high levels in the livers of prey species. Due to low levels of Δ6- and Δ5-desaturases in their livers, cats have a dietary requirement for the fatty acid arachidonic acid.

The horse has several anatomical and digestive differences that may complicate extrapolation of data collected in humans and laboratory animals, including the following:

1. Nonruminant with extensive hindgut fermentation: Despite the relatively similar layout of the foregut to that of humans and carnivores (i.e., nonruminant), the horse's hindgut differs in its size and function. The large intestine makes up more than 65 percent of the horse's digestive capacity. The microorganisms residing in the equine hindgut, although fewer in number, are similar to those found in the rumen of ruminants and are capable of extensive fermentation of fibrous feeds. The expansive hindgut of the horse also functions to slow the rate of passage of ingesta, with most feeds taking 24–36 hours to traverse the equine gastrointestinal tract (> 85 percent of that time spent in the

TABLE 4-8 Adaptations in Nutrient Metabolism of the Cat

Nutrient	Nutritional Adaptation	Mechanism	Comment
Protein	High protein requirement	Lack of down-regulating control over aminotransferase and urea-cycle enzymes	Carnivorous diet is consistently high in protein.
Amino acids	Rats, chickens, and pigs respond to an amino acid imbalance by decreasing consumption of the imbalanced diet. Cats do not decrease food intake when consuming an amino acid imbalanced diet.	—	Carnivorous diet has a relatively consistent amino acid pattern that meets the amino acid requirements of the cat. Cats have no need to seek alternate protein sources to meet their amino acid requirements.
	Cats do not synthesize arginine and can die if they consume a single meal containing a source of protein/amino acids, but devoid of arginine.	Lack of pyrroline-5-carboxylase and ornthine amino transferase activity results in insufficient ornithine and citrulline synthesis.	Carnivorous diet is a rich source of arginine. A natural carnivore diet would not be deficient in arginine.
	Cats do not synthesize taurine and have a higher requirement when consuming retorted food than when consuming extruded dry food.	1) Lack of cysteine dioxygenase and cysteine sulphinic acid decarboxylase activity results in insufficient taurine synthesis	Carnivorous diet is a rich source of taurine.
		2) Decreased enterohepatic circulation of taurine due to bacterial hydrolysis of taurocholic acid in cats consuming retorted food	
		3) Obligatory conjugation of bile acids with taurine	
		4) Production of felinine	
	Low tolerance for excess glutamic acid	—	—
Vitamins	Cats have a high tolerance to excess vitamin D and do not synthesize vitamin D.	High activity of 7-dehydrocholesterol Δ7-reductase	Carnivorous diet is a rich source of vitamin D.
	Cats do not convert β-carotene to vitamin A.	Lack of dioxygenase activity to convert β-carotene to vitamin A	Carnivorous diet would not contain β-carotene.
	Plasma retinyl compounds are largely present as retinyl esters rather than as retinol-binding protein.	—	—
	Niacin is not synthesized from tryptophan.	High levels of picolinic acid carboxylase shunt tryptophan toward picolinic acid synthesis rather than niacin synthesis.	Carnivorous diet is a rich source of niacin.
Carbohydrates	Glucokinase activity is low in the liver and red blood cells.	—	Carnivorous diet is naturally low in carbohydrate.
	Fructosemia/fructosuria from ingestion of large quantities of sucrose	Aldolase B may be low in feline liver.	Carnivorous diet does not contain sucrose.
	Cats lack a sweet taste receptor.	Ineffective Tas 1r2 receptor	Carnivorous diet is a poor source of glucose.
Fatty acids	Have a dietary requirement for arachidonic acid	Low Δ6-desaturase in liver	Carnivorous diet contains sufficient arachidonic acid.

hindgut). The reliance on fermentation to meet its nutrient needs also means the horse may be subjected to toxins and harmful metabolites generated when the health of the microbial population is upset.

2. No gallbladder: Similar to the rat, the horse does not have a gallbladder. Instead, bile is secreted continuously from the liver. Bile secreted from a gallbladder is much more concentrated than that secreted by the liver due to reabsorption of water and inorganic salts by the mucosal cells of the gallbladder viscus (Ullrey, 1972). Differences in bile composition may affect the emulsification of dietary fats and fat-soluble vitamins, interactions with pancreatic lipase, and the formation of micelles. Despite these differences in bile secretion and composition, horses seem to be very adept at digesting and absorbing dietary fats (Kronfeld et al., 2004).

3. Activity of pancreatic enzymes: The concentrations of pancreatic enzymes are also different in the horse compared to other nonruminant species. Lorenzo-Figueras et al. (2007) reported the activities of pancreatic amylase, elastase, trypsin, and chymotrypsin were lower in the adult horse compared to adult pigs and rats. In contrast, the authors found that the activity of pancreatic lipase was similar between adult horses, pigs, and rats. These findings might explain, in part, why horses seem to have an upper limit to starch digestion in the small intestine, as well as why horses are fairly tolerant of large amounts of fat added the diet.

4. Efficient intestinal conversion of β-carotene to retinol: As an herbivore, the horse evolved to subsist predominantly on forages. Fresh, growing forages can contain high concentrations of β-carotene, which can be oxidized in the equine intestine (and to a smaller extent in the liver) to retinol, thereby supplying the horse with an active source of vitamin A. The conversion rate for pregnant mares and growing horses has been estimated to be 555 and 333 international units (IU) vitamin A per 1 mg β-carotene, respectively (NRC, 2007). These conversion efficiencies are higher than those reported for other nonruminant species, such as the pig (267 IU vitamin A/mg β-carotene) and human (275 IU vitamin A/mg β-carotene) (McDowell, 2000), but much lower than in the rat at about 33 percent as efficient as the rat (NRC, 2007).

Excretion

Species differences in renal excretion of animal dietary supplements may be less likely to impact safety compared to hepatic metabolism. In general, water-soluble, rather than lipid-soluble compounds are renally excreted; lipid-soluble compounds tend to be passively resorbed as compound concentration increases in the tubular lumen. Glomerular filtration and active tubular secretion parallel cardiac output and thus should be predictable among species based on allometric scaling (Riviere et al., 1997). However, differences in active transport and passive resorption, the latter influenced by differences in urinary pH, may result in differential excretion among species (e.g., horses normally have a neutral to slightly alkaline urinary pH compared to cats and dogs for which urine pH tends to be acidic). Little information is available regarding specific differences in renal excretion of xenobiotics among the dog, cat, horse, or human.

Extrapolation of Disposition Data among Species

The more physiologically and metabolically similar two species are, the more similar the disposition of a given xenobiotic or nutrient and the greater the likelihood that similar supplementation levels can be used (Vessey, 1982). This is perhaps more true for water-soluble xenobiotics because they tend to be distributed to extracellular fluid and are renally excreted, thus removing the impact of many factors that might influence the disposition of a lipid-soluble compound. The disposition of these compounds is more likely to be predictable when standardized among species based on allometric scaling (Lin, 1995; Riviere et al., 1997).

Extrapolation of human dosing regimens to animals is complicated by the tendency to describe human dosing regimens in terms of total dose rather than dose per unit weight (i.e., kg). Dividing human total doses by the standard 70 kg person offers an acceptable initial mg/kg dose upon which further dosing modifications might be made. Feline blood volume more closely approximates humans than does canine blood volume (70 ml/kg in cats and humans versus 90 ml/kg in dogs). The blood volume of a healthy horse represents approximately 6–10 percent of its body weight. However, extrapolation is complicated beyond simply dosing patterns as has been revealed by several studies that have attempted to comprehensively compare kinetics among the species. A review of pharmacokinetic data of 103 drugs in preclinical drug approval laboratory animals (dog, rat, monkey) found only an 18–53 percent predictive success rate for allometric scaling of volume of distribution, clearance, and mean residence time among the species (Nagilla and Ward, 2004; Ward and Smith, 2004a,b). Dog and monkey allometry was least predictive of human pharmacokinetics (32 percent correct), followed by rat and monkey allometry (44 percent correct), rat and dog allometry (61 percent correct), and standard three-species allometric scaling (64 percent correct). However, a later study of 21 drugs (Evans et al., 2006) demonstrated that pharmacokinetic data modified based on a two-dimensional molecular structure yielded reasonable predictability among the dog, rat, or monkey data, with the dog most predictive of human volume of distribution, but monkey hepatic flow most predictive of human clearance and mean residence time. The drugs were generally characterized by a large volume of distribution (15 drugs had a volume of distribution > 3 L/kg). Two-dimensional physicochemical and topological properties were computed based on molecular weight, octanol-water partition, chemical bonds (e.g., hydrogen or rotational), and polar surface area. The predictability of these algorithms when applying human or monkey data to dogs, and subsequently cats and other species, warrants consideration. Species differences in gastrointestinal absorption are dramatic and have been extensively reviewed elsewhere (Martinez et al., 2002). Gastrointestinal transit times, pH, and intrinsic intestinal permeability are all species dependent. In fact, it has been demonstrated that the oral absorption of many xenobiotics by the dog is greater than that by humans and rodents. This may reflect differences in physiology of the gastrointestinal tract (e.g., permeability, pH, and motility) or greater hepatic first pass for xenobiotics in dogs compared to humans (Chiou, 2000). These factors make extrapolation of human data to dogs problematic for both drugs and animal dietary supplements.

Breed Differences

Human polymorphisms in CYP metabolic enzymes have been associated with both therapeutic failure resulting from extremely rapid metabolism of a xenobiotic and with toxic effects, due to decreased metabolism (Ingelman-Sundberg, 2002). Among the animal species, differential kinetics or response of breeds to xenobiotics is increasingly being understood through the discipline of pharmacogenomics. Polymorphism of the MDR1 gene and P-gp has been reported in humans and are associated with altered disposition and thus susceptibility to adverse events. Polymorphism reflecting a mutation deletion of MDR1 that causes nonfunctional P-gp has been documented in Collies and related working breed dogs. The incidence of the deletion is impressively high: 35 percent of Collies were homozygous and another 42 percent heterozygous for the mutation deletion (Mealey et al., 2002; Hugnet et al., 2004). The impact of this mutation on compound safety in afflicted animals has been profound. Because substrate specificity for P-gp seems to be similar among species, human data might be relevant to other animals (Mealey, 2006).

As in humans, polymorphism in xenobiotic metabolizing enzymes also has been reported in other animals. That breed differences in xenobiotic metabolism may be clinically relevant has been established for some canine breeds. For example, Court et al. (1999) demonstrated that propofol metabolism was about 3-fold less in Greyhounds compared to Beagles. Celecoxib metabolism was attributed to CYP2D15, for which three canine variants were found (Paulson et al., 1999). Polymorphism also has been described for CYP2C isoenzymes, again in Beagle dogs (Blaisdell et al., 1998). Other examples thus far demonstrated include variable thiopurine methyltransferase (TPMT) activity in Giant Schnauzers (less) and Alaskan Malamutes (more) compared to other canine breeds (Kidd et al., 2004). Polymorphisms have also been described in cats: three variants of CYP2E were described by Tanaka et al. (2005), although breeds were not cited.

As mentioned earlier in this chapter, the activity levels and energy requirements of different dog breeds vary considerably. As a result, food and animal dietary supplement intake will vary if the animal dietary supplement is incorporated into the food.

Response (Dynamics)

Pharmacodynamic responses may be profoundly different not only between but within species. These differences may reflect polymorphism resulting in altered kinetics, differential responses to enantiomers or differences in physiology of health, or pathophysiology of disease. An example of differences in physiology among species that might alter response to animal dietary supplements is the structure of hemoglobin that might render it more susceptible to oxidative damage. As such, Heinz-body hemolytic anemia may emerge in some species. Feline hemoglobin in particular is predisposed to oxidative damage because of its unique structure, which includes a greater number of sulfhydryl bonds that provide opportunity for oxidation (Stolk and Smith, 1966). Japanese canine breeds may likewise be at risk (Yamoto and Maede, 1992). Other unique considerations for the cat might include its propensity for drug-induced retinal damage, hepatic lipidosis associated with anorexia, and potentially an increased risk of nephrotoxicity. Horses have been documented to have an increased sensitivity to doxycycline-induced cardiotoxicity compared to other animals including cats and dogs (Riond et al., 1992).

Interactions of Dietary Supplement with Diets or Drugs

Interactions occur whenever the action of one compound is modified by the presence of another, concurrently administered compound. The incidence of interactions and the risk of adversity increase with the number simultaneously administered, whether in the same or different preparations (Griffin and D'Arcy, 1979). Interactions may occur during any aspect of diet or drug movement (Table 4-9), although more might be anticipated prior to (pharmaceutic) or during absorption (pharmacokinetic; "kinetic"). Kinetic interactions occur when one alters the disposition of another, and thus occur not only during absorption (probably the most common for human dietary supplements), but also involve the other three drug movements of distribution, metabolism, and excretion. Pharmacodynamic ("dynamic") interactions occur when one compound alters body (physiologic) response to another. Interactions might occur between active ingredients, additives or excipients, carriers, or other components of an animal dietary supplement, or with storage containers or the environment. Interactions may occur between animal dietary supplements and drugs or nutrients. Few, if any, interactions have been described specifically for animal dietary supplements. As such, much of the information must be extrapolated from interactions described for

TABLE 4-9 Potential Types of Interactions Involving Animal Dietary Supplements

Phase	Interaction	Sequela
Pharmaceutic	Binding to luminal contents	Decreased rate or extent of absorption
(Pharmaco)kinetic (Disposition)	**Absorption**	
	Increased splanchnic blood flow (nutrients)	Increased rate of absorption
	Gastric motility	Altered rate or ectent of absorption
	Gastric pH	Ionization decreases rate and extent of aborption. Degree of ionization dependent on compound pKa.
	Competition for transport proteins	Altered rate or extent
	Inhibition or induction of drug metabolizing enzymes	Altered rate or extent
	Distribution	
	Competition for transport proteins in circulation	Altered concentration of free drug
	Competition for transport proteins in tissues	Altered concentration of free drug
	Altered regional blood flow	Altered drug delivery
	Metabolism	
	Competition for transport proteins	Altered clearance
	Induction of phase I enzymes (CYP 450)	Increased clearance of other compounds Increased risk of toxic metabolites
	Inhibition of phase I enzymes (CYP 450)	Decreased clearance of other compounds
	Increased phase II enzymes (glutathione)	Increased clearance, especially toxic metabolites
	Excretion	
	Competition for transport proteins	Altered renal clearance
	Altered renal blood flow	Altered renal clearance
	Altered urinary pH	Altered passive resorption and clearance
(Pharmaco)dynamic (Response)	Additive or synergistic interaction	Enhanced response
	Competitive or irreversible inhibition	Decreased response

dietary supplements intended for use in humans. Those dietary supplements that are most popular, or have been studied more in depth for therapeutic benefits, generally are more likely to be supported scientifically in regards to potential interactions that may lead to adverse events. This is particularly true for herbal supplements (Hu et al., 2005), in part because of their popularity as well as long history of Eastern use. Among the herbs for which interactions are best described (albeit, information remains limited) is garlic. Reports, unfortunately, are often unsubstantiated, or presented in the form of case reports, limiting extrapolation to animals.

Pharmaceutical Interactions

Because both foods and drugs can interact and alter the absorption of one another (Schmidt and Dalhoff, 2002), interactions involving animal dietary supplements that alter the absorption of the supplement, drugs, or food should be anticipated. The effects may reflect a direct chemical reaction, generally occurring in the gastrointestinal tract, that precludes absorption. Either the rate or extent of absorption may be impacted. For example, dietary fiber markedly decreases the absorption of lutein (Riedl et al., 1999). Although limited information is available regarding direct interactions, caution is advised when predicting xenobiotic-diet interactions based on chemical structure (Schmidt and Dalhoff, 2002).

Pharmacokinetic Interactions

Xenobiotic interactions that occur inside the body may lead to life-threatening adversities either due to therapeutic failure or increased side effects. Pharmacokinetic interactions occur when one xenobiotic alters the disposition of another xenobiotic (Pond, 1984). Each xenobiotic movement (absorption, distribution, metabolism, or excretion) might be altered by another xenobiotic. Over 50 percent of recent drug withdrawals in the United States have occurred because of serious drug-drug interactions, emphasizing the increasing recognition of the role of interactions in adversity. The majority of xenobiotic interactions involve either transport proteins or xenobiotic metabolizing enzymes (Huang and Lesko, 2004). Accordingly, interactions involving absorption and metabolism are probably best described and of most importance. This high incidence suggests that these types of interactions should be actively investigated for animal dietary supplements. Examples of dietary supplements with known drug interactions (Hu et al., 2005) include St. John's Wort (induction of CYP3A4, particularly intestinal), echinacea (induction and inhibition of intestinal CYP), ginkgo biloba (induction of CYP 219A), and grapefruit (inhibition of CYP3A4 and inhibition of P-glycoprotein). Flavonoids are inhibitors of several P-glycoprotein substrates, which increase the risk of diet-diet or diet-drug interactions (Zhang and Morris, 2003). Characterization of the xenobiotic interactions as a cause of adverse effects is difficult because large numbers of subjects generally must be studied to identify even common interactions. The use of models to predict xenobiotic interactions is complicated by the complex interactions among the factors influencing compound disposition. Of potential xenobiotic-nutrient interactions affecting absorption, competition among substrates for transport proteins have probably been the best described (Zhang and Morris, 2003; Huang and Lesko, 2004).

Pharmacokinetic xenobiotic interactions frequently alter the metabolism of a concurrently administered xenobiotic. Most of the interactions result from modulation of hepatic (phase I) xenobiotic metabolizing enzymes. Induction of xenobiotic metabolizing enzymes is a protective mechanism that facilitates excretion of potentially toxic compounds. However, induction is a double-edged sword: although inducers generally increase the elimination of a potentially toxic xenobiotic, increased formation of toxic or carcinogenic metabolites may also occur. Most CYP enzymes are inducible, although the response to inducers varies within and among species. Human CYP known to be influenced by inducers include CYP 1A1/2, 2A6, 2C9, 2C19, 2E1, and 3A4. Inducers are substrates for the enzymes that they induce, and induction generally is dose dependent. Induction is accompanied by an increase in the intracellular concentration of the induced enzyme, often because of increased transcription. Although inducers tend to exhibit enzyme specificity, they may induce more than one CYP. Inducers may result in significant activity of an enzyme that otherwise (constitutively) is either present in very low concentrations or altogether absent. Maximal transcription in response to an inducer generally requires 10 to 12 hours of exposure to a xenobiotic with activity returning to baseline by 18 hours (dependent on dose) following discontinuation of exposure to the inducer. However, the impact of the inducer may persist, depending on the rate of CYP degradation (Hollenberg, 2002). The impact of induction on the metabolism of selected substrates varies with the extent being dose dependent (Kawalek et al., 2003).

Inhibition of CYP enzymes also occurs, with some inhibitors exhibiting broad-enzyme interactions toward a number of different CYPs and others selective for a single enzyme (Hollenberg, 2002). Most inhibitory interactions are transient, resolving when therapy with the inhibitor is discontinued. Like induction, reversible inhibition seems to be dose-dependent (Hollenberg, 2002; Levy et al., 2003).

Despite the lack of mandated quality assurance or adverse event surveillance, several reviews have described interactions between drugs and botanicals or herbs (Hu et al., 2005) and foods (Schmidt and Dalhoff, 2002). Most reports involving herbs or botanicals reflect case reports, case series, or open, uncontrolled studies rather than randomized, controlled studies (Hu et al., 2005). Mechanisms are often difficult to identify, in part because of broad substrate specificity. Those most commonly identified involve altered pharmacokinetics of the xenobiotic due to interference with either P-glycoprotein or xenobiotic metabolizing enzymes, particularly CYP3A4. Food-drug interactions most commonly occur in the gastrointestinal tract (Schmidt and Dalhoff, 2002) and reflect therapeutic failure due to reduced bioavailability of the drug. Less commonly, increased drug concentrations reflect altered appetite or gastrointestinal acidity.

Pharmacodynamic Interactions

Pharmacodynamic xenobiotic interactions occur when one xenobiotic directly alters the chemical or physiologic response to another xenobiotic. Pharmacodynamic interactions can enhance the response of a xenobiotic due to additive or synergistic effects at the same receptor or at different sites but with the same physiologic reaction. Pharmacodynamic interactions may decrease the response of some xenobiotics due to competitive antagonism at the same receptor site or due to antagonistic responses mediated at distant, but physiologically related sites. Antagonistic pharmacodynamic interactions have been used therapeutically to mute the response of xenobiotics. A number of pharmacodynamic interactions have been documented between herbs or botanicals and drugs. For example, as reviewed by Hu et al. (2005), selected organosulfur components of garlic act as anticoagulants, contributing to increased bleeding times when garlic is administered with warfarin compared to bleeding times in the presence of warfarin alone.

SUMMARY

As this chapter demonstrates, numerous intrinsic and extrinsic factors influence the potential safety of an animal dietary supplement. These factors need to be evaluated thoroughly when evaluating the safety of each animal dietary supplement. They formed the scientific basis of factors the committee considered to be important when evaluating the safety of specific animal dietary supplements (lutein, evening primrose oil, and garlic). The factors that determine the disposition of nutrients and xenobiotics are complex. The movements (absorption, distribution, metabolism, and excretion) that determine compound disposition are dynamic, each in turn, influenced by a number of factors. Differences reflect compound chemistry, with major criteria being molecular weight, lipid versus water solubility, and compound pKa. Differences also reflect animal factors. These include "normal" changes such as aging or pregnancy, abnormal changes such as those induced by disease, nutrient or xenobiotic interactions, and differences associated with gender or species differences. The more foreign the compound, the more complex the factors determining the disposition of a compound. Not surprisingly, predicting the disposition of any compound comprising an animal dietary supplement in a target species will be difficult without supportive scientific data in normal target animals or in samples of populations at risk. Less ideally, studies might be extrapolated from a closely related species.

REFERENCES

Abadia, A. R., J. J. Aramayona, and M. J. Munoz. 1995. Ciprofloxacin pharmacokinetics in dogs following oral administration. J. Vet. Med. Assoc. 42:505–511.

Abo El-Sooud, K. 2003. Comparative disposition kinetics and plasma protein binding of gentamicin sulphate in three juvenile animal species. J. Vet. Med. Series A: Physiol. Pathol. Clin. Med. 50:196–200.

Albarellos, G. A., V. E. Kreil, and M. F. Landoni. 2004. Pharmacokinetics of ciprofloxacin after single intravenous and repeat oral administration to cats. J. Vet. Pharmacol. Ther. 27:155–162.

Andersone, Z., and J. Ozolins. 2004. Food habits of wolves Canis lupus in Latvia. Acta Theriol. 49:357–367.

Ansorge, H., G. Kluth, and S. Hahne. 2006. Feeding ecology of wolves Canis lupus returning to Germany. Acta Theriol. 51:99–106.

Archer, M. 1973. The species preference of grazing horses. J. Br. Grassl. Soc. 28:123–128.

Archer, M. 1978. Further studies on palatability of grasses to horses. J. Br. Grassl. Soc. 33:329–243.

Arnold, G. W. 1984. Comparison of the time budgets and circadian patterns of maintenance activities in sheep, cattle and horses grouped together. Appl. Anim. Behav. Sci. 13:19–30.

Arthur, G. H. 1996. The development of the conceptus. Pp. 51–62 in Veterinary Reproduction and Obstetrics, 7th Edition, G. H. Arthur, D. E. Noakes, H. Pearson, and T. J. Parkinson, eds. Philadelphia: W.B. Saunders Co., Ltd.

Autio, K., K. M. Rassnick, and S. J. Bedford-Guaus. 2007. Chemotherapy during pregnancy: A review of the literature. Vet. Comp. Oncol. 5:61–75.

Baggott, J. D. 1977. Principles of Drug Disposition in Domestic Animals: The Basis of Veterinary Clinical Pharmacology. Philadelphia: W. B. Saunders Co., Ltd.

Baggott, J. D. 2000. Principles of Antimicrobial bioavailability and disposition. Pp. 50–87 in Antimicrobial Therapy in Veterinary Medicine, 3rd edition, J. F. Prescott, J. D. Baggot, and R. D. Walker, eds. Ames, IA: Blackwell Publishing.

Bailey, C. A., and B. H. Chen. 1988. Research note: Carotene and zanthophyll changes during growth and processing of turf bermudagrass. Poult. Sci. 67:1644–1646.

Baker, D. H. 2006. Comparative species utilization and toxicity of sulfur amino acids. J. Nutr. 136:1670S–1675S.

Benno, Y., H. Nakao, K. Uchida, and T. Mitsuoka. 1992. Impact of the advances in age on the gastrointestinal microflora of beagle dogs. J. Vet. Med. Sci. 54:703–706.

Berlin, C. M. 1981. Pharmacologic considerations of drug use in the lactating mother. Obstet. Gynecol. 58:17S–23S.

Blaisdell, J., J. A. Goldstein, and S. A. Bai. 1998. Isolation of a new canine cytochrome P450 CDNA from the cytochrome P4502C subfamily (CYP2C41) and evidence for polymorphic differences in its expression. Drug Metab. Dispos. 26:278–283.

Blood, D. C., V. P. Studdert, and C. C. Gay, eds. 2007. Saunders Comprehensive Veterinary Dictionary, 3rd Edition. Philadelphia, PA: W B Saunders Co., Ltd.

Bogaards, J. J. P., M. Bertrand, P. Jackson, M. J. Oudshoorn, R. J. Weaver, P. J. van Bladeren, and B. Walther. 2000. Determining the best animal model for human cytochrome P450 activities: A comparison of mouse, rat, rabbit, dog, micropig, monkey and man. Xenobiotica 30:1131–1152.

Boyd, L., and N. Bandi. 2002. Reintroduction of takhi, Equus ferus przewalskii, to Hustai National Park, Mongolia: Time budget and synchrony of activity pre- and post-release. Appl. Anim. Behav. Sci. 78:87–102.

Breves, G., F. Geburek, M. Burmester, and K. Feige. 2007. Electrophysiological characterization of electrolyte and nutrient transport in the small intestine of horses. P. 64 in Proc. 11th Cong. Eur. Soc. Vet. Comp. Nutr., Leipzig, Germany.

Byers, F. M., and G. T. Schelling. 1988. Lipids in ruminant nutrition. Pp. 298–312 in The Ruminant Animal, Digestive Physiology and Nutrition, D. C. Church, ed. Prospect Heights, IL: Waveland Press, Inc.

Carter, A. M. 2007. Animal models of human placentation: A review. Trophoblast Res. (Placenta 28, Supplement A) 21:S41–S47.

Chavez, A. S., and E. M. Gese. 2005. Food habits of wolves in relation to livestock depredations in northwestern Minnesota. Am. Midl. Nat. 154:253–263.

Chiou, W. L., H. Y. Jeong, S. M, Chung, and T. C. Wu. 2000. Evaluation of using dog as an animal model to study the fraction of oral dose absorbed of 43 drugs in humans. Pharm. Res. 17:135–140.

Churchwell, M. D., and B. A. Mueller. 2007. Selected pharmacokinetic issues in patients with chronic kidney disease. Blood Purif. 25:133–138.

Clewell, H. J., J. Teeguarden, T. McDonald, R. Sarangapani, G. Lawrence, T. Covington, R. Gentry, and A. Shipp. 2002. Review and evaluation of the potential impact of age- and gender-specific pharmacokinetic differences on tissue dosimetry. Crit. Rev. Toxicol. 32:329–389.

Coman, B. J., and H. Brunner. 1972. Food habits of the feral house cat in Victoria. J. Wildl. Manag. 36:848–853.

Court, M. H., B. L. Hay-Kraus, D. W. Hill, A. J. Kind, and D. J. Greenblatt. 1999. Propofol hydroxylation by dog liver microsomes: Assay development and dog breed differences. Drug Metab. Dispos. 27:1293–1299.

Cowan, R. H., A. F. Jukkola, and B. S. Arant. 1980. Pathophysiologic evidence of gentamicin nephrotoxicity in neonatal puppies. Pediatr. Res. 14:1204–1211.

Crane, K. K., M. A. Smith, and D. Reynolds. 1997. Habitat selection patterns of feral horses in southcentral Wyoming. J. Range Manage. 50:374–380.

Crowell-Davis, S. L., K. A. Houpt, and J. Carnevale. 1985. Feeding and drinking behavior of mares and foals with free access to pasture and water. J. Anim. Sci. 60:883–889.

Cullison, R. F. 1984. Acetaminophen toxicosis in small animals: Clinical signs, mode of action and treatment. Compend. Cont. Educ. Pract. Vet. 6:315–323.

Dayton, P. G., S. A. Cucinell, M. Weiss, and J. M. Perel. 1967. Dose-dependence of drug plasma level decline in dogs. J. Pharmacol. Exp. Ther. 158:305–316.

Delco, F., L. Tchambaz, R. Schlienger, J. Drewe, and S. Krahenbuhl. 2005. Dose adjustment in patients with liver disease. Drug Saf. 28:529–545.

Doreau, M., W. Martin-Rosset, and D. Petit. 1980. Nocturnal feeding activities of horses at pasture. Ann. Zootech. 29:299–304.

Dowling, P. 2005. Geriatric pharmacology. Veterinary Clinics of North America: Small Animal Practice 35(3):557–569.

Driscoll, C. A., M. Menotti-Raymond, A. L. Roca, K. Hupe, W. E. Johnson, E. Geffen, E. H. Harley, M. Delibes, D. Pontier, A. C. Kitchener, N. Yamaguchi, S. J. O'Brien, and D. W. Macdonald. 2007. The Near Eastern origin of cat domestication. Science 317(5837):519–523.

Duncan, P. 1985. Time-budgets of Camargue horses. III. Environmental influences. Behaviour 92:188–208.

Ecobichon, D. J., A. S. D'Ver, and W. Ehrhart. 1988. Drug disposition and biotransformation in the developing Beagle dog. Fundam. Appl. Toxicol. 11:29–37.

Evans, C. A., L. J. Jolivette, R. Nagilla, and K. W. Ward. 2006. Extrapolation of preclinical pharmacokinetics and molecular feature analysis of "discovery-like" molecules to predict human pharmacokinetics. Drug Metab. Dispos. 34:1255–1265.

Farrar, H. C., and J. L. Blume. 1991. Fetal effects of maternal drug exposure. Annu. Rev. Pharmacol. Toxicol. 31:525–547.

Fitzgerald, B. M., and B. J. Karl. 1979. Foods of feral house cats (*Felis catus* L.) in forest of the Orongorongo Valley, Wellington. N. Z. J. Zool. 6:107–126.

Fowden, A. L. 1997. Comparative aspects of fetal carbohydrate metabolism. Equine Vet. J. Supplement (24):19–25.

Gade-Jørgensen, I., and R. Stagegaard. 2000. Diet composition of wolves Canis lupus in east-central Finland. Acta Theriol. 45:537–547.

Gandhi, M., F. Aweeka, R. M. Greenblatt, and T. F. Blaschke. 2004. Sex differences in pharmacokinetics and pharmacodynamics. Annu. Rev. Pharmacol. Toxicol. 44:499–523.

Ginsberg, G., D. Hattis, A. Russ, and B. Sonawane. 2005. Pharmacokinetic and pharmacodynamic factors that can affect sensitivity to neurotoxic sequelae in elderly individuals. Environ. Health Perspect. 113:1243–1249.

Goldstein, R., E. Lavy, M. Shem-Tov, A. Glickman, H. Bark, and G. Ziv. 1995. Pharmacokinetics of ampicillin administered intravenously and intraosseously to kittens. Res. Vet. Sci. 59:186–187.

Goodwin, D. 2002. Horse behavior: Evolution, domestication and feralisation. Pp. 1–18 in The Welfare of Horses, Volume 1, N. Waran, ed. Dordrecht, The Netherlands: Kluwer Academic Publishers.

Goodwin, D., H. P. Davidson, and P. Harris. 2002. Foraging enrichment for stabled horses: Effects on behavior and selection. Equine Vet. J. 34:686–691.

Griffin, J. P., and P. F. D'Arcy. 1979. A Manual of Adverse Drug Interactions, 2nd ed. Chicago: Billing and Sons.

Guengerich, F. P. 2008. Cytochrome P450 and chemical toxicology. Chem. Res. Toxicol. 21:70–83.

Gurr, M. I., J. L. Harwood, and K. N. Frayn. 2002. Lipid Biochemistry: An Introduction, 5th Edition. Oxford, UK: Blackwell Science Ltd.

Halbert, M. K., and J. C. Archer. 2007. Dioxin and furan contamination of deodorizer distillates and natural vitamin E supplements. J. Food Comp. Anal. 20:506–514.

Hansen, R. M., R. C. Clark, and W. Lawhorn. 1977. Foods of wild horses, deer, and cattle in the Douglas Mountain area, Colorado. J. Range Manage. 30:116–118.

Harper, E. J. 1998. Changing perspectives on aging and energy requirements: Aging and digestive function in humans, dogs and cats. J. Nutr. 128:2632S–2635S.

Harper, E. J., and C. L. Turner. 2000. Age-related changes in apparent digestibility in growing kittens. Reprod. Nutr. Dev. 40:249–260.

He, Y.-L, S. Murby, G. Warhurst, L. Gifford, D. Walker, J. Ayrton, R. Eastmond, and M. Rowland. 1998. Species differences in size discrimination in the paracellular pathway reflected by oral bioavailability of poly(ethylene glycol) and D-peptides. J. Pharm. Sci. 87:626–633.

Hickman, M. A., M. L. Bruss, J. G. Morris, and Q. R. Rogers. 1992. Dietary-protein source (soybean vs casein) and taurine status affect kinetics of the enterohepatic circulation of taurocholic acid in cats. J. Nutr. 122:1019–1028.

Hinchcliff, K.W., G. A. Reinhart, R. DiSilvestro, A. Reynolds, A. Blostein-Fujii, and R. A. Swenson. 2000. Oxidant stress in sled dogs subjected to repetitive endurance exercise. Am. J. Vet. Res. 61:512–517.

Hollenberg, P. F. 2002. Characteristics and common properties of inhibitors, inducers, and activators of CYP enzymes. Drug Metab. Rev. 34(1-2):17–35.

Houpt, K. A. 2006. Mastication and feeding in horses. Pp. 195–209 in Feeding in Domestic Vertebrates: From Structure to Behavior, V. L. Bels, ed. Wallingford, UK: CABI Publishing.

Hu, Z., X. Yang, P. C. L. Ho, S. Y. Chan, P. W. S. Heng, E. Chan, W. Duan, H. L. Kohl, and S. Zhou1. 2005. Herb-drug interactions. Drugs 65:1239–1282.

Huang, S.-M., and L. J. Lesko. 2004. Drug-drug, drug-dietary supplement, and drug-citrus fruit and other food interactions: What have we learned? J. Clin. Pharmacol. 44:559–569.

Hubbard, R. E., and R. M. Hansen. 1976. Diets of wild horses, cattle and mule deer in the Piceance Basin, Colorado. J. Range Manage. 29:389–392.

Huggett, D. B., I. A. Khan, J. C. Allgood, D. S. Block, and D. Schlenk. 2001. Organochlorine Pesticides and Metals in Select Botanical Dietary Supplements. Bull. Environ. Contam. Toxicol. 66:150–155.

Hugnet, C., S. A. Bentjen, and K. L. Mealey. 2004. Frequency of the mutant MDR1 allele associated with multidrug sensitivity in a sample of Collies from France. J. Vet. Pharmacol. Therap. 27:227–229.

Hurria, A., and S. M. Lichtman. 2007. Pharmacokinetics of chemotherapy in the older patient. Cancer Control 14:32–43.

Ingelman-Sundberg, M. 2002. Polymorphism of cytochrome P450 and xenobiotic toxicity. Toxicology 181–182:447–452.

IOM (Institute of Medicine). 2005. Dietary Supplements: A Framework for Evaluating Safety. Washington, DC: The National Academies Press.

Janis, C. 1976. The evolutionary strategy of the Equidae and the origins of rumen and cecal digestion. Evolution 30:757–774.

Jedrzejewski, W., B. Jedrzejewska, H. Okarma, K. Schmidt, K. Zub, and M. Musiani. 2000. Prey selection and predation by wolves in Bialowieza Primeval Forest, Poland. J. Mammal. 81:197–212.

Jolivette, L. J., and K.W. Ward. 2005. Extrapolation of human pharmacokinetic parameters from rat, dog, and monkey data: Molecular properties associated with extrapolative success or failure. J. Pharm. Sci. 94:1467–1483.

Jones, E. H., and B. J. Coman. 1981. Ecology of the feral cat, Felis catus (L.), in South-Eastern Australia; I, diet. Aust. Wildl. Res. 8:537–547.

Kararli, T. T. 1995. Comparison of the gastrointestinal anatomy, physiology and biochemistry of humans and commonly used laboratory animals. Biopharm. Drug Dispos. 16:351–380.

Kawalek, J. C., K. D. Howard, D. E. Farrell, J. Derr, C. V. Cope, J. D. Jackson, and M. J. Myers. 2003. Effect of oral administration of low doses of pentobarbital on the induction of cytochrome P450 isoforms and cytochrome P450-mediated reactions in immature Beagles. Am. J. Vet. Res. 64:1167–1175.

Kondo, T., S. Naruse, T. Hayakawa, and T. Shibata. 1994. Effect of exercise on gastroduodenal functions in untrained dogs. Int. J. Sports Med. 15:186–191.

Kidd, L. B., O. E. Salavaggione, C. L. Szumlanski, J. L. Miller, R. M. Weinshilboum, and L. T. Trepanier. 2004. Thiopurine Methyltransferase Activity in Red Blood Cells of Dogs. J. Vet. Int. Med. 18:214–218.

Kienzle, E., and A. Rainbird. 1991. Maintenance energy requirement of dogs: what is the correct value for the calculation of metabolic body weight in dogs? J. Nutr. 121(11 Suppl):S39–S40.

Krauer, B., and F. Krauer. 1991. Drug kinetics in pregnancy. Pp. 1–17 in Handbook of Clinical Pharmacokinetics, M. Gibaldi, and L. Prescott, eds. New York: ADIS Health Science Press.

Kronfeld, D. S., J. L. Holland, G. A. Rich, T. N. Meacham, J. P. Fontenot, D. J. Sklan, and P. A. Harris. 2004. Fat digestibility in Equus caballus follows increasing first-order kinetics. J. Anim. Sci. 82:1773–1780.

Krysyl, L. J., M. E. Hubbert, B. F. Sowell, G.E. Plumb, T. K. Jewett, M. A. Smith, and J. W. Waggoner. 1984. Horses and cattle grazing in the Wyoming Red Desert, I. Food habits and dietary overlap. J. Range Manage. 37:72–76.

Kunta, J. R., and P. J. Sinko. 2004. Intestinal drug transporters: In vivo function and clinical importance. Curr. Drug Metab. 5:109–124.

Landoni, M. F., A. L. Soraci, P. Delatour, and P. Lees. 1997. Enantioselective behaviour of drugs used in domestic animals: A review. J. Vet. Pharmacol. Therap. 20:1–16.

Langston V. C., S. Sedrish, and D. M. Boothe. 1996. Disposition of single-dose oral enrofloxacin in the horse. J. Vet. Pharmacol. Ther. 19:316–319.

Lavy, E., R. Goldstein, M. Shem-Tov, A. Glickman, G. Ziv, and H. Bark. 1995. Disposition kinetics of ampicillin administered intravenously and intraosseously to canine puppies. J. Vet. Pharmacol. Ther. 18:379–381.

Lawler, D. E., R. H. Evans, B. T. Larson, E. L. Spitznagel, M. R. Ellersieck, and R. D. Kealy. 2005. Influence of lifetime food restriction on causes, time, and predictors of death in dogs. J. Am. Vet. Med. Assoc. 226:225–231.

Levy, R. H., H. Hachad, C. Yao, and I. Ragueneau-Majlessi. 2003. Relationship between extent of inhibition and inhibitor dose: Literature evaluation based on the metabolism and transport drug interaction database. Curr. Drug Metab. 4:371–380.

Lin, J. H. 1995. Species similarities and differences in pharmacokinetics. Drug Metab. Dispos. 23:1008–1021.

Lorenzo-Figueras, M., S. M. Morisset, J. Morisset, J. Laine, and A. M. Merrit. 2007. Digestive enzyme concentrations and activities in healthy pancreatic tissues of horses. Am. J. Vet. Res. 68:1070–1072.

MacFadden, B. J. 2005. Fossil horses—evidence for evolution. Science 307:1728–1730.

Marchello, E. V., W. A. Shurg, J. A. Marchello, and S. P. Cuneo. 2000. Changes in lipoprotein composition in horses fed a fat-supplemented diet. J. Equine Vet. Sci. 20:453–458.

Martin-Rosset, W., M. Doreau, and J. Cloix. 1978. Activities of a herd of draught brood mares and their foals on pasture. Ann. Zootech. 27:33–45.

Martinez, M., G. Amidon, L. Clark, W. W. Jones, A. Mitra, and J. E. Riviere. 2002. Applying the biopharmaceutics classification system to veterinary pharmaceutical products: Part II. Physiological considerations. Adv. Drug Delivery Rev. 54:825–850.

Mayes, E., and P. Duncan. 1986. Temporal patterns of feeding behavior in free-ranging horses. Behaviour 96:105–129.

McDowell, L. R. 2000. Vitamins in Animal and Human Nutrition, second edition. Ames, IA: Iowa State University Press.

McInnis, M. L., and M. Vavra. 1987. Dietary relationships among feral horses, cattle, and pronghorn in southeastern Oregon. J. Range Manage. 40:60–66.

Mealey, K. 2006. Veterinary Clinics of North America: Small Animal Practice. Pharmacogenetics 36:961–973.

Mealey, K. L., S. A. Bentjen, and D. K. Waiting. 2002. Frequency of the mutant MDR1 allele associated with ivermectin sensitivity in a sample population of Collies from the northwestern United States. Am. J. Vet. Res. 63:479–481.

Medina, M. F., and R. García. 2007. Predation of insects by feral cats (Felis silvestris catus L., 1758) on an oceanic island (La Palma, Canary Island). J. Insect Conserv. 11:203–207.

Menard, C., P. Duncan, G. Fleurance, J. Y. Georges, and M. Lila. 2002. Comparative foraging and nutrition of horses and cattle in European wetlands. J. Appl. Ecol. 39:120–133.

Morita, T., Y. Mizutani, M. Sawada, and A. Shimada. 2005. Immunohistochemical and Ultrastructural Findings Related to the Blood–Brain Barrier in the Blood Vessels of the Cerebral White Matter in Aged Dogs. J. Comp. Path. 133:14–22.

Nagilla, R., and K. W. Ward. 2004. A comprehensive analysis of the role of correction factors in the allometric predictivity of clearance from rat, dog, and monkey to humans. J. Pharm. Sci. 93:2522–2534.

Nouws, J. F. M. 1992. Pharmacokinetics in immature animals: A review. J. Anim. Sci. 70:3627–3634.

NRC (National Research Council). 2005. Mineral Tolerance of Animals. Washington, DC: The National Academies Press.

NRC. 2006. Nutrient Requirements of Dogs and Cats. Washington, DC: The National Academies Press.

NRC. 2007. Nutrient Requirements of Horses, 6th Revised Edition. Washington, DC: The National Academies Press.

Odberg, F. O., and K. Francis-Smith. 1976. A study on eliminative and grazing behavior—the use of the field by captive horses. Equine Vet. J. 8:147–149.

Ostrander, E. A., and R. K. Wayne. 2005. The canine genome. Genome Res. 15:1706–1716.

Papich, M. G., and L. E. Davis. 1986. Drug therapy during pregnancy and in the neonate. Vet. Clin. North Am. Small Anim. Pract. 16:525–538.

Patil, A. R., and T. M. Bisby. 2002. Comparison of maintenance energy requirements of client-owned dogs and kennel dogs. Supplement to Compendium on Continuing Education for the Practicing Veterinarian. 24 (9A):81.

Patil, A. R., G. L. Czarnecki-Maulden, and K. E. Dowling. 2000. Effect of advances in age on fecal microflora of cats. FASEB J. 14(4):A488.

Paulson, S. K., L. Engel, B. Reitz, S. Bolten, E. G. Burton, T. J. Maziasz, B. Yan, and G. L. Schoenhard. 1999. Evidence for polymorphism in the canine metabolism of the cyclooxygenase 2 inhibitor, Celecoxib. Drug Metab. Dispos. 27:1133–1142.

Peachey, S. E., J. M. Dawson, and E. J. Harper. 1999. The effect of ageing on nutrient digestibility by cats fed beef tallow-, sunflower oil- or olive oil-enriched diet. Growth Dev. Aging 63(1-2):61–70.

Pearre Jr., S., and R. Maass. 1998. Trends in the prey size-based trophic niches of feral and house cats *Felis catus* L. Mammal. Rev. 28:125–139.

Perez-Camargo, G. 2004. Cat nutrition: What is new in the old? Compend. Cont. Educ. Pract. Vet. 26, No 2(A):5–14.

Pond, S. M. 1984. Pharmacokinetic drug interactions. Pp. 49–62 in Pharmacokinetic Basis for Drug Treatment, L. Z. Benet, N. Massoud, and J. G. Gambertoglio, eds. New York: Raven Press.

Putnam, R. J., R. M. Pratt, J. R. Ekins, and P. J. Edwards. 1987. Food and feeding behavior of cattle and ponies in the New Forest, Hampshire. J. Appl. Ecol. 24:369–380.

Raman, P., L. Patino, and M. Nair. 2004. Evaluation of metal and microbial contamination in botanical supplements. J Agric. Food Chem. 52:7822–7827.

Renfree, M. B. 1982. Implantation and placentation. Pp. 26–69 in Reproduction in Mammals 2. Embryonic and Fetal Development, Second edition, C. R. Austin and R. V. Short, eds. Cambridge: Cambridge University Press.

Reynoso, C. R., O. Mora, V. Nieves, A. Shimada, and E. González de Mejía. 2004. β-carotene and lutein in forage and bovine adipose tissue in two tropical regions of Mexico. Anim. Feed Sci. Technol. 113:183–190.

Riedl, J., J. Linseisen, J. Hoffmann, and G. Wolfram. 1999. Some dietary fibers reduce the absorption of carotenoids in women. J. Nutr. 129:2170–2176.

Riond, J. L., J. E. Riviere, W. M. Duckett, C. E. Atkins, A. D. Jernigan, J. Rikihisa, and S. L. Spurlock. 1992. Cardiovascular effects and fatalities associated with intravenous administration of doxycycline to horses and ponies. Equine Vet. J. 24:41–45.

Riviere, J. E. 2003. Comparative Pharmacokinetics: Principles, Techniques and Applications. Ames, IA: Blackwell Publishing.

Riviere, J. E., G. L. Coppoc, E. J. Hinsman, W. W. Carlton, and D. S. Traver. 1983. Species dependent gentamicine pharmacokinetics and nephrotoxicity in the young horse. Toxicol. Sci. 3: 448–457.

Riviere, J. E., T. Martin-Jimenez, S. F. Sundlof, and A. L. Craigmill. 1997. Interspecies allometric analysis of the comparative pharmacokinetics of 44 drugs across veterinary and laboratory animal species. J. Vet. Pharmacol. Therp. 20:453–463.

Sagir, A., M. Schmitta, K. Dilgerb, and D. Häussingera. 2003. Inhibition of Cytochrome P450 3A: Relevant drug interactions in gastroenterology. Digestion 68:41–48.

Salter, R. E., and R. J. Hudson. 1979. Feeding ecology of feral horses in western Alberta. J. Range Manage. 32:221–225.

Salter, R. E., and R. J. Hudson. 1980. Range relationships of feral horses with wild ungulates and cattle in western Alberta. J. Range Manage. 33:266–271.

Santschi, E. M., and M. G. Papich. 2000. Pharmacokinetics of gentamicin in mares in late pregnancy and early lactation. J. Vet. Pharmacol. Ther. 23:359–363.

Savides, M. C., F. W. Oehme, and H. W. Leipold. 1985. Effect of various antidotal treatments on acetaminophen toxicosis and biotransformation in cats. Am. J. Vet. Res. 46:1485–1489.

Schmidt, L. E., and K. Dalhoff. 2002. Food-drug interactions. Drugs 62:1481–1502.

Schofield, E., ed. 2005. Feed Manufacturing Technology V. Arlington, VA: American Feed Industry Association, Inc.

Sequin, M. A., M. G. Papich, K. J. Sigle, N. M. Gibson, and J. K. Levy. 2004. Pharmacokinetics of enrofloxacin in neonatal kittens. Am. J. Vet. Res. 65:350–356.

Shah, S. S., S. Sanda, N. L. Regmi, K. Sasaki, and M. Shimoda. 2007. Characterization of cytochorme P450-mediated drug metabolism in cats. J. Vet. Pharmacol. Ther. 30:422–428.

Sidorovich, V. E., L. L. Tikhomirova, and B. Jedrzejewksa. 2003. Wolf Canis lupus numbers, diet and damage to livestock in relation to hunting and ungulate abundance in northeastern Belarus during 1990–2000. Wildl. Biol. 9:103–111.

Speakman, J. R., A. van Acker, and E. J. Harper. 2003. Age-related changes in the metabolism and body composition of three dog breeds and their relationship to life expectancy. Aging Cell 2:265–275.

Stolk, J. M., and R. P. Smith. 1966. Species differences in methemoglobin reductase activity. Biochem. Pharmacol. 15:343–351.

Syme, M. R., J. W. Paxton, and J. A. Keelan. 2004. Drug transfer and metabolism by the human placenta. Clin. Pharmacokinet. 43:487–514.

Tanaka, T. 1999. Gender-related differences in pharmacokinetics and their clinical significance. J. Clin. Pharm. Ther. 24:339–346.

Tanaka, N., R. Shinkyo, T. Sakaki, M. Kasamastu, S. Imaoka, Y. Funae, and H. Yokota. 2005. Cytochrome P450 2E polymorphism in feline liver. Biochim. Biophys. Acta–General Subjects 1726:194–205.

Tasler, J., W. Obtulowicz, M. Cieszkowski, and S. Konturek. 1974. Gastrointestinal secretory function during physical exercise. Acta Physiol. Pol. 25:215–226.

Taylor, E. J., C. Adams, and R. Neville. 1995. Some nutritional aspects of aging in dogs and cats. Proc. Nutr. Soc. 54:645–656.

Tidemann, C. R., H. D. Yorkston, and A. J. Russack. 1994. The diet of cats, *Felis catus*, on Christmas Island, Indian Ocean. Wildl. Res. 21:279–286.

Tran, Q. D., C. G. J. M. van Lin, W. H. Hendriks, and A. F. B. van der Poel. 2007. Lysine reactivity and starch gelatinization in extruded and pelleted canine diets. Anim. Feed Sci. Technol. 138:162–168.

Traver, D. S., and J. E. Riviere. 1982. Ampicillin in mares: A comparison of intramuscular sodium ampicillin or sodium ampicillin-amipcillin trihydrate injections. Am. J. Vet. Res. 43:402–404.

Trepanier, L. A. 2006. Cytochrome P450 and its role in veterinary drug interactions. Vet. Clin. N. Am. Small Anim. Pract. 36:975–985.

Tyden, E., L. Olsen, J. Tallkvist, P. Larsson, and H. Tjalve. 2004. CYP3A in horse intestines. Toxicol. Appl. Pharmacol. 201:112–119.

Ullrey, D. E. 1972. Biological availability of fat-soluble vitamins: vitamin A and carotene. J. Anim. Sci. 35:648–657.

van Dijk, S., and T. Wensing. 1989. Comparison of the lipoprotein pattern of the horse, the pony and the lactating and non-lactating cow obtained by a combination of an ultracentrifugation and a precipitation technique. Comp. Biochem. Physiol. B. 94:735–738.

Vessey, D. A. 1982. Hepatic metabolism of drugs and toxins. Pp. 197–230 in A Textbook of Liver Disease, D. Zakim and T. Boyer, eds. Philadelphia, PA: W. B. Saunders Publishing Ltd.

Vestal, R. 2000. Aging and pharmacology. Cancer 80:1302–1310.

Vila, C., J. Seddon, and H. Ellegren. 2005. Genes of domestic mammals augmented by backcrossing with wild ancestors. Trends Genet. 21:214–218.

Ward, K. W., and B. R. Smith. 2004a. A comprehensive quantitative and qualitative evaluation of extrapolation of intravenous pharmacokinetic parameters from rat, dog, and monkey to humans. I. Clearance. Drug Metab. Dispos. 32:603–611.

Ward, K. W., and B. R. Smith. 2004b. A comprehensive quantitative and qualitative evaluation of extrapolation of intravenous pharmacokinetic parameters from rat, dog, and monkey to humans. II. Volume of distribution and mean residence time. Drug Metab. Dispos. 32:612–619.

Watson, T. D. G. 1991. Lipoprotein Metabolism in the Horse. Ph.D. Thesis, University of Glasgow.

Watson, T. D. G., C. J. Packard, and J. Shepherd. 1993. Plasma lipid transport in the horse (Equus caballus). Comp. Biochem. Physiol. Part B Biochem. Mol. Biol. 106:27–34.

Welch, R. M., A. H. Conney, and J. J. Burns. 1966. The metabolism of acetophenetidin and N-acetyl-p-aminophenol in the cat. Biochem. Pharmacol. 15:521–532.

Welsch, F. 1982. Placental transfer and fetal uptake of drugs. J. Vet. Pharmacol. Ther. 5:91–104.

Xia, C. Q., G. Xiao, N. Liu, S. Pimprale, L. Fox, C. J. Patten, C. L. Crespi, G. Miwa, and L.-S. Gan. 2005. Comparison of species differences of P-glycoproteins in Beagle dog, rhesus monkey, and human using ATPase activity assays. Mol. Pharm. 3:78–86.

Yamoto, O., and Y. Maede. 1992. Susceptibility to onion-induced hemolysis in dogs with hereditary high erythrocyte reduced glutathione and potassium concentrations. Am. J. Vet. Res. 53:134–137.

Zhang, S., and M. E. Morris. 2003. Effects of the flavonoids biochanin A, morin, phloretin, and silymarinon P-glycoprotein-mediated transport. J. Pharmacol. Exp. Ther. 304:1258–1267.

5

Categories of Scientific Evidence

In any assessment of the safety of a dietary compound intended to support health, there are several potential sources of information. These sources range from carefully controlled experiments with the specific substance to anecdotal evidence about a related compound. Although randomized, placebo-controlled, clinical and/or research trials in the target species (i.e., horses, dogs, and cats) are most desirable, they are not always available and consequently other types of evidence are used. This chapter discusses the strategies used for evaluation of the individual supplements and the various categories of evidence available.

EVALUATION STRATEGY

The Model

The charge of the committee was to evaluate the safety of specific animal dietary supplements, not to determine efficacy. The evaluation was initiated proactively, not in response to a signal or adverse event. The committee's initial review evaluated the available literature and established a concern level where appropriate. The integrative evaluation process consisted of data acquisition, determination of the strength of evidence, assessment of risk, and monograph preparation. The committee reviewed available information for each of the target supplements in a systematic fashion and focused attention to assess numerous characteristics (Box 5-1). This outline formed the basis of the approach used in the assessment of the safety of lutein, evening primrose oil, and garlic, but was adapted slightly for each supplement.

Data Source

To ensure the best available information was used to assess safety and/or risk, a broad-based evaluation of the worldwide scientific literature was conducted. The search was largely restricted to documents whose text or translated summaries were written in English. Although this may represent a limitation for common and historical usage for certain ingredients (e.g., garlic), most of the scientific data were available or abstracted in English. A few papers of particular interest that were in other languages were translated for review. The search paid particular attention to the pharmacologic or toxicological studies of the target compound. Data of adequate quality were limited for certain compounds (i.e., garlic and evening primrose oil), necessitating a broader review of available reports. Although not all were peer-reviewed, available industry and government reports, scientific abstracts, and published proceedings were evaluated. Industry and government monographs, the U.S. Pharmacopeia, patents, regulatory actions, and reports of adverse events were assessed. Credible reports of adverse events, postmarketing surveillance, and historical and contemporaneous usage were factored into the overall assessment. The potential for bias was considered when weighing the importance of the information.

Factors Considered When Weighing Strength of Evidence

Criteria to evaluate safety of animal dietary supplements have not been established. Several models from traditional toxicology testing to classic feeding trials may be available for supplement evaluation. The quality and application of different methodologies to dietary supplement evaluation were considered by the committee in determining the best evidence for safety. In determining which categories of evidence would be accepted and how to weigh their relative importance, the committee carefully considered its desire for scientific rigor while acknowledging the practical value of nontraditional data for safety assessment. The committee noted unique considerations in the following categories:

- Toxicity testing. The goal of toxicity testing is to identify possible adverse effects, develop a dose response relationship, and predict the level of risk to an exposed

BOX 5-1
An Outline for Safety Assessment of Animal Dietary Supplements

1) Description
   a) Common names and synonyms
   b) Source and botanical characteristics
   c) Composition
      i) Nutrient analysis
      ii) Contamination
      iii) Variation of composition
   d) Putative active compounds
   e) Proposed biological activity
   f) Method of analysis
   g) Related compounds
      i) Compounds with similar active ingredients
      ii) Compounds with similar biological activity
2) Effects of Manufacturing, Processing, and Storage on Composition
   a) Manufacturing and processing information
   b) Stability and storage characteristics
3) Potential for Contamination or Adulteration
   a) Potential for contamination
   b) Potential for adulteration
4) Biology: ADME (Absorption, Distribution, Metabolism, Excretion)
   a) Absorption
   b) Distribution
   c) Metabolism
   d) Excretion
5) Purported Role in Health and Disease
6) Drug Interactions
7) Diet Interactions
8) Impact of Disease and Vulnerable Populations
   a) Disease
   b) Vulnerable populations (breed, gender, disease, life stage, etc.)
9) Safety
   a) Toxicity studies
      i) Target species (horse, dog, and cat)
      ii) Nontarget species
      iii) Ex vivo studies
      iv) In vitro studies
   b) Safety Studies
      i) Target species (horse, dog, and cat)
      ii) Nontarget species
      iii) Ex vivo studies
      iv) In vitro studies
   c) Nonsafety Studies
      i) Target species (horse, dog, and cat)
      ii) Nontarget species
      iii) Ex vivo studies
      iv) In vitro studies
   d) Use, Risk, and Exposure as a Supplement
      i) Consumption as part of the normal diet
      ii) Safety of similar compounds
10) Current Regulatory Status
11) Limitations to the Assessment of Safety
12) Risk Assessment
13) Other Recommendations
14) References

population (NRC, 2006). It would therefore appear that toxicity testing paradigms proposed for nutrients, drugs, and food additives would be most useful in evaluating the safety of animal dietary supplements. Although various methods of toxicity testing are certain to provide valuable information toward risk assessment, key limitations were identified. Acute toxicity studies and establishment of the median lethal dose of a population (LD_{50}) have certain limitations when evaluating animal dietary supplements. In these studies, dosing occurs for a short period of time (e.g., single dosing) at doses higher than occurs clinically. Adverse events may be overlooked when the study endpoint is lethality. More useful are subchronic and chronic toxicity testing where dose response and chronic intake studies may identify adverse effects based on common usage. Chronic intake studies evaluate both duration of exposure and total or cumulative dose. Study outcomes using acute toxicity studies compared to methods using chronic intake may be quite different. Dose response studies in the target species and determination of the NOAEL (no observed adverse event level), LOAEL (lowest observed adverse event level), or safe upper limit (SUL) can be established by these methods (see Chapter 3). Such information, generated from scientifically sound studies, is considered high quality and most desirable for risk assessment. However, the committee noted this approach may be impractical for many animal dietary supplements. Many supplements occur in the natural state as combinations of compounds. Natural ingredients have variable concentrations of active compounds based on the source, plant parts, preparation method, and combination with other ingredients. Without a standardized compound, traditional dose response and toxicology testing are complicated by an inability to establish a standard testing dose. Practical limitations of using standard toxicity testing methodology exist. For example, standard cat foods include approximately one-third protein. Thus, a special protein source could not be tested in this manner as it is impossible to feed it at a 4 X level. Even at 3-fold the standard intake, other nutritional deficiencies would occur, confounding the safety interpretation of such a study. Therefore, the committee recognized that LD_{50} studies are not always possible due to practical considerations of study design or ethical concerns.

• Ingredient and food feeding trials. Safety evaluation of new ingredients or foods destined for pet foods often rely on feeding trials with test ingredients included at 1, 3, and 5 times the intended use and fed over a period of 3 months to 1 or more years in the life stage of the animal intended for use (FDA, 1989). While specific protocols are not standardized, assessment of animal health requires regular monitoring of food intake, body weight, biochemical and hematologic data, and in some cases histopathologic evaluation of certain target tissue samples based on expected adverse effects. These studies, when well designed, provide strong evidence of ingredient safety or risk at the level of intended use. Nevertheless, certain adverse events may go undetected in these feeding studies, and, as such, the studies do not provide definitive proof of safety. For example, automated hematology analyzers would not detect increased Heinz body formation in cats fed garlic unless resulting in anemia. While increased Heinz bodies in and of themselves may not be considered a serious adverse event, they do point to the impact of chronic oxidative stress within the patient. Over the course of months to years, chronic oxidative stress could promote other health effects. These effects would go undetected. Because animals in feeding studies are typically on several feeding trials throughout life, the long-term effect (increased rate of cancer or thyroid disease, for example) would be difficult to detect and trace to an individual feeding trial. Unfortunately, published studies of this nature are uncommon due to length and cost of testing, lack of perceived need, public objection, or more often because they are proprietary. Horse feed, pet food, and supplement manufacturers were contacted and requested to provide data from any such studies. Irrespective of the limitations stated above, these data were invaluable in establishing a history of use, dose, and outcome for certain supplements. Without this cooperation and access to proprietary data, the task of evaluating these supplements would have been even more challenging.

• Ingredient regulatory status. The committee considered an ingredient's regulatory designation as not relevant. Certain feed additives used as processing aids or as flavoring components may be designated as GRAS (generally regarded as safe) by FDA (FDA, 1958). Ingredients with official GRAS designation are typically flavoring agents or additives that were in common use prior to 1958 and have a reasonable certainty of safety. Regulations allow manufacturers to define ingredients as GRAS by self-affirmation (FDA, 1997), and FDA notification or review is not required. Due to the variable nature of GRAS determination and the fact that the levels often supplemented are greater than those defined by regulations, GRAS-designated ingredients cannot be assumed safe at higher doses and for all use.

• Other data included in the safety assessment include the following:

— Knowledge of an ingredient. Extensive characterization and knowledge of an ingredient (e.g., composition, active compounds, bioavailability, route of elimination, and contamination risk) are considered of importance when evaluating ingredients. These data can sometimes help predict an adverse event or define a target organ of interest.

— Knowledge of related substances. Related ingredients that are considered to have similar active compounds and properties were assessed. For example, reports of adverse events from onions were considered when evaluating the risk of garlic.

— Historical use. The committee agreed historical use of a supplement in the species of interest provided value, particularly when the level consumed was known. Historical or common use included known intake or exposure in the natural food supply, current or past use in manufactured or prepared foods, and recommended intake and dosing for supplement intake by suppliers or from popular books and websites. In some cases, the description of a supplement dose was similar to that of a drug, given as a range per body weight or size. An example would be the therapeutic use of fatty acids described for evening primrose oil. In other examples, the level of intake was less defined and an average intake could only be estimated (e.g., garlic intake in cats). This resulted in reporting historical levels as a range in some cases or mean intake in others. The lack of reported adverse events with common usage was considered important but still low grade evidence. There are significant limitations to any self-reporting system. Underreporting of adverse human events is known to be extensive with estimates that less than 1 percent of actual events are reported (FDA, 2006). The lack of accurate reporting is likely amplified in veterinary medicine where a centralized reporting agency is not generally recognized, data from poison center hotlines are not open for public search, doses may be unknown, and many adverse effects may be clinically unapparent or unnoticed by owners (e.g., Heinz body anemia with garlic toxicity or nausea). Nonetheless, when adverse events are recognized, especially if it is a significant health issue, the data may provide the best evidence available. For this evaluation, historical use included not only common usage as a supplement but also population exposure from the natural diet or environment.

— Signals. Reports of adverse events in response to consumption of a dietary supplement are considered an important source of information in risk assessment (IOM-NRC, 2005). Although anecdotal claims and case reports are typically low strength of evidence, these were considered significant if well documented in the target species and consistent with purported mechanism of action or known interaction.

— Research trials. Studies that include clinical populations, research animals, efficacy (utility) studies, or case reports may be of high quality depending on design and available information. For the supplements evaluated by this committee, these utility trials often represented the best level of information available. When doses, form, frequency, and route of administration were provided, the committee could estimate safety or risk if adverse effects were reported. More frequently, these studies are not designed to evaluate safety and the value may be limited. For example, a study evaluating the effect of evening primrose oil on crusting dermatitis may not have evaluated blood work, stool quality, appetite, reproductive performance, or other features of normal health. In this example, bleeding disorders, reduced seizure threshold, drug interactions, or less obvious adverse effects would go unnoticed since the investigators were focused only on changes in the skin. It can not be assumed that simply because no problems were reported that none existed. Preferred safety studies are those that are specifically designed to assess effects expected based on biologic activity of the compound.

— Data from other related species are also of importance. Predictions of toxicity may be possible in species with similar physiology or among supplements with like or related compounds. While limited data are available for garlic in cats, data from onion ingestion, a known toxin, were considered more strongly in the absence of specific information on garlic in cats. Similarly, if garlic data had been available for the ferret (an obligate carnivore similar to the cat), they would have been strongly considered.

QUALITATIVE EVALUATION

In a scientific approach it is important to evaluate factors (clarity of the data, replication by others, consistency with results arrived at by alternative methods, and consistency with plausible theories) useful for determination if facts rise to the level of scientific evidence (Bechtel, 1990). Guiding principles for evaluating data as outlined by the IOM-NRC report (2005) on dietary supplements were utilized. These guidelines are in keeping with principles of evidence-based medicine (EBM) and qualitative assessment of data.

Evidence-based medicine originally developed as a guide to help physicians translate results of scientific literature into clinical practice. Evidence-based medicine now integrates the best available research, clinical expertise, and patient factors into clinical decision-making to optimize clinical outcome (Roudebush et al., 2004; Figure 5-1). While EBM does not adequately address factors of supplement safety, the guidelines for ranking strength of evidence apply. Philosophically, these concepts were embraced in determining the importance of individual reports or available data.

DATA FROM THE TARGET SPECIES

Data obtained from the target species are key elements in the evaluation of the safety of dietary supplements. However, animal studies vary considerably in quality and rigor. Quality studies consist of randomized trials specifically designed for safety assessment in the target species, using sufficient numbers of animals to achieve statistically validity. Similar to drug safety studies, they would ideally allow determination of NOAEL and LOAEL and prediction of expected adverse events. The most reliable are those that follow national and international protocols and are conducted by qualified investigators (NRC, 2006). Because of expense and ethical issues, traditional safety/toxicity studies, such as median lethal dose (LD_{50}) tests (both classic

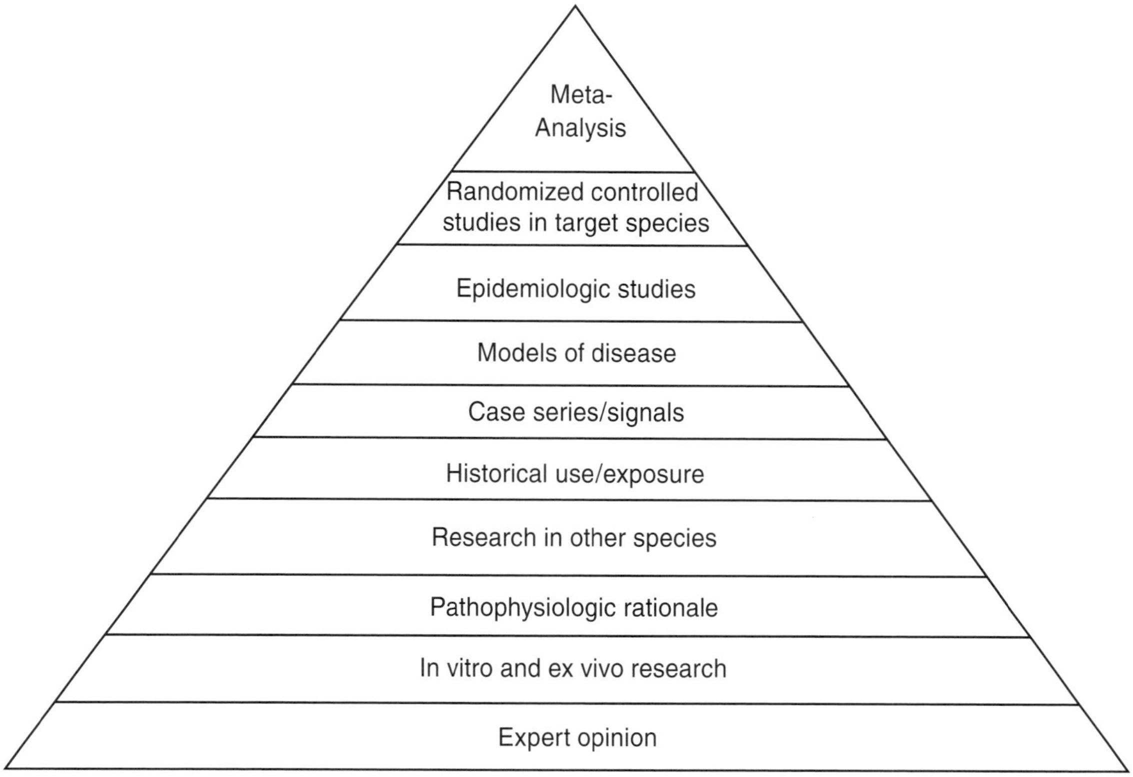

FIGURE 5-1 Evidence pyramid.
NOTE: The strength of evidence increases in progression from bottom to top.
SOURCE: Adapted from Roudebush et al. (2004).

and up-and-down), are rarely conducted with companion animals. Consequently, other types of experiments have to be evaluated. A variety of other types of experiments can provide valuable data provided established standards are followed (e.g., ILSI, 2003; FDA, 2006) and the experiments have adequate statistical power. Examples of these types of experiments are dose-response efficacy studies and measurements of the effects on feed intake. Trials designed to measure efficacy must be interpreted with caution when determining safety because they generally have inadequate sensitivity for safety. The efficacy study design often fails to determine a dosage endpoint and may not report adverse events in sufficient detail to determine a risk assessment. Nevertheless, when adverse events are observed in efficacy trials, they provide valuable information and, when evaluating safety of dietary supplements, are often the only well-controlled data available.

Studies that are poorly conducted (e.g., with inadequate controls, poor statistical design, and invalid measurements) received less attention than well-conducted studies but cannot be ignored completely. This is particularly important if adverse events are reported.

"Case studies" that describe adverse effects associated with the ingestion of substances usually involve a small number of animals and describe acute effects. Although rarely helpful in providing quantitative data, these reports help establish which organs and physiological systems may be affected and serve as a signal of potential risk.

Comprehensive databases of spontaneously reported adverse events are another category of evidence. Databases are maintained by organizations such as the National Animal Supplement Council, feed and supplement food manufacturers, and the Poison Control Center of the American Society for the Prevention of Cruelty to Animals. The strengths of such systems are that they can be large scale and can enable contributions by both professionals and consumers. Weaknesses include underreporting, lack of sufficient detail, subjectivity, and variability in report quality. The same strengths and weaknesses apply to other databases of adverse events.

Finally, evidence obtained from historical feeding practices can aid in the evaluation of safety of a dietary supplement. When a dietary component has a long and widespread history of being fed to the target species, it is unlikely that it produces acute toxic effects. For example, garlic has been fed at low levels to horses for hundreds of years in many countries (see Chapter 8). This suggests that at these levels adverse events are relatively unlikely under normal circumstances. Indeed, garlic is listed in the Federal Food Drug and Cosmetic Act (FFDCA) as GRAS when used as a seasoning or flavoring. Of course, GRAS is not the same as "without any toxic effects," and safety at low levels does not ensure safety at higher levels. If the level of intake is significantly higher than traditional practice, safety can not be assumed. The committee noted that consumption over many years does not necessarily mean that the substance was consumed without adverse effects. A key question to consider when determining the relevance of historical use to current application: Are the route, dose, duration, and compound truly similar to historical use?

DATA FROM OTHER ANIMAL SPECIES

In reviewing the value of animal data in the assessment of safety of dietary supplements for humans, the IOM-NRC (2005) established the following "guiding principle":

> *Even in the absence of information on adverse effects in humans, evidence of harm from animal studies is often indicative of potential harm to humans. This indication assumes greatest importance when the route of exposure is oral, the formulation tested is identical or highly similar to that consumed by humans, and more than one species show the same or similar toxicity.*

The same guiding principle applies to between-species comparisons in animals—evidence of harm in one animal species is often indicative of potential harm in another. This is a key issue because almost 90 percent of animals used in toxicity research are rats and mice (Weideman, 1993), and there are very few controlled safety/toxicity studies in horses, dogs, and cats.

Rodents have numerous advantages as test animals and there are well-defined protocols for using them in determining the safety of ingested substances (OFAS, 2003; NTP, 2006; OECD, 2007). In some cases, however, there are important pharmacokinetic and pharmacodynamic differences between species that make it invalid to extrapolate data directly from rodents (or other species) to horses, dogs, and cats. These data serve as a risk indicator only. Nevertheless, the following principles (adapted from IOM-NRC, 2005) apply:

- In the absence of specific evidence that certain animal study findings are irrelevant to the target species, such evidence should be used to evaluate potential risk to the target species.
- A lack of observed or reported detrimental effect in another animal species is not evidence that a particular substance is "safe" in the target species.
- When there is no detailed understanding of pharmacokinetics to make an interspecies comparison possible, it is appropriate to assume that the most experimental studies in highly susceptible animal species are relevant to the target species.
- Studies with other animals that predict possible serious harm or death warrant more attention than those that predict mild, self-limiting effects in the target species.

Data from closely related species are generally more predictive of effects in the target species than are data from more genetically distant species. Thus, data from other members of the family *Equidae* (e.g., donkeys, asses, and zebras) would be most predictive for horses, data from the family *Canidae* (e.g., wolves, foxes, and coyotes) for dogs, and data from the family *Felidae* (e.g., lions, tigers, and leopards) or closely related carnivores such as the mink and ferrets for cats. However, it is important to recognize that even within closely related species, marked differences in metabolism or molecular structure may alter a compound's toxic potential. For example, the structure of feline hemoglobin and the red blood cell (RBC) membrane structure in Japanese breed dogs result in greater RBC susceptibility to oxidative damage and hemolysis.

Just as for data from the target species, quality of studies conducted with other species of animals varies considerably. Careful evaluation of the quality of the study needs to be considered along with all the other factors.

> Guiding Principle: A credible report or study of an adverse event in an animal species that is associated with dietary supplements raises concern about the safety of use in the target animal species. More attention should be paid to events in closely related species or similar events across several species.

DATA FROM HUMANS

Like data from other species, information about use of dietary supplements in humans can prove valuable. Information may be in the form of clinical trials, epidemiologic data, case reports, historical use, and self reports of adverse events. Within each category, of evidence the quality of the information must be evaluated to determine the level of importance the data will provide in the overall assessment. Similarly, the weighted level of concern is higher with reports of serious adverse effect compared to mild or reversible adverse effects.

Cases with large numbers, potential for significant morbidity, temporal association with the supplement, laboratory test response, and biologically plausible mechanisms that are applicable across species should be strongly considered. The strength of spontaneous reports and case reports are limited by subjectivity, lack of detailed description of the supplement, lack of precise exposure data, and significant confounding factors associated with everyday use. Further limitations in animal studies include the ability to only report obvious clinical signs, whereas humans can describe symptoms like headache, visual disturbances, or nausea. Well-documented reports serve as a signal of risk for use in other species. Conversely, lack of adverse effects in humans does not imply safety in the target species. For example, human RBC do not seem to be significantly affected by the toxic compounds in garlic or onions at the intake levels evaluated. Red blood cells from cats and dogs readily undergo oxidation and hemolysis upon consumption of relatively low amounts of these sulfur compounds. Lifestyle differences are also notable between species. Confounding factors such as smoking and alcohol use may modify the response in people, whereas subgroups of animal may have exposure to a variety of parasiticides (e.g., flea, nematode, and heartworm preventative products). Finally, reliability of data collection is a significant limitation in human studies, and underreporting is extensive with an estimate that only 1 percent of adverse events are reported to the FDA (2006).

Historical use in humans requires careful consideration. Several questions must be asked when determining the relevance of historical use to current applications. Are the current route and levels of use similar to traditional levels? How do these levels relate to target species exposure? How similar are the preparations to historical use? For example, alcohol or water extracts may be more concentrated and contain secondary metabolites compared to whole plant use. Are duration of exposure, the intended population, and rationale for use the same? Species differences and the variation between traditional and current usage patterns make the value of historical use in people lower strength of evidence to assess safety.

As noted from principles of EBM, double-masked clinical studies are usually considered of high design quality when randomized and controlled (Roudebush et al., 2004). However, human randomized clinical trials have limitations. Clinical studies are often of small size, limited duration, and study a narrow population focus.

Furthermore, the endpoint in most trials is efficacy rather than safety. Adverse effects may not be recognized because they are not observed due to the study design, they are not reported, there is a prolonged latency period, or rare events are unrecognized due to low statistical power. Nonetheless, quality clinical trials can clearly ascribe an adverse event to a supplement treatment as opposed to confounding factors in uncontrolled reports. The utility of clinical trials is enhanced by clear descriptions of the study population, the inclusion and exclusion criteria, the study conditions, the intervention, and the adverse event and its temporal associations.

Epidemiological studies capture information of common usage and typically contain sample size sufficient to identify adverse effects. The ability to monitor adverse events typically relies on the endpoint monitored. For example, if cancer is an endpoint, the study may have overlooked the development of anemia if hemograms were not evaluated. Epidemiologic studies are not typically designed to establish causality. Epidemiologic studies are helpful in defining signals, establishing a level of concern for target animal exposure, and developing a hypothesis for further testing. Because these studies do not establish causality, they are of moderate to low quality when determining risk.

> Guiding Principle: A credible report or study of an adverse event in humans that is associated with dietary supplements raises concern about the safety of use in the target animal species.

ACTIVE COMPOUNDS

Knowledge of the composition, pharmacology, bioavailability, metabolism, and bioactivity of a compound is appropriate information to be used to predict risk associated with a supplement. It is expected that active compounds will have a similar biologic behavior and safety profile regardless of the source. Less commonly, preparation method, secondary metabolites, contaminants, and other factors can alter response to an active component of a supplement. As an example, the variability in forms and preparations of garlic as well as the differing effects of processing may influence its biological effects postadministration. Thus, it will be unlikely that a single dose can be established that will imply safety for all compounds and preparations. Quality studies of the active compound in the target species are considered of significant importance when determining safety or risk.

DATA FROM RELATED SUBSTANCES

In the absence of data on the active compounds, data from related compounds may be useful to assess the risk associated with a dietary supplement. Limited information may be available for a new ingredient or compound. It is prudent to consider other substances that are genetically (e.g., plants), structurally, or functionally (e.g., vitamin A vs. lutein) related. Certain limitations exist. Plants of different species may contain compounds at different strengths, have secondary metabolites, or concentrate compounds in different parts of the plant. Minor differences in structure can alter binding properties and chemical behavior very substantially. Preparation methods can inactivate toxic compounds or may result in secondary metabolites of increased toxicity. When assessing the strength of association, important considerations are:

- Chemical relatedness: Is the chemical structure highly similar to a chemical associated with potential adverse effect?

• Taxonomic relatedness: Is the ingredient from the same family or genus of plants with known toxicity? For example, onions and garlic are within the same family of plants and contain similar active compounds, thus adverse effects documented with onions should raise concern for the use of garlic.

• Functional relatedness: Compounds not structurally or taxonomically related may still act at the same site or by a similar mechanism of action as a known class of compounds. Where known compounds are linked to adverse health events, it is reasonable to expect a similar outcome from like-functioning compounds.

> Guiding principle: Evaluating related compounds can help predict the potential hazard of a compound.

EX VIVO DATA

Ex vivo experiments are those done in or on living tissue in an artificial environment outside the organism. The most common "ex vivo" procedures involve cell culture or isolated organ perfusion studies. These methods allow experimentation under highly controlled conditions impossible in the intact organism. Ex vivo studies can be used to isolate organs or pathways, define mechanisms of action, or isolate a specific cellular response. As such, ex vivo studies are commonly the initial mode of toxicity and safety evaluation of compounds. Biotransformation of compounds, production of metabolic byproducts, and intact systems regulation (e.g., neural control and hormonal release) may be partially preserved in some models to more closely represent the in vivo processes. More often, ex vivo studies do not evaluate tissues in their "natural" environment. Whole body counterregulatory systems, elimination pathways, and/or other routes of biotransformation are eliminated, which lowers the strength of evidence from such studies compared to whole animal studies. The limitations and points of evaluation are similar to those of in vivo studies. While ex vivo studies are usually performed in vitro, the use of these two terms is not synonymous. Examples of ex vivo studies used to assess the safety of animal dietary supplements include descriptions of the use of isolated rat uterus and guinea pig ilium to study the hypotensive effect of garlic in living tissues (Rashid and Khan, 1985).

IN VITRO DATA

In vitro trials refer to the technique of performing a given experiment in a controlled environment outside of a living organism, such as in a test tube. An example of an in vitro study evaluated by the committee was a trial in which isolated platelets from canine whole blood were incubation with sodium 2-propenyl thiosulfate from garlic to assess the compound's anti-aggregatory effect on canine platelets (Chang et al., 2005). Because the test conditions may not correspond to the conditions inside of the organism, results may not represent the response that would occur in a living organism; however, they certainly provide useful information on possible mechanisms of activity and function.

In vitro studies are valuable in that they can provide information on toxicity and mechanism of action not easily available from whole-animal studies. In vitro studies are typically targeted to a specific outcome. Assays may evaluate the impact of a compound on receptor binding, cell function, enzyme activity, or alterations in genes, to name a few. In vitro models may use body fluids, cultures, or isolated cells. Newer assays employ genomics, metabolomics, and proteomics. Key factors used to assess the validity of both ex vivo and in vitro assays compared to in vivo response are:

• Biological plausibility: Does the assay accurately mimic the biologic system? In vitro studies vary in their accuracy in predicting harm because they can not mimic the interrelated physiology of the whole animal system.

• Predictive value: Can the assay be validated to assure that assay outcomes predict biologic behavior and risk?

• Severity: Can the severity of adverse events be predicted by the assay?

• Consistent mechanism of action: Does the assay describe mechanism of action consistent with the effects noted?

• Relevance: What is the relevance of the in vitro concentration of the compound? Is it supraphysiological and not achievable in natural systems?

• Consistent results: Is there consistency in results across assay results?

> Guiding Principle: Evaluation of in vitro studies is valuable in describing the potential for toxic effects, mechanism of action, and biological plausibility, but these studies may have variable predictability to the whole animal.

LIMITATIONS

Determination of the safety of a compound is hampered by several factors associated with the evaluation approach described in this chapter. The most significant limitation is the lack of available data considered to be of high quality. Animal dietary supplements are marketed without regulatory definition, which means that premarket approval or assessment, standard toxicology testing, dose response analysis, and product characterization are rarely available.

Secondly, evaluation primarily of English-language literature limits the scope of data available. Because many supplement compounds have been used in traditional medicine from China and other regions that do not use English, the committee acknowledges important information may be overlooked. Nonetheless, key non-English studies were translated and reviewed. The committee does not believe it has overlooked data that would significantly alter conclusions generated in this report.

This evaluation approach may not adequately evaluate unique categories of compounds. For example, ingredients that are obtained from genetically modified organisms (GMO), probiotics, prion contamination within animal products, or nanoformulation may require unique studies or assays to detect and/or define hazards or prove safety. An adverse response caused by unique compounds may go undetected due to lack of recognition of the compound with the associated event.

Incomplete ingredient characterization can limit the evaluation of similar or related compounds contained within the ingredient. Within the complex nature of natural substances, hundreds of chemicals are present. Secondary metabolites are often formed secondary to processing. The number of unknown compounds limits the scope of investigation as well as limits the ability to standardize a product. Because botanical products are produced from different regions, soils, growing conditions, and processing methods, the variability of product content is often large. This variability in ingredient often limits determination of safe levels of use or concentrations that are associated with risk. Future efforts to standardize supplements and encourage production under good manufacturing practice will aid in this interpretation. Nonetheless, data currently available have often been generated with varied and unstandardized compounds making dose determination difficult and safety assessment difficult.

REFERENCES

Bechtel, W. 1990. Scientific evidence: Creating and evaluating experimental instruments and research techniques. PSA: Proc. Biennial Meet. Philos. Sci. Assoc. Vol. 1:561.

Chang, H. S., O. Yamato, M. Yamasaki, and Y. Maede. 2005. Modulatory influence of sodium 2-propenyl thiosulfate from garlic on cyclooxygenase activity in canine platelets: Prossible mechanism for anti-aggregatory effect. Prostaglandins Leukot. Essent. Fatty Acids 72:351–355.

FDA (Food and Drug Administration). 1958. Food Additive Amendment to the FFDCA of 1938. PL 85-929, 72 Stat 184.

FDA. 1989. Target Animal Safety Guidelines for New Animal Drugs. Online at: http://www.fda.gov/cvm/Guidance/Guideline33.htm. Accessed May 15, 2008.

FDA. 1997. Substances Generally Recognized as Safe. Federal Register 62(No. 74):18938–18964.

FDA. 2006. Good Laboratory Practice for Nonclinical Laboratory Studies. Online at: http://www.accessdata.fda.gov/scripts/cdrh/cfdocs/cfCFR/CFRSearch.cfm?CFRPart=58&showFR=1. Accessed September 21, 2007.

ILSI (International Life Sciences Institute). 2003. Best Practices for the Conduct of Animal Studies to Evaluate Crops Genetically Modified for Input Traits. Washington, DC: International Life Sciences Institute.

IOM-NRC (Institute of Medicine-National Research Council). 2005. Dietary Supplements: A Framework for Evaluating Safety. Washington, DC: The National Academies Press.

NRC (National Research Council). 2006. Toxicity Testing for Assessment of Environmental Agents: Interim Report. Board on Environmental Studies and Toxicology Washington, DC: The National Academies Press.

NTP (National Toxicology Program). 2006. Specifications for the Conduct of Studies to Evaluate the Toxic and Carcinogenic Potential of Chemical, Biological and Physical Agents in Laboratory Animals for the National Toxicology Program (NTP). Online at: http://ntp.niehs.nih.gov/files/Specifications_2006Oct1.pdf. Accessed September 20, 2007.

OECD (Organisation for Economic Co-operation and Development). 2007. Draft Updated Test Guideline 407: Repeated Dose 28-Day Oral Toxicity Study in Rodents. Paris, France: OECD. Online at: http://www.oecd.org/dataoecd/22/27/39791889.pdf. Accessed January 22, 2008.

OFAS (Office of Food Additive Safety). 2003. Redbook 2000. Toxicological Principles for the Safety Assessment of Food Ingredients. Online. CFSAN Food and Drug Administration. Online at: http://www.cfsan.fda.gov/~redbook/red-toca.html. Accessed January 22, 2008.

Rashid, A., and H. H. Khan. 1985. The mechanism of hypotensive effect of garlic extract. J. Pak. Med. Assoc. 35:357–362.

Roudebush, P., T. A. Allen, C. E. Dodd, B. J. Novotny, and J. E. Bauer. 2004. Application of evidence-based medicine to veterinary clinical nutrition. J. Am. Vet. Med. Assoc. 224:1766–1771.

Weideman, M. 1993. Toxicity tests in animals: historical perspectives and new opportunities. Environ. Health Perspect. 101:222–225.

6

Lutein

DESCRIPTION

Common Names and Synonyms

The name lutein originates from the Latin word lūteum (the neuter of lūteus) or yellow, from lūtum. Other synonyms have included lutein ester, trans-lutein, beta and epsilon-Carotene-3-3′-diol, and xanthophyll.

Source

Natural Sources

Lutein was first discovered in the corpus luteum and was first prepared as a dried preparation of corpus luteum. Neither mammals nor birds can synthesize lutein de novo, and, as such, its appearance in these species reflects consumption and accumulation of lutein in selected tissues. Lutein is commonly found associated with its "sister" xanthophyll, zeaxanthin. Lutein, along with β-carotene, is one of the most widely distributed carotenoids. In plants, carotenoids are located in chloroplasts, where they are associated with proteins, in chromoplasts as oil droplets, or in crystalline form.

Lutein is abundant in green and yellow fruits and vegetables. Vegetable sources considered high in lutein content include green leafy vegetables such as spinach, kale, and collard greens, corn, kiwis, zucchini, pumpkins, squash, peas, and cucumbers; fruits with lutein include green peppers (Khachik et al., 1995). Lutein is covalently bound to fatty acids in fruits and flowers (especially marigold) (Table 6-1) (Khachik et al., 1995; Alves-Rodrigues and Shao, 2004). Lutein is the major pigment of marigold (Table 6-1) (Sowbhagya et al., 2004).

Forages seem to be a rich source of lutein for herbivores, including the horse (Table 6-1). The amount of lutein present in fresh forages seems to be affected by stage of maturity, season, and climatic conditions. Prache et al. (2003) found that the lutein content of cool-season, native-grass pasture in France (consisting predominantly of *Lolium perenne, Dactylis glomerata*, and *Festuca arundinacea*) declined from 415 mg/kg dry matter (DM) in early May to 252 mg/kg DM in early August. Reynoso et al. (2004) reported that fresh warm-season grasses (*Cynodon dactylon* and *Digitaria decumbens*) growing in dry tropical conditions in Mexico contained less lutein (45–87 mg/kg DM) than the same grasses growing in humid tropical conditions (120–295 mg/kg DM). In contrast, Calderón et al. (2006) reported very little variation in the lutein concentration of mixed forage over two growth cycles in a natural mountain grassland in the French Massif Central (lutein averaged 172 mg/kg DM). However, this study employed strip- and rotational-grazing management, which likely would have maintained forage in a relative vegetative state. The authors also commented that the ambient temperature was hotter than the 35-year norm. Ambient temperature and the amount of sunlight contribute to the daily and seasonal variability in the level of β-carotene in forage (Livingston et al., 1968; Park et al., 1983) and will likely affect lutein concentration similarly. In addition, leaves contain 5–10 times the carotenoid concentration found in stems (Livingston et al., 1968). As a result, the decline in leaf-to-stem ratio with increasing forage maturity results in a lower carotenoid concentration (Park et al., 1983). Grass hay described as "medium quality" (12.8 percent crude protein, 60.5 percent neutral detergent fiber (NDF)) was reported to contain 60 mg lutein/kg DM (Prache et al., 2003), whereas a more mature grass hay (5.6 percent crude protein, 70.9 percent NDF) fed to lactating dairy cows contained 18 mg lutein/kg DM (Calderón et al., 2007).

Fresh legumes also contain a high level of lutein, although apparently less than grass forages. For example, Cardinault et al. (2006) reported that fresh red clover (*Trifolium pretense*) harvested at 50 percent bud (17.0 percent crude protein, 49.2 percent NDF) contained 136 mg lutein/kg DM. This level of lutein is almost half that reported for fresh

TABLE 6-1 Lutein Content of Select Feeds and Feed Sources

Source	Lutein (mg/kg DM)
Fruits and Vegetables[a]	
Broccoli	15.1
Collards	51.2
Green beans	4.2
Kale	150
Lettuce, romaine	17
Mango	0.1
Orange	3.5
Peach	0.2
Peas	3.3
Spinach	91.6
Squash, acorn	0.5
Squash, butternut	24
Tomatoes	0.13
Forages[b]	
Alfalfa, meal	143
Red clover	136
Cool-season grass, fresh	252–415
Cool-season grass, hay	18–60
Warm-season grass, fresh	45–295
Silage, cool-season grass	250
Silage, corn	25
Cereal Grains and Oil Seeds[c,d]	
Corn	0–29.7
Corn gluten (as pet food ingredient)	154
Wheat	0.5–2.6
Triticale	0.05–0.35
Barley, hulled	1.6[e]
Oats, whole	1.8[e]
Soybean meal	0.3
Flaxseed	6.5[e]
Egg Yolk[d]	
Corn-soybean meal chicken diet	7.2
Corn-soybean meal-lutein chicken diet	36.1
Corn-soybean meal-corn gluten-alfalfa chicken diet	53
Processed Pet Foods[d]	
Dog food, dried "high" content	27.5
Dog food, dried "mid" content	9.6–25
Dog food, dried "low" content	3.7–7.3
Cat food, dried "high" content	32.6–44.8
Dog food, canned	5.2–21.7
Cat food, canned	11.8–21.8
Marigold[f]	
Dark orange	869
Orange-brown	701
Orange	323–378
Yellow	175
Bright yellow	6
Green-yellow	4

[a]Sources: Khachik et al. (1995); Humphries and Khachik (2003).
[b]Sources: NRC (1994), Prache et al. (2003), Reynoso et al. (2004), Calderón et al. (2007).
[c]Sources: Berardo et al. (2004), Humphries et al. (2004), USDA (2006), Calderón et al. (2007).
[d]Source: Kemin Nutrisurance (2007).
[e]Value includes lutein and zeaxanthin.
[f]Source: Sowbhagya et al. (2004).

grass forages in early- to mid-maturity (Prache et al., 2003; Reynoso et al., 2004; Calderón et al., 2006). Season and climatic conditions during growth, as well as forage handling and storage, could potentially override the effect of forage species on carotenoid composition.

With the exception of corn, data on the lutein content of cereal grains and plant protein sources are relatively scarce. Nonetheless, most cereal grains and oilseed meals seem to contain low concentrations of carotenoids (Table 6-1). Berardo et al. (2004) reported the lutein content of 24 corn genotypes ranged from 0 to 29.7 mg/kg DM (mean 13.1 mg/kg DM). Carotenoid analyses of the whole-meal fraction of more than 100 varieties of wheat and triticale demonstrated that durum wheat varieties contained more lutein (0.5–2.6 mg/kg DM) than bread wheat varieties (0.05–1.6 mg/kg DM) and triticale (0.05–0.35 mg/kg DM) (Humphries et al., 2004). Soybean meal fed to lactating dairy cows was reported to contain 0.3 mg lutein/kg DM (Calderón et al., 2007). Although intended to serve as a resource for human food composition, the National Nutrient Database of the U.S. Department of Agriculture (USDA) provides the combined lutein+zeaxanthin for some feedstuffs that have common application in the equine feed and pet food industries. The lutein+zeaxanthin concentration of hulled barley, whole oats, and various varieties of wheat grain was listed as 1.6, 1.8, and 2.2 mg/kg DM, respectively (USDA, 2006). In the same database, flaxseed was listed as containing 6.5 mg/kg DM lutein+zeaxanthin, but no value was listed for flaxseed oil. Similarly, corn oil, canola oil, soybean oil, and olive oil were also listed as containing "0" lutein+zeaxanthin, but it is unclear whether these oils are devoid of lutein or they have simply not yet been measured (USDA, 2006).

Animals cannot synthesize lutein. However, dried marigold petals and concentrate are added to feed (33 mg/kg of a low-pigment diet) to improve color of poultry skin and eggs yolks and, more recently, to increase the lutein content of eggs (Lee and Caston, 2004; Breithaupt, 2007). Accordingly, egg yolks might be a rich source of lutein.

Processed Sources

Crystalline lutein and lutein esters are the most common forms of lutein supplements. The major commercial source of processed lutein is the marigold (*Tagetes erecta* sp., family Asteraceae) flower of the Compositae family. India is a major source of commercial marigold production. The two common species of marigold are the African Aztec (*T. erecta*) and French Marigold (*T. patula*), the latter native to Mexico and Guatemala. Lutein provides the main coloring for marigold. Approximately 60–90 percent of carotenoid esters comprising marigold pigment are lutein, with concentrations greatest in the petals (Piccaglia et al., 1998), which are approximately 40–50 percent of the flower (Sowbhagya et al., 2004). The deeper the color of marigold, the greater the lutein content (Piccaglia et al., 1998). Marigold contains 0.77 percent lutein (saponified mixture, on a dry basis) (Tsao and Yang, 2006) varying in concentration from 4 µg/mg in greenish yellow flowers to 800 µg/g in orange brown colors (Sowbhagya et al., 2004) (Table 6-1).

The recent surge in popularity of lutein, reflecting, in part, the increasing interest in possible therapeutic benefits for a number of disorders, has led to searches for alternative sources of lutein. The interest in alternative sources also reflects the existence of patents for extraction of lutein from natural products; the patents limit access of manufacturers to pure (e.g., free-form, crystallized) lutein. Alfalfa has long been a recognized source of lutein (Gugliemelli et al., 1954; Philip et al., 1976). The use of dehydrated alfalfa meal in poultry diets as a source of xanthophylls is common (Table 6-1) (NRC, 1994). Alfalfa meal containing 17 percent crude protein was listed as containing 143 mg lutein/kg DM (NRC, 1994). Recent efforts in genetic manipulation of alfalfa germplasm may yield more cost-effective sources for extraction. Another newer potential source of lutein is a green microalga (Cisneros et al., 2004).

Composition

The chemical formula of lutein is $C_{40}H_{56}O_2$. Its molecular weight is 568. The designated International Union of Pure and Applied Chemistry (IUPAC) name is 4-[18-(4-hydroxy-2,6,6-trimethyl-1-cyclohexenyl)-3,7,12,16-tetramethyl-octadeca-1,3,5,7,9,11,13,15,17-nonaenyl]-3,5,5-trimethyl-cyclohex-2-en-1-ol. Additional identifiers include CAS number of 27-40-2; Food additive E number of E161b.

Structure

Lutein is a carotenoid, the term used to refer to a group of natural fat-soluble plant pigments. The term carotenoid reflects their original extraction from carrots (Johnson, 2007). Carotenoids are comprised of isoprenoids, also referred to as terpenoids, which are 5-carbon unit building blocks (Johnson, 2007). Carotenoids vary in chain length, with the majority containing 40 carbons or 8 isoprenoid units. The carbons are highly conjugated, with most molecules containing 9 to 13 double bonds. Over 600 carotenoids occur naturally in two major groups: (1) the carotenes (2) and their oxygenated counterparts (oxycarotenoids), also referred to as xanthophylls, which include lutein and zeaxanthin. The colors of carotenoids range from yellow to red. The carotenes are more lipid soluble and darker in color, and the xanthophylls are more polar and yellow (e.g., autumn leaves).

Synthesis

Carotenoids are synthesized primarily by photosynthetic plants and selected non-photosynthetic Eubacteria. Mammals cannot synthesize carotenoids from the isoprenoid molecules. However, subsequent metabolism of ingested carotenoids may occur via phase I metabolic enzymes. Biosynthetic pathways of carotenoids involve di-iron proteins, common among fatty acid desaturases, and cytochrome P450 pathways, commonly involved in sterol synthesis.

Kim and DellaPenna (2006) have described the primary path of lutein synthesis. As a xanthophyll, the synthesis of lutein is a lengthy process, which currently precludes its commercial synthetic manufacturing (Breithaupt, 2007). Lutein synthesis begins with the red carotenoid lycopene (Figure 6-1). Synthesis involves at least four enzymatic steps, beginning with cyclization of both ends of lycopene such that two rings are yielded. Two isoforms may be produced: if the rings are symmetrical and identical (β, β), the product is β-carotene, whereas rings that are symmetrical but not identical (β, ε) yield α-carotene (Figure 6-1). Both α and β carotene are retinoids, meaning that each can be converted to retinol, the animal form of vitamin A. However, conversion of β-carotene is much more efficient than conversion of α-carotene. In addition to retinol, α- and β-carotene are further metabolized through hydroxylation of both end rings, yielding the respective oxygenated carotenoid, that is, the respective xanthophylls. It is the substitution in the end rings of the carotenoids that contribute to their marked diversity and numbers. Hydroxylation of α-carotene yields lutein, whereas hydroxylation of β-carotene yields zeaxanthin. The end rings of lutein are hydroxylated at the 3 and 3′ positions, resulting in a designation of beta (β, double bond between C5=C6) and epsilon (ε, double bond between C4=C5) for each ring, respectively. Enzymes involved in the conversion of lycopene to the xanthophylls include two non-heme hydroxylases, one cytochrome P450 hydroxylase, and a second cytochrome P450 monooxygenase (Kim and DellaPenna, 2006).

Because of their terminal rings (Figure 6-1) (Granado et al., 2003), neither lutein nor zeaxanthin are substrates for the 15, 15″ monooxygenase enzyme that cleaves α or β-carotene into vitamin A (retinal). As such, lutein does not possess provitamin A activity (Alves-Rodrigues and Shao, 2004; Shao and Hathcock, 2006) and side effects typical of vitamin A should not be expected (Alves-Rodrigues and Shao, 2004; Shao and Hathcock, 2006).

The combination of chiral centers (a carbon with 4 different groups attached) and *cis* versus *trans* positions can yield tens of thousands of different carotenoids, although steric hindrance reduces the numbers to those that are thermocodynamically and sterically favorable (Johnson, 2007). Lutein contains three enantiomeric chiral-carbons (C3, C3′ and C6′), which are designated as the S enantiomers. In its natural state, lutein is present in different isomeric forms, with *trans* (also referred to as E) predominating at 60–90 percent, leaving the remaining 10–40 percent to be 9-, 13-, or 15-*cis* (also referred to as Z) (Sowbhagya et al., 2004). The different isomers present in lutein are the 9-*cis*, 13-*cis*, and 15-*cis* and the all *trans*, the latter presumably being more stable

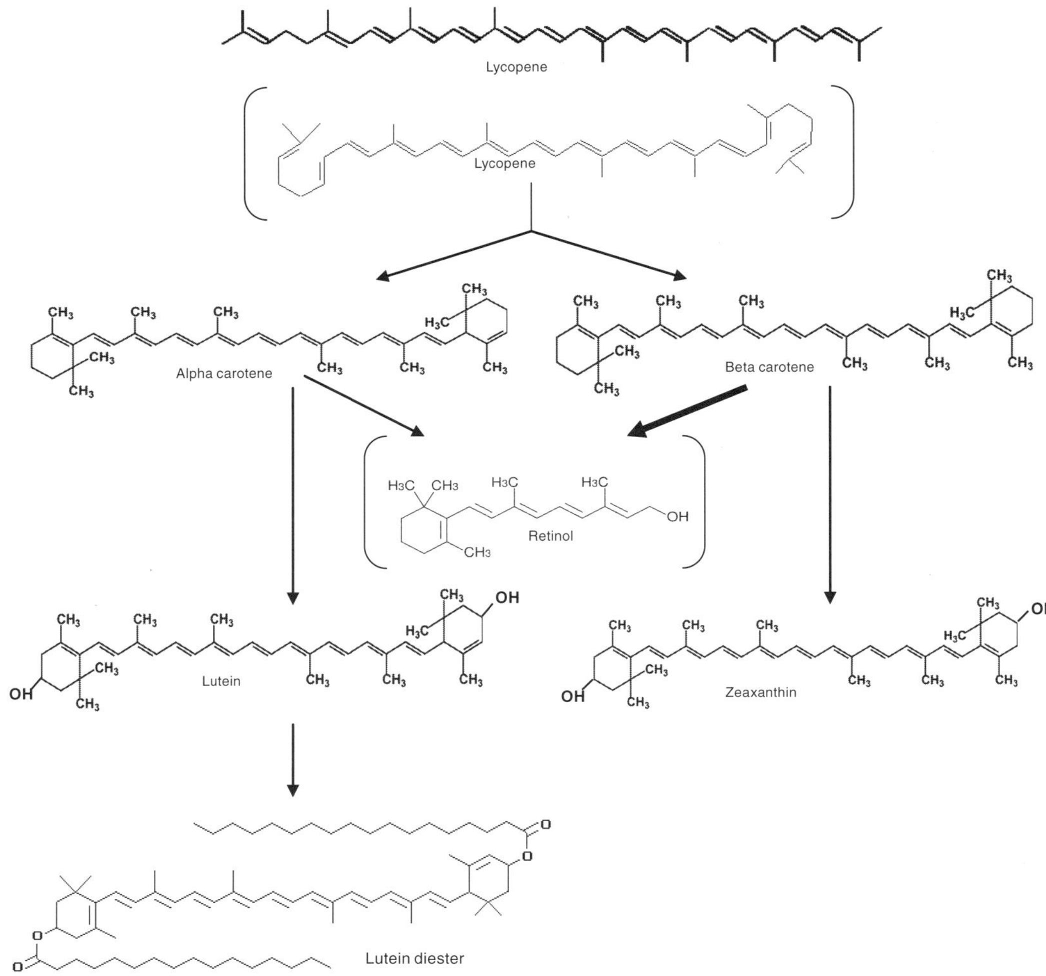

FIGURE 6-1 Synthesis of the xanthophylls, lutein and its sister isomer zeaxanthin.
NOTE: Synthesis of these substances begins with cyclization of the carotenoid, lycopene. Formation of two end rings yields the provitamin A carotenes, because they each can be synthesized to retinol, the animal form of vitamin A, these carotenes are also called retinoids. Formation of two beta rings (double bond between C5=C6) yields the β-carotene whereas formation of a beta and epsilon ring (C4=C5) yields the α-carotene. Conversion of β-carotene to retinol is twice as efficient (larger arrow) than that of α-carotene. In addition to retinol, subsequent hydroxylation of each carotene yields the two xanthophylls (oxygenated carotenes). Oxygenation of α-carotene yields lutein whereas oxygenation of β-carotene yields zeaxanthin. Because animals lack the enzyme necessary to remove the hydroxyl groups, the xanthophylls cannot be converted to retinol and as such, neither are provitamin A. Accordingly, there should be no risk of adverse events associated with toxicity of vitamin A compounds.

and effective (Sowbhagya et al., 2004). The principal stereoisomer of lutein is (3R, 3′R, 6′R)-β, ε-Carotene-3, 3′-diol. Despite being more hydrophilic than carotenes due to its di-hydroxylation, lutein is nonetheless more lipophilic than hydrophilic. Solubility of lutein esters in cold oil is less than 25 percent; this compares to 35 percent in hot (80°C) corn oil (Sowbhagya et al., 2004).

In its natural state, lutein is present in the diet either bound to plant proteins or esterified as mono- or diesters and combined with saturated fatty acids (Figure 6-1) (Granado et al., 2003; Alves-Rodrigues and Shao, 2004). Lutein esters seem to represent only a small proportion of total lutein in fruits and vegetables, with small amounts present in yellow-orange fruits such as peaches and oranges (Alves-Rodrigues and Shao, 2004). The predominant ester is dipalmitate; others include dimysristate, myristate palmitate, palmitate stearate, and distererate (Sowbhagya et al., 2004). Cleaved fragments are referred to as apocarotenoids. Cleavage might be nonspecific (i.e., the result of lipoxygenase activity, photo-oxidation, or radical oxidation) or may reflect directed, specific enzymatic degradation (dioxygenases) (Johnson, 2007).

Putative Active Compound

The active ingredient of lutein is the parent compound, in the free form, with the *trans* isomer generally recognized to be more bioactive than the *cis* isomer (Sowbhagya et al., 2004), although bioactivity has been attributed to both. The purported biological activity of lutein is protection of lipid components.

Analytical Methods

The process of lutein extraction for analysis has been reviewed by Sowbhagya et al. (2004). Extraction of lutein (e.g., from marigolds) involves large amounts of organic solvents, contributing to the difficulty in purifying lutein. Extraction from marigold petals generally is accomplished using an acetone:hexane solvent mixture followed by crystallization, purification, and saponification.

Analysis of lutein is limited by the lack of a suitable reference standard. This reflects, in part, its lipophilic nature, which complicates its separation from other carotenoids (Aman et al., 2005). Generally, standards are guaranteed to be no more than 70 percent pure (Tsao and Yang, 2006). The Food and Agriculture Organization of the United Nations has offered specifications for Tagetes extract (a synonym for xanthophylls, which includes lutein and zeaxanthin) extracted with hexane from dried petals (Sowbhagya et al., 2004; JECFA, 2005). More recently, the U.S. Pharmacopeia (USP) has generated standards for lutein (USP, 2007) based on the purified fraction obtained from saponification of the oleoresin of the marigold, *Tagetes erecta* L. Specifications include that the product not contain less than 80.0 percent of total cartotenoids calculated as lutein ($C_{40}H_{56}O_2$), not less than 74.0 percent of lutein, and not more than 8.5 percent of zeaxanthin, both calculated as ($C_{40}H_{56}O_2$) on the anhydrous basis. Its spectral range is 300 to 700 nm.

Several methods for detection of lutein have been described. Gas and thin layer chromatography with ultraviolet spectrophotometry have been used to confirm the absence of free lutein in marigolds and to detect and quantitate the proportion of methyl esters, including palmitic (including dipalmitic), myristic (and dimyristate), stearic, and lauric esters (Sowbhagya et al., 2004). Traditionally, the analytical method of choice for lutein quantification is high-performance liquid chromatography (HPLC), using reverse phase, using a C-18 column and ultraviolet detection (446 nm) (Jiang et al., 2005). With HPLC analysis, thus far 8 lutein esters have been separated and identified in marigolds (Sowbhagya et al., 2004). A method has also been published for the chiral separation of carotenoids, again based on HPLC analysis (Bhosale et al., 2007a).

More recently, high-speed, counter-current chromatography (HSCCC) has allowed purification of lutein (Wei et al., 2003) and facilitated direct measurement of crude extracts of plants while simultaneously providing broad separation (Wei et al., 2003; Aman et al., 2005). Using HSCCC, lutein from marigold can be purified to 97 percent (Tsao and Yang, 2006).

In addition, to the lack of standard HPLC methods, other analytical factors impact the reliability of data dependent upon lutein quantitation (e.g., quantitation in foods, bioavailability, or other pharmacokinetic studies). Analysis often includes combination of lutein and zeaxanthin, and inclusion of their metabolites, including ketokeratonoids. Accordingly, lutein content may be overestimated. Methods also often fail to identify lutein as either free or total (e.g., including free and that which is bound to proteins or esters).

Interestingly, several methods have been developed that allow measurement of retinal pigment (cartotenoids) in living tissues (Bhosale et al., 2007b). These include heterochromotic flicker photometry, autofluorescence, dual wave length reflectometry, and resonance Raman spectroscopy.

Related Compounds

Carotenoids are also closely related to sterols, ubiquinones, terpenes, and vitamin K (all terpenoids). However, of the more than 600 naturally occurring carotenoids, only a few are acquired by animals (Johnson, 2007). Because they are precursors of lutein, lycopene and α-carotene (the immediate precursor) should be considered related (Figure 6-1). Because of their common source, lutein and zeaxanthin generally are associated with one another in plants and animals. Zeaxanthin is synthesized from the β-carotene and is often referred to as a "cousin" or "sister" carotenoid. Lutein and zeaxanthin differ only by the position of a single bond in the peripheral ring, resulting in the ε-ring for lutein (Figure 6-1), compared to the two β-rings of zeaxanthin. As such, lutein and zeaxanthin are geometric isomers, with lutein referred to as a diol of α-carotene and zeaxanthin a diol of β-carotene (Sowbhagya et al., 2004). Both occur naturally as all-*trans* (all-*E*). Like lutein, zeaxanthin is a food dye (E number E161h). Lutein has three chiral centers; zeaxanthin has two. The close structural, physical, and biological association of lutein and zeaxanthin renders their analytical and functional separation difficult. For this reason, they often are referred to together as xanthophylls.

Effects of Manufacturing, Processing, and Storage on Composition

Preparations

Two sources of lutein currently are available for supplementation: crystalline (pure, free) lutein and lutein esters (Alves-Rodrigues and Shao, 2004). Studies of lutein largely have involved the pure crystalline form, derived from marigolds, and prepared as capsules or solutions in some type of oral vehicle. Often supplementation is accomplished by the addition of the pure crystalline form mixed into a diet. The lutein is often predissolved in an oil base prior to addition to the diet. A few commercial products are available that contain pure, free crystalline lutein. However, most commercial dietary supplement products exist as lutein esters (several available) due to patent protections that preclude extraction of purified lutein from natural products (especially marigolds; patent carried by OmniActive Health Technologies and Kemin).

Alternative preparations of lutein are available in Europe. These include a sublingual spray (New Focus®, Good Health Naturally), characterized by unknown oral bioavailability, and an ophthalmic ointment containing purified extract of marigold petals (as xanthophylls dipalmitate) (Adaptinol®; Bayer) (Sowbhagya et al., 2004).

Processing and Stability

Processing

Marigold pigmentation is a cheaper and more readily available source of natural yellow to orange pigmentation compared to other natural sources (e.g., turmeric and saffron). Processing from marigolds has been reviewed by Sowbhagya et al. (2004). Full flowers with minimal calyx are harvested. Because availability is seasonal, flowers are stored (70 to 80 tons) in a well-drained room during peak season. The flowers are compressed, sprayed with a lactic bacterial culture, and covered with lime and a tarp. Excess water is drained during storage, with negligible pigment in the waste. Lactic acid fermentation occurs anaerobically, stabilizing the stored flowers for 3 to 4 months. Neither lactic fermentation nor the anaerobic environment seems to negatively impact stability (Sowbhagya et al., 2004). Further processing involves drying at temperatures below 60 to 65°C until dehydrated to a moisture level of 8–10 percent. The quality of the starting material and the conditions of dehydration are described as the two critical factors that influence the retention of xanthophylls during processing (Sowbhagya et al., 2004). The dry yield of flowers approximates 10 percent, which contains 1 to 2 percent xanthophylls (Sowbhagya et al., 2004). The dried flowers are then powdered and pelleted. Pellets are subjected to extraction with hexane. Different techniques for extracting pigments have been studied for their impact on pigment content. For example, ethanol extraction in a more alkaline pH yields a darker extract compared to extraction at a lower pH (Sowbhagya et al., 2004). The xanthophyll yield can be increased by re-extraction and extraction at higher temperatures (45°C). The final oleoresin contains 8–10 percent xanthophylls. The extract can be purified with a propanol extraction followed by precipitation. The precipitated fraction may contain close to 50 percent lutein esters; a second precipitation can increase the yield to 65 percent purity. The lutein esters in the oleoresin can be solubilized up to 20 percent weight/weight (w/w) in vegetable oil. The xanthophylls are de-esterified (freed) from the oleoresin by saponification with potassium hydroxide followed by a hexane extraction, generally yielding about 1–4 percent xanthophyll. Saponification of marigold oleoresin yields lutein and lutein esters at a ratio of 2:1 (w/w). The freed xanthophyll can then be used directly in animal feeds or it can be modified into a dry powder by adsorption onto calcium silicate, gum, starch, or other compounds. Food colorings may contain lutein that has been extracted and purified from marigolds, but cannot contain unpurified lutein.

Extraction of lutein from plants is covered by patents, with a patent currently existing for processing from marigolds and others pending for extraction from other plants. Processing from other plants is based on methods similar to those used for marigolds. A number of patents are pending for the processing of lutein from other natural sources or oleoresin; patents include processing of different portions of the plants in order to increase lutein yield (Sowbhagya et al., 2004). The use of enzymes such as cellulase, glycanase, and glucosidase also is being considered (Delgado-Vargas and Paredes-López, 1997). Lu et al. (2005) demonstrated that enzymes increased lutein extraction from corn gluten approximately 60 percent.

Stability

Stability information is available for lutein when stored in its natural, unprocessed state or following extraction and/or concentration from lutein-rich plants.

Nonextracted State

Solar radiation and heat influences lutein concentration of sun-cured forage or hay, with concentration tending to be lower compared to fresh forage. For example, Bailey and Chen (1988) reported the concentration of xanthophylls in *Cynodon dactylon* to be over 800 mg/kg DM when the grass was freshly cut, but the content declined to 55 mg/kg DM after the same forage was dried to make hay. The xanthophyll content of *Dactylis glomerata, Lolium perenne*, and *Trifolium pretense* declined an average of 83 percent between direct cut forage and hay (Chauveau-Duriot et al., 2005). Beta-carotene can be dramatically affected by forage harvesting and storage conditions (McDowell, 2000), and presumably, these factors also significantly affect the lutein concentration of forages. For example, green hay curing in the swath may lose half its β-carotene content in one day's exposure to sunlight and almost all of it if left exposed to rain as well as sunlight.

Extracted State

Stability of the extracted lutein products generally is assessed by the amount of color lost during processing, with darkest colors reflecting greater xanthophyll retention (Table 6-1) (Sowbhagya et al., 2004). Lutein occurs naturally as an acetylated ester. The *trans* isomers reportedly are more stable and effective than the *cis* forms, although *cis* isomers seem to be biologically active (Sowbhagya et al., 2004). The conjugated structure of lutein that determines its biologic activity also renders it susceptible to oxidation and isomerization of all-*trans* configuration to the *cis* form. Mitigating factors facilitating oxidation and isomerization include light, presence of metals, and degradative enzymes (Sowbhagya et al., 2004; de Oliveira and Rodriguez-Amaya, 2007). Exposure to oxygen in air results in color loss. Oxidative enzymes (e.g., lipoxygenase) will hasten degradation, yielding peroxides. Extracted lutein also seems to be light sensitive (Lopez-Hernandez et al., 2001), although it is not clear if the extent of degradation is impacted by the plant source of the xanthophyll or the process by which it is extracted. Regardless, light and oxygen sensitivity mandate the need for packaging in tin or opaque containers. Lutein stability also is negatively impacted by the combination of extreme pH and light (Sowbhagya et al., 2004). Lutein is chemically stable in a pH range of 3 to 9, and unstable in acids of pH < 2 (Sowbhagya et al., 2004). Thermal processing increases conversion from all-*trans* to *cis* isomers by 22 percent (Updike and Schwartz, 2003), although the pigment is stable at 80 to 100°C for 3 minutes (Sowbhagya et al., 2004). However, thermal processing also increases antioxidant activity of carotenoids, including lutein, extracted from cactus pear (Jaramillo-Flores et al., 2003). Saponification results in hydrolysis of esters, increasing polarity and thereby reducing lipophilicity (potentially impacting compound movement in the body), but this can be reversed by resterification with acetic anhydride/pyridine. Processing should be designed such that the fraction of unsaponified lutein is minimized (Sowbhagya et al., 2004). Partial saponification of lutein esters increases stability if followed by neutralization with a weak acid (final pH of 8 with 10 to 20 percent weight of unsaponified xanthophyll esters) (Sowbhagya et al., 2004).

The addition of stabilizing factors to products intended as food colorants has been studied (Sowbhagya et al., 2004). Examples include mesquite or Arabic gum added to oil-in-water emulsions. The composition of the emulsifying agent (and pH) influence stability, with mesquite appearing to provide more stability than Arabic gum (Sowbhagya et al., 2004).

Processing seems to impact commercial preparations of lutein. For example, different preparations containing corn have varying amounts of lutein, including different brands of the same preparation. Reasons proposed by the authors for variations in lutein content reflect differences in the carotenoid composition, losses during processing, and losses during preparation for consumption (e.g., cooking) (de Oliveira and Rodriguez-Amaya, 2007). The potential impact of food preparation on lutein oral absorption also is addressed in the Biology section of this chapter.

Conditions that alter stability of lutein may impact validity of studies because of improper sample handling. Care must be taken in handling of tissue samples following collection from animals as well as following extraction of the carotenoid of interest from the tissue, prior to analysis. Su et al. (1999) demonstrated that carotenoids generally remained stable following exposure to fluorescent lighting for 72 hours, but that stability tended to be impacted more by storage at room temperature compared to storage in the refrigerator (4°C) or freezing (–20°C).

Potential for Contamination or Adulteration

Although as a plant, contaminants might be expected, no information was found related to potential contaminants of lutein products with herbicides, microorganisms, or heavy metals. Marigold contains natural insecticides (Wells et al., 1993), antimicrobials, and antiparasitic compounds (Sturz and Kimpinski, 2004), which may complicate detection of contaminants acquired during processing or storage. However, natural insecticides also may reduce the need for and risk of contamination by applied insecticides. A review of lutein approvals at the website www.consumerlab.com found that of 23 products reviewed for contaminants none contained any.

BIOLOGY

Absorption, Distribution, Metabolism, and Excretion

The disposition (absorption, distribution, metabolism, and excretion) of lutein has been described in rats and humans following intravenous or oral administration. Limited information is available regarding lutein concentrations in target species. Although the disposition of other carotenoids might be available in target species (e.g., lycopene in dogs [Korytko et al., 2003]; β-carotene in dogs, cats, and horses [Fonnesbeck and Symons, 1967; Greiwe-Crandell et al., 1997; Kienzle et al., 2003; Gay et al., 2004]), the di-hydroxy substitutions on the β-rings and epsilon rings of lutein render it more polar than lycopene or its metabolites, α- and β-carotene. This difference in polarity can contribute to marked differences in the disposition of lutein compared to the carotenes (Granado et al., 2003).

Absorption

Target Species

No information is available (other than serum concentrations; see below) regarding absorption of lutein from horses, dogs, or cats.

Nontarget Species

Humans

The absorption of lutein seems to follow the same pathway as that of dietary fat. The factors influencing bioavailability of carotenoids have been reviewed (Alves-Rodrigues and Shao, 2004). In its natural state in food, lutein is either bound to proteins or esterified as either a mono- or diester and combined with saturated fatty acids. Absorption requires release from the matrix in which the carotenoid is contained (release from protein), dispersion into a lipid phase, formation of micelles (involving bile salts), and movement to the brush border of the small intestine. This is then followed by passive absorption and transport into the lymphatic circulation. No active transport systems have been identified for carotenoids in the gastrointestinal tract. Location and physical form of carotenoids are more important to absorption of lutein than is the chemical state. Absorption is influenced by the state of the food and the presence of enzymes or other degradative molecules. Lutein bioavailability in particular has been demonstrated to be impacted by the food matrix, and the amount and type of food processing (i.e., raw versus cooked, natural versus processed) (Molldrem et al., 2004). For example, Bowen et al. (2002) noted that lutein is very bioavailable in eggs but less so in leafy vegetables; the digestible lipid matrix of the egg yolk was proposed to facilitate lutein absorption. Absorption of lutein seems to be facilitated when ingested in an oil preparation, perhaps due to better dissolution in the delivery vehicle (Bowen et al., 2002; Alves-Rodrigues and Shao, 2004). Relative bioavailability in mixed vegetables in humans is 67 percent compared to 45 to 54 percent in spinach. Mechanical disruption (e.g., homogenization or chopping) increases bioavailability from raw leafy vegetables (McEligot et al., 1999; van het Hof et al., 1999b).

Lutein diesters contain fatty acids at either end that must be removed by gastrointestinal enzymes (lipases or esterases) prior to absorption (Alves-Rodrigues and Shao, 2004). Gastrointestinal de-esterification of lutein does not seem to occur in the stomach. De-esterification seems to be inefficient, with the extent dependent upon dietary fat content as well as the food matrix. As such, crystalline (free) lutein might be expected to be more orally bioavailable because de-esterification is not necessary. However, the impact of esterification on lutein absorption is not clear. For example, Bowen et al. (2002) compared bioavailability of lutein when ingested as an unesterified crystalline lutein (extracted from marigolds; 20 g unesterified lutein/100g total lutein) suspension in safflower oil, or as an esterified preparation (marigold powder; 36.7 g esterified lutein/100 g total lutein). Using a crossover study for each preparation, paralleled by two doses (0.5 and 0.67 micromole/kg body weight), diesters were 62 percent more bioavailable than unesterified lutein. However, comparison with studies of others led the authors to conclude that it was the lack of dissolution of the unesterified product in the vehicle that limited its bioavailability. Nonetheless, the authors concluded the esterification did not present an impediment to oral absorption. This study demonstrates the importance of standardizing all aspects of the supplemented product, in addition to standardization of other study methods, when dealing with dietary supplements.

Isomerization of the freed carotenoids does not seem to take place in the stomach, despite low pH. However, preferential appearance of the 13-*cis* isomer over the 9-*cis* isomer in the plasma of monkeys suggests either isomerization does occur in monkeys, or the 13-*cis* isomer is preferentially absorbed to the 9-*cis* isomer (Snodderly et al., 1990).

Once freed from its dietary matrix, lutein is incorporated into micelles, absorbed by enterocytes, and incorporated along with other lipids (including other carotenoids) into chylomicrons. From the enterocyte, chylomicrons are absorbed into the lymphatic system first and eventually empty into the systemic circulation where they are delivered to tissues, including the liver. In the liver, the chylomicrons are processed such that the carotenoids are incorporated into lipoproteins (principally low and high density) and then re-released into systemic circulation (Alves-Rodrigues and Shao, 2004). In human single-dose studies, lutein seems to peak in chylomicrons and serum, respectively, at 2 or 16 hours post ingestion. Efficiency of absorption of lutein seems to be inversely related with concentration, perhaps reflecting solubility or availability of chylomicrons.

Forage Animals

A very thorough investigation of the digestion and absorption of carotenoids in sheep given fresh red clover was recently performed by Cardinault et al. (2006). Six mature Texel wethers were surgically fitted with three canulas, one each in the rumen, proximal duodenum, and distal ileum. Digestive flow (mg/day) of lutein and other carotenoids through each segment of the digestive tract was assessed using a double-marker technique involving continuous infusion of ^{51}Cr-EDTA (marker of liquid phase) and ^{103}Ru-phenanthroline (marker of solid phase). The flow of lutein increased about 17 percent from an intake of 174 mg/day in red clover to 204 mg/day in the duodenum. A net disappearance of lutein was observed from the duodenum to the ileum (ileal lutein flow 172 mg/day), resulting in an apparent absorption of 16 percent. Fecal lutein flow (181 mg/day) was ≈ 5 percent greater than the lutein concentration of digesta passing from the ileum through the large intestine. These results demonstrate that absorption of lutein occurs primarily in the small intestine of ruminants, as has been found in other mammals. This study also confirmed the earlier work of Tucker et al.

(1967) that suggested the cecum and colon are not major absorption sites of carotenoids. Studies on the in vitro and in situ disappearance of lutein from alfalfa hay in cattle and goats have found very little degradation of lutein by rumen microorganisms even after 64 hours of incubation (Mora et al., 1999). The greater flow of lutein going out of than into the rumen and large intestine observed by Cardinault et al. (2006) indicates that microorganisms residing in these segments may have the ability to synthesize lutein; however, they acknowledged that the synthesis of lutein by ruminal bacteria has never been shown. Alternatively, it is possible that production of free xanthophyll forms may be generated by the release of conjugated forms of xanthophylls after the action of ruminal microorganisms. An earlier study by Cardinault et al. (2004) demonstrated that free xanthophylls increased in media when ruminal fluid was incubated with carotenoid-enriched food, but not purified xanthophylls.

Although horses are not ruminants, the small intestine is likely the predominant site of lutein absorption in all herbivores. Microbial activity in the equine stomach and the small intestine is thought to affect the digestive process in the horse, although to a lesser extent than that found in the hindgut. The impact of fermentation on the degradation of dietary carotenoids or microbial synthesis of carotenoids has not been addressed in the horse, but evidence of microbial influence on dietary lutein content in sheep (Cardinault et al., 2006) warrants further investigation regarding a like impact in the horse.

Although it is widely agreed that carotenoids are absorbed from the gastrointestinal tract into the lymphatic system, the potential for direct absorption of carotenoids has only recently been addressed. Cardinault et al. (2006) surgically fitted five wethers with catheters in the portal and mesenteric veins and mesenteric artery to ascertain the contribution of carotenoid flux across the portal-drained viscera after consumption of fresh red clover. Carotenoids in the red clover consisted of lutein (136 mg/kg), epilutein (40 mg/kg), trans-β-carotene (16 mg/kg), and 13-*cis*-β-carotene (13 mg/kg). Among these carotenoids, only lutein and epilutein were recovered in the portal system. Arterio-venous differences were positive, but not significantly different from zero, indicating that this absorption process is very low. The authors estimated direct absorption of lutein into portal blood may only account for 8 percent of that apparently absorbed from the small intestine.

Distribution

Target Species

Specific information is not available (other than serum concentrations; see below) regarding distribution of lutein from horses, dogs, or cats.

Nontarget Species

Humans and Rats

Lutein is the second most common carotenoid in human serum. Distribution of carotenoids is largely dependent on lipoproteins, with even distribution among the various lipoprotein fractions. For lutein, its polarity should result in lutein being positioned at the surface of the lipoproteins facilitating easy transfer to tissues. As with other carotenoids, tissue concentration of lutein is determined, in part, by the concentration of low-density lipoprotein receptors (Granado et al., 2003). Organs of preferential distribution in the rat include the lung (ng/mg protein) (1.59 ± 0.52), liver (36 ± 4), and spleen (12.8 ± 4.9) (Itagaki et al., 2006), with peak accumulation occurring at approximately 4 hours. Accumulation in red blood cells (RBC) results in higher concentrations compared to plasma, suggesting preferential distribution to erythrocytes. Khachik et al. (1997a) have demonstrated the presence of lutein in human milk. In the rat, lutein distributes poorly to the brain and fat (Itagaki et al., 2006). Distribution to the brain may reflect structural similarities between lutein and vitamin A, a known substrate for P-glycoprotein-mediated efflux (Itagaki et al., 2006).

Lutein and zeaxanthin accumulate in the retina preferentially to other carotenoids; indeed, lutein and zeaxanthin are the only dietary carotenoids present in both the retina and the lens of humans. A xanthophyll-binding protein has been isolated from membrane extracts of the human macula (Yemelyanov et al., 2001). Because lutein and zeaxanthin are the major human retinal carotenoids, they are referred to as macular pigments (Bhosale et al., 2007a). However, the distributions of lutein and zeaxanthin throughout the retina are uneven. In human adult retinas, the concentrations of lutein and zeaxanthin in the young and older adult macula approximate 9 and 10 ng (ratio of 1.7:1; 4 mm diameter specimen), respectively, compared to 2.2 and 1 ng (ratio of 2.2, 8 mm diameter specimen) in the periphery and 0.5 and 0.4, respectively (ratio of 1.75), in the entire lens (Bhosale et al., 2007a). Accumulation in the retina reflects, in part, highly specific binding proteins (Alves-Rodrigues and Shao, 2004). Supplementation with lutein seems to correlate with an increase in retinal concentrations. In human cadaver studies, long-term supplementation with lutein is associated with a 3- to 10-fold increase in ocular lutein concentrations (Bhosale et al., 2007a).

Forage Animals

In sheep and cattle, circulating and adipose levels of β-carotene and lutein seems to have an inverse relationship. Sheep have been described to preferentially accumulate lutein rather than β-carotene in plasma and fat, whereas cattle have lower lutein concentrations in plasma and fat compared to β-carotene (Prache et al., 2003; Cardinault et al., 2006; Nozière et al., 2006). To the committee's knowledge, circulating or tissue levels of lutein have not been reported for the horse.

Biotransformation

Target Species

The synthetic pathway from lycopene to lutein and zeaxanthin seems to occur only in plants and selected algae. However, as was previously discussed, it has been suggested, although not confirmed, that gastrointestinal microflora may synthesize lutein or release conjugated lutein in free form (see Cardinault et al., 2006). Animals do not seem to possess enzymes necessary for synthesis of either oxygenated carotenoid from their precursors. This discussion will therefore focus on biotransformation of absorbed lutein in animals. The biotransformation of carotenoids, including lutein, is not well understood, but use of isotopes and other methods, including deductive reasoning based on the appearance of metabolites, has provided some information.

Nontarget Species

Dehydration products (anhydrolutein) and oxidative metabolites of lutein (also referred to as ketocarotenoids, including epilutein), which normally are absent in food, have been detected in human serum and tissues, including milk (Khachik et al., 1995, 1997a,b, 2006b). A dose-dependent appearance of nondietary lutein metabolites has been described in the human retina (Granado et al., 2003; Khachik et al., 2006b). Their appearance suggests retinal biotransformation of both lutein and zeaxanthin (Bhosale et al., 2007a). Because of the large concentrations of lutein found in its retina, the Japanese quail has been promoted as a possible small animal model for the disposition—and specifically—biotransformation of retinal lutein (Bhosale et al., 2007b). Isomers and esters of lutein also have been detected in a variety of other tissues, suggesting that metabolism is more extensive than simple degradation.

Summary of Concentration Versus Time Course

Target Species

In Beagle dogs receiving 0.45, 0.9, and 1.9 mg/kg BW of crystalline lutein suspended in soybean oil and added to the diet for 12 weeks, maximum lutein concentrations were approximately 25.5, 27, and 30 nmol/L, respectively (0.025, 0.027, and 0.03 μmol/L), at 12 weeks (Figure 6-2a). Interestingly, concentrations in the dog are approximately 5-fold less (when compared on a mg/kg BW dose basis) to that reported in the cat (Kim et al., 2000a). In Tabby cats receiving 0.71, 3.6, and 7.2 mg/kg BW crystalline lutein (apparently not suspended in oil) added to the diet for 12 weeks, maximum lutein concentrations approximated 0.04, 0.12, and 0.14 μmol/L, respectively, at 12 weeks (Figure 6-2b). Differences between the results from dog and cat studies may reflect, in part, different lutein preparations and concentrations used in the various studies (e.g., concentrations might be expected to be higher in dogs because of the use of products containing lutein suspended in oil compared to cats, in which lutein was mixed into the core diet). Differences, however, more likely reflect differences in elimination half-life. In the dog studies mentioned above plasma lutein concentrations increased less than 10 percent from week 2 to week 12, suggesting steady-state occurs rapidly (Kim et al., 2000b). In contrast, in cats, plasma lutein concentrations increased from week 2 to week 12 by 25 percent and did not seem to have reached steady-state at study end (Kim et al., 2000a). These data suggest a longer half-life of lutein in cats compared to dogs, and thus a greater accumulation ratio. Plasma lutein concentrations in both the dog and cat appear to be substantially lower than concentrations achieved in humans following ingestion of similar doses (Table 6-2); this difference also may reflect a longer half-life and thus greater accumulation in humans compared to dogs and cats. In both the dog and cat, changes in lutein dose did not result in direct proportional changes in plasma lutein concentrations (Figures 6-2a and 6-2b), an observation also made in humans (Table 6-2).

No information is available regarding lutein concentrations in horses.

Nontarget Species

Humans

The 63rd report of the FAO/WHO Joint Expert Committee on Food Additives (JECFA, 2005) promulgated specifications for preparations with high (> 80 percent) lutein content, based on a summary of lutein data in rats and monkeys. Based on their review, which may include data that are either unpublished or not available for public or peer review, the JECFA found that lutein absorption is rapid, bioavailability is low at 30 to 40 percent, and increases in doses up to 200-fold resulted in only a 2- to 3-fold increase in plasma concentrations. Radioisotope (^{14}C) studies of lutein in humans receiving 125 nmole lutein-^{14}C orally indicate plasma concentrations of ^{14}C peak at about 15 hours and do not approach baseline until close to 500–600 hours (25 days) postdosing (Burri and Clifford, 2004). Granado et al. (2003) reported the concentration of lutein in humans receiving a variety of lutein supplements based on several studies in five European countries. Concentrations (μmol/L) in these studies ranged from 0.25 to 2.5 (median 1.15); 1.25 to 3.0 (median 1.65) with lutein esters (n = 56); and 0.15 to 0.5 (median 0.25). Doses were not provided in the summary data, but might be gleaned from review of the original report. A dose-concentration response was docu-

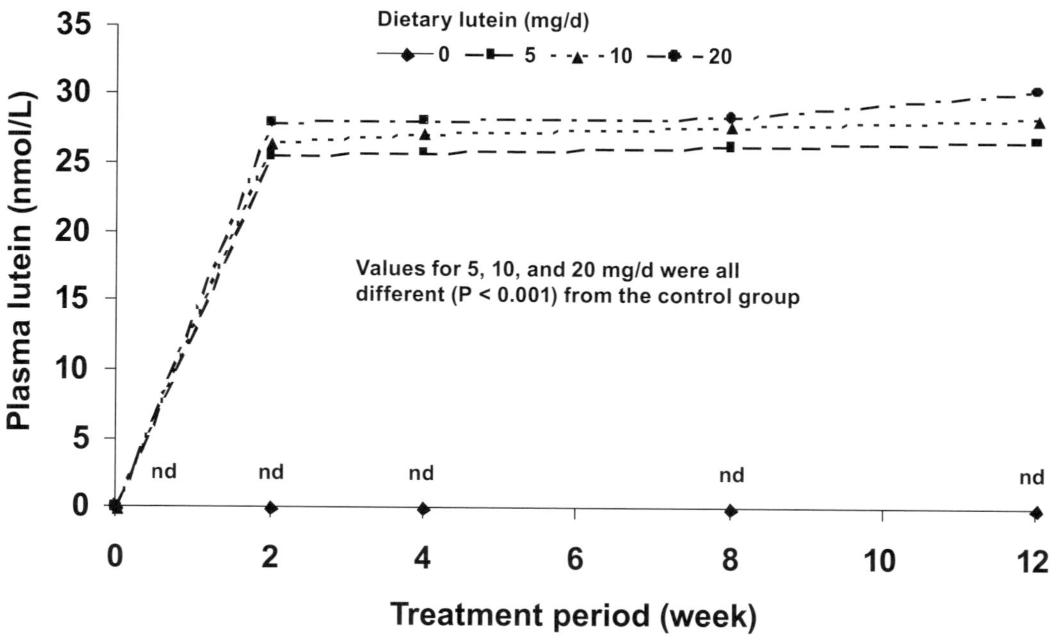

FIGURE 6-2a Concentrations of plasma lutein + zeaxanthin in dogs fed diets containing 0, 5, 10, or 20 mg of lutein for 12 weeks.
NOTE: Values are means (n = 14); nd: undetected.
SOURCE: Redrawn from *Veterinary Immunology and Pathology*, 74/3–4, H. W. Kim, B. P. Chew, T. S. Wong, J. S. Park, B. B.C. Weng, K. M. Byrne, M. G. Hayek, and G. A. Reinhart, Dietary lutein stimulates immune response in the canine, 315–327, Copyright (2000), with permission from Elsevier.

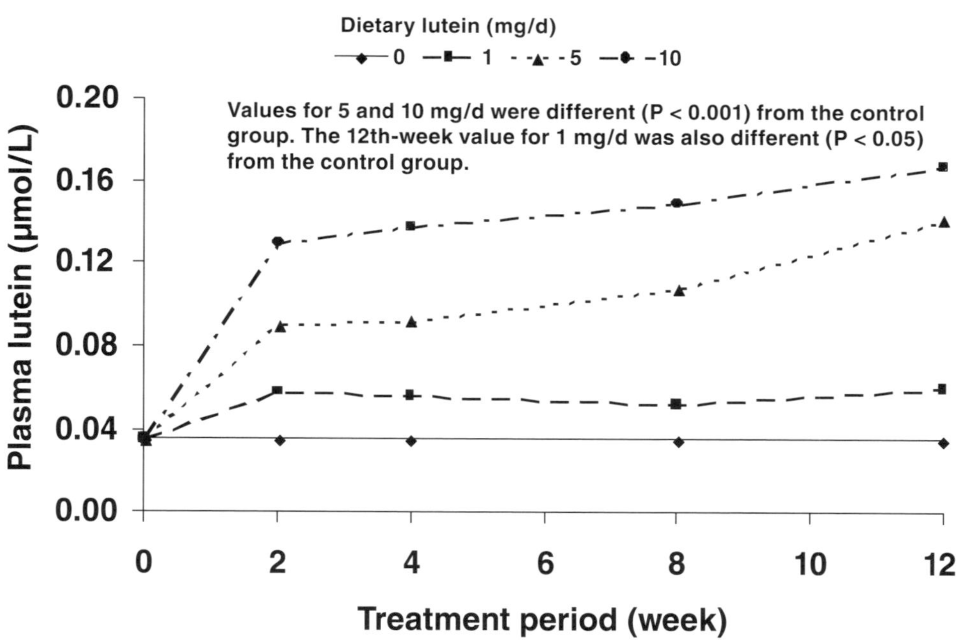

FIGURE 6-2b Concentrations of plasma lutein + zeaxanthin in cats fed diets containing 0, 1, 5, or 10 mg of lutein for 12 weeks.
NOTE: Values are means (n = 14).
SOURCE: Redrawn from *Veterinary Immunology and Pathology*, 74/3–4, H. W. Kim, B. P. Chew, T. S. Wong, J. S. Park, B. B.C. Weng, K. M. Byrne, M. G. Hayek, and G. A. Reinhart, Dietary lutein stimulates immune response in the canine, 315–327, Copyright (2000), with permission from Elsevier.

TABLE 6-2 Lutein Dose and Plasma Concentration Relationship Among Different Species

Species	Dose (mg/kg BW)	Plasma Lutein (μmol/L)
Dog[a,b]	0.45	0.025
	0.9	0.027
	1.9	0.03
Cat[c,d]	0.71	0.04
	3.6	0.12
	7.3	0.14
Human[e,f]	20.5 (0.29)	1.32
	20 (0.29)	1.06
	15 (0.21)	0.6–1.75
	12 (0.17)	1.5
	8 (0.11)	0.37

[a]In soybean oil, administered orally.
[b]Source: Kim and DellaPenna (2006a).
[c]Mixed in base food.
[d]Source: Kim and DellaPenna (2006b).
[e]Source: Shao and Hathcock (2006).
[f]Total daily dose with dose/70 kg in parentheses.

mented in humans receiving either 4.1 or 20 mg/day (0.06 or 0.28 mg/kg BW/day). The elimination (disappearance) half-life was much longer in humans compared to rats, approximating 5 to 7 days, with an accumulation ratio of 7 (low dose) to 10 (high dose). Steady state occurred at 15 to 30 days (compared to 2 to 3 days in rats) (Thurmann et al., 2005). The JECFA (2005) findings on human disposition of lutein were similar, indicating peak absorption at 11 to 16 hours postintake, steady state reached at approximately 30 days, and an elimination half-life of about 5 to 7 days. In contrast, kinetic studies in men and women (Rock et al., 1992; Burri et al., 2001) found lutein elimination half-life to be between 33 to 76 days. More recent studies focusing on the role of lutein in treatment or prevention of acute macular degeneration in humans have been accompanied by measurement of serum lutein concentration in elderly (> age 60) human patients (Khachik et al., 2006b; Rosenthal et al., 2006). Following administration of 2.5 to 10 mg/day (approximating 0.035 to 0.14 mg/kg BW/day), concentrations ranged from 210 to 1,000 nmol/L (0.2 to 10 μmol/L) in one study (Khachik et al., 2006b) and 35.1 to 66.8 μg/dl (618–1176 nmol/L; 0.62–1.18 μmol/L) in a second (Rosenthal et al., 2006). Although differences in preparations are likely to contribute to differences in absorption, these data suggest that lutein concentrations in humans are substantially higher than those achieved in either dogs or cats, and higher in cats compared to dogs, when lutein intake is compared on a mg/kg BW basis. Further, in all species, dose-concentration relationship of lutein seems to be limited, probably by absorption.

Purported Role in Health and Disease

Physiology

Plants

Carotenoids function to protect the lipid components of plants, whereas their water-soluble counterparts, flavenoids, protect the water components. As such, carotenoids are found throughout the plant kingdom and, because of consumption of plants, in the animal kingdom. From an evolutionary standpoint, carotenoids are among the oldest of molecules, dating back at least 3 billion years (Johnson, 2007). Over 600 carotenoids occur in nature. As a group, carotenoids are characterized by a marked structural diversity that seems to have evolved in response to their diverse biologic functions. These include structural support of cell membranes and photosystems, harvesting of light, photoprotection, and substrates for hormone synthesis (Kim and DellaPenna, 2006). Beta-carotene is the most biologically active of the carotenoids (Hinds et al., 1997). Synthesis occurs primarily in photosynthetic plants, reflecting their natural function.

Two primary functions are attributed to lutein and zeaxanthin: filtration of high-energy blue light and quenching of photo-induced reactive oxygen radicals (Alves-Rodrigues and Shao, 2004). In photosynthetic plants, lutein and zeaxanthin are located in chloroplasts where they are integrated with light-harvesting chlorophyll proteins. They facilitate photosynthesis by helping to regulate harvesting of light, in part by controlling distribution of the light-harvesting proteins (Johnson, 2004, 2007). Lutein facilitates folding of the protein and, along with zeaxanthin, quenches excessive light. As a light-absorption pigment, lutein increases the efficiency of light transfer to chlorophyll and acts as a photoprotectant (Schieber and Carle, 2005). Blue light (440 nm) is the highest energy form of visible light and is capable of generating reactive oxygen species (ROS) that cause photo-oxidation (Alves-Rodrigues and Shao, 2004). Orange light (590 nm) requires 100 times more energy than blue light to cause an equivalent level of cellular damage. As lipophilic, polyene chromophores, both lutein and zeaxanthin absorb blue light (peak absorption is 446 nm). The absorption of blue light protects plants from damage but does not prevent photosynthesis. The ability of lutein and zeaxanthin to absorb blue light contributes to their ability to protect the retina in animals. Absorption of blue light also is responsible for the color of lutein and zeaxanthin, causing yellow pigmentation at low concentrations and orange-red at high concentrations.

In addition to their light-harvesting (photosynthetic and protective) responsibilities, carotenoids are associated with biomembranes where they serve as antioxidant or membrane stabilizers (Johnson, 2007). Their antioxidant activity is closely related to their photoprotection. However, carotenoid activity is dependent upon its highly delocalized polyene backbone. End ring oxidation (Figure 6-1), which distinguishes xanthophylls from carotenes, is a basis for their antioxidant activity, allowing carotenoids to quench chlorophyll as well as radical oxygen species. Quenching occurs through vibration of the molecule, such that excessive light energy is absorbed rather than harming the plant. Radical oxidation of carotenoids has been referred to as "sacrificial radical scavenging" because it often causes destruction of the carotenoid (Johnson, 2007). However, in doing so, lipid peroxidation of the host is avoided. Substitutions on the cyclohexene rings at each end strongly influence the properties of the carotenoid. For example, for lutein, ketonization of the fourth ring carbon elongates the double bonds of the polyene, causing its spectrum to shift from yellow to red.

Animals

The major plant-origin carotenoids in human plasma are β-carotene, α-carotene, lycopene, β-cryptoxanthin, lutein, and zeaxanthin (Aman et al., 2005); similar data do not appear to be available in dogs, cats, or horses. Among the most well-known functions of many carotenoids (but not lutein) in mammals is conversion to vitamin A. Retinoids are molecules related to vitamin A, being comprised of a cyclic end group, polyene side chain, and polar end group (Figure 6-1). It is the polyene system that generates the color typical of retinoids (generally, yellow, orange, or red); as such, retinoids are chromophores. Variations in side chains and end groups yield different classes or generations of retinoids. However, of the over 600 carotenoids, less than 10 percent can be converted to vitamin A (Hinds et al., 1997). The oxygenated carotenoids, lutein and zeaxathin cannot be converted to vitamin A in mammals because they lack the appropriate enzymes and are not retinoids.

Retinoids are of either plant or animal origin. Of those predominating in human plasma, β-carotene is converted to retinol 2-fold more efficiently than α-carotene and β-cryptoxanthin. Retinol is a retinoid of animal origin, absorbed as a precursor retinyl ester from animal sources such as liver and eggs. Hydrolysis of the ester yields retinol. Plant sources of retinoids are pro-vitamin A carotenoids that are cleaved to yield retinal (also known as retinaldehyde). Irreversible oxidation of retinal yields retinoic acid. Retinol, retinal, and retinoic acid occur as either *trans* or *cis* configurations. The *cis* configuration is less stable and easily converted to the *trans* configuration. However, the *cis* configuration can occur naturally and has a critical role in physiology in that 11-*cis*-retinal is covalently linked with an opsin protein (rod, or blue, red, or green cone opsins) to yield rhodopsin.

The impact of retinoids in normal mammalian physiology is diverse and important. Formation of rhodopsin is one of their more important roles. Located in rod (photoreceptors) cells of the eye, it is the molecule involved in the initial step of vision. The long unsaturated electron network provided by the polyene of retinal renders is a powerful absorber of light. Light causes an immediate shift in configuration from a *cis* to a *trans* position, forces separation of retinal and ospin, triggering G-protein signals and electrical impulses to the optic nerve. In addition to vision, roles for retinoids have been identified in regulation of cell proliferation and differentiation, immune modulation, growth of tissues including bone, activation of tumor suppressor genes, and vision.

Carotenoids also act as chromophobes, contributing to up to five colors of songbirds. Further oxidation by animal metabolism yields the variable colors that lead to species sexual dimorphism, with the colors depending upon the enzymes present (Kim and DellaPenna, 2006; Johnson, 2007). A similar effect does not occur in mammals, which lost their ability to develop different coat colors from carotenoids when driven into nocturnal habitats by (dinosaur) predators (Johnson, 2007). Inclusion in oil droplets of the retinas of birds renders the bird tetrachromatic (able to discriminate colors).

Humans

The potential roles of lutein in human health have been reviewed by Alves-Rodrigues and Shao (2004) and Shao and Hathcock (2006). Two primary biologic activities contribute to the purported benefits of lutein: absorption of high-energy light and scavenging of oxygen radicals. Some studies have attempted to correlate outcome measures (for example, reduced incidence of age-related macular degeneration, increased response of tumors to chemotherapeutic agents, or decreased incidence of cancer) to dietary intake of natural forms of lutein (i.e., dark or orange vegetables such as spinach and maize (Granado et al., 2003)), whereas others are based on clinical trials in animal models or humans supplemented with lutein in the diet.

Purported benefits include:

1. Treatment or prevention of age-related macular degeneration (AMD);
2. Antioxidant effects through scavenging of oxygen radicals;
3. Immunomodulation, specifically of T-cells;
4. Anticancer effects;
5. Reduced risk of atherosclerosis;
6. Protection against UV radiation, e.g., in the skin;
7. Anti-aging; and
8. Coloration of foods of animal origin and as a natural food colorant.

Landrum and Bone (2000), Krinsky et al. (2003), and Alves-Rodrigues and Shao (2004) have reviewed the science supporting the beneficial effects of lutein in the human eye due to light absorption and antioxidant activity, particularly with respect to the treatment or prevention of macular degeneration. Photoprotection, including protection of the retina from phototoxicity and reduction in cataracts, are more universally recognized potential benefits of lutein. Lutein and zeaxanthin are the predominant carotenoids in the retina and, in particular, the macula. Both areas of the retina contain a high proportion of polyunsaturated fats, rendering the retina vulnerable to peroxidation by radical oxygen. Retinal accumulation of lutein and zeaxanthin, at the exclusion of other carotenoids, implies a specific role of these two xanthophylls in retinal photoprotection. Lutein is accumulated particularly in the macula fovea of humans, which is particularly sensitive to damage, whereas zeaxanthin is more diffusely distributed (Schalch et al., 2007). Photoprotection includes absorption of light, and blue light in particular, that otherwise would be absorbed by the retina, potentially causing retinal oxidation. In addition to retinal distribution, lutein and zeaxanthin are the exclusive carotenoids in the lens, suggesting a protective effect in cataract formation.

The antioxidant effects of carotenoids occur in vitro and in vivo. Those with at least 11 conjugated double bonds, including lutein, are 5-fold more effective as antioxidants than retinol (Jaramillo-Flores et al., 2003). More recently, Wang et al. (2006) described a dose-dependent antimutagenic effect of lutein based on Ames testing. Immunomodulatory effects of lutein are supported by a number of studies, including in cats (Kim et al., 2000a) and dogs (Kim et al., 2000b), targeting both humoral and cellular responses. Examples of immunomodulatory effects of lutein include its influence on the evolutionary development of animals, particularly birds (Blount, 2004). Lutein also seems to have a role in sexual dimorphism that is linked to sexual attractiveness among the species. Evidence for specific immunomodulation by lutein in dogs and cats is based on increased CD4-T and CD21+B cells in cats receiving 10 mg of lutein daily for 12 weeks and dogs treated for 12 weeks (Kim et al., 2000a,b).

Moss (2006) has reviewed the potential role of carotenoids, including lutein, in treatment of human patients undergoing chemotherapy. Anticancer effects have been proposed for carotenoids, including lutein (Khachik et al., 1995; Le Marchand et al., 1995; Kim et al., 1998). Clinical trials have focused on prevention of cancer, with findings suggesting that daily consumption of approximately 6 to > 7.5 mg per person is associated with a decreased incidence of endometrial, lung (not statistically significant), and breast cancer.

Purported cardiovascular effects of lutein in humans include reduction of the risk of atherosclerosis as reviewed by Alves-Rodrigues and Shao (2004). Proposed evidence includes epidemiologic studies correlating incidence with foods high in lutein (Bradbury, 2001), as well as more specific cardiovascular disease outcome measures in persons ingesting lutein (Dwyer et al., 2001).

Lutein in the skin purportedly reduces ultraviolet irradiation damage, immunosuppression, and other negative sequelae based on a mouse sunburn model (Lee et al., 2004). This effect, along with the potential role of lutein in slowing the progression of macular degenerationa and other purported benefits, may support the role that lutein might have in slowing aging.

In addition to potential health benefits, lutein, along with other xanthophylls, is used in either powder form or as an extract to improve the color of skin and eggs. Petals are also fed to birds as a source of pigment (Sowbhagya et al., 2004; Breithaupt, 2007). When mixed with vegetable oil (20 to 30 percent w/w), the xanthophylls can be used as food colorants. However, FDA restrictions require that lutein can be added as a colorant only in a purified extract form. Increasingly, lutein and other xanthophylls are being used as an alternate source of natural, rather than synthetic, dyes as food colorants (Sowbhagya et al., 2004).

Drug Interactions

Limited information is available regarding the potential impact of lutein on drug-metabolizing enzymes. Using substrates as markers of CYP450 enzyme activity, Gradelet et al. (1996) demonstrated that lutein did not increase the metabolism of markers of P4501A, 1A2, 2B1/2, 2E1, or 3A1/2 activity whereas several other non-pro vitamin-A carotenoids were marked inducers of CYP450 1A1 and 1A2. Lutein does not appear to significantly alter glutathione-S-transferase activity in the liver, lung, kidney, or small intestine of male Wistar rats following 16 days of supplementation at 45 mg/kg BW (Jewell and O'Brien, 1999). Cytochrome P-450 activity also was studied, based on metabolism of substrates by microsomes. The only significant substrate impacted by lutein was metabolism of benzyloxyresorufin-O-dearylation (BROD), which was decreased in the lutein supplement group. However, the demethylation of several other resorufin compounds was not impacted, leading the authors to include that lutein had no significant impact on drug metabolizing enzymes (Jewell and O'Brien, 1999).

Diet Interactions

Absorption

The absorption of carotenoids from the gastrointestinal tract is impacted by multiple factors, including the physiochemical properties of the carotenoid itself, the food matrix in which it is incorporated, and the meal with which it is eaten (Pullakhandam and Failla, 2007). In general, absorption of lutein in humans as part of a diet supplemented with crystalline lutein is almost double that of lutein obtained from natural sources (Alves-Rodrigues and Shao, 2004). Cooking or other processing seems to increase bioavailability.

Carotenoids appear to compete with one another for absorption, perhaps explaining the inverse relationship between concentration or dose of intake and absorption (see previous discussion). Kostic et al. (1995) demonstrated the combination of β-carotene and lutein reduced the area under the curve of both compounds when administered simultaneously to humans compared to the area under the curve when each was given individually. The appearance of lutein versus β-carotenes or other carotenoids in chylomicrons (rather than appearance in plasma) has been suggested as the most relevant measure of interaction between the compounds (Alves-Rodrigues and Shao, 2004). That carotenoids compete with one another for inclusion in chylomicrons was supported using in vitro methods (Pullakhandam and Failla, 2007), but the degree of interaction may vary with preparation. Lutein may be absorbed preferentially to β-carotenes, particularly in the presence of high concentrations of β-carotene (Gartner et al., 1996; van den Berg and van Vliet, 1998), although inconsistencies in methodologies complicate consensus of results (Alves-Rodrigues and Shao, 2004). Whereas one study demonstrated β-carotene was absorbed to a greater extent than lutein (O'Neill and Thurnham, 1998), another demonstrated an almost 5-fold greater bioavailability of lutein compared to β-carotene (van het Hof et al., 1999a). Further, lutein administered in its natural form as yellow carrots seems to have decreased gastrointestinal absorption of β-carotene (Molldrem et al., 2004). In contrast to absorption, lutein does not appear to influence β-carotene metabolism. Fat seems to increase oral bioavailability of lutein, whereas alcohol may decrease oral absorption (Molldrem et al., 2004; Pullakhandam and Failla, 2007).

Several studies have studied the impact of the combination of lutein with other vitamins on absorption of either compound. In humans, although the sample size was small, vitamin C appeared to facilitate the absorption of lutein (Tanumihardjo et al., 2005). In Beagle dogs (n = 56) and Tabby cats (n = 56) receiving 1.9 mg/kg BW and 7.1 mg/kg BW of lutein respectively, absorption of vitamin A was not impacted (Kim et al., 2000a,b). Dietary fiber may have a profound impact on absorption of carotenoids, including lutein. A study in women (Riedl et al., 1999) demonstrated that the area under the curve (AUC) of lutein was decreased by 40 to 74 percent by pectin, guar, alginate, or cellulose. Physical properties of fibers proposed to negatively impact lutein absorption included binding capacity of bile acids or water and subsequent impact on viscosity and luminal content volume, or altered small intestinal morphology, such as enhanced enterocyte turnover.

Distribution

Lutein and vitamin E or its congeners may share mechanisms of gastrointestinal absorption or, more likely, distribution to tissues by lipoproteins. One study demonstrated a dose effect of lutein on the ratio and possible distribution of tocopherols in rats (Jenkins et al., 2000). However, the effect could not be attributed to lutein alone, indicating a need for additional studies.

Impact of Disease and Vulnerable Populations

Species Differences

The absorption of carotenoids from the gastrointestinal tract is impacted by the physiologic and nutritional status of the consumer, the matrix of the preparation, and, in humans, the genotype (Pullakhandam and Failla, 2007). Because species diets are markedly variable, species differences in absorption of lutein are likely to be profoundly different. Some of these differences were addressed under Biology (ADME). Although few direct comparison data are available to demonstrate these differences, comparative review of intake dose and plasma lutein concentrations (Table 6-2) suggest differences do occur and may profoundly impact plasma concentrations. Relevance to safety, however, is not known.

In most other animals, including dogs and horses, β-carotene is oxidized in the enterocyte to retinol following absorption. However, domestic cats cannot convert β-carotene to vitamin A (NRC, 2006). As a result, domestic cats are strictly dependent upon preformed vitamin A in their diets to meet their requirements. Schweigert et al. (2002) demonstrated that although cats exhibit little to no intestinal conversion of β-carotene to vitamin A, they do have the ability to absorb β-carotene when administered at a physiological dose. However, the authors noted that the postadministration pattern of β-carotene in plasma appeared to be different from that reported in humans in that the rise in plasma β-carotene was slower and elevated levels persisted for a longer period of time. The delayed increase in plasma β-carotene levels and the lack of conversion to vitamin A suggest the cat differs from other mammals in the absorption and metabolism of β-carotene. Whether similar digestive and metabolic differences for lutein and other carotenoids exist in cats remains to be determined, but caution is warranted when extrapolating physiologic handling of carotenoids from other species to cats.

The lack of a gallbladder in horses might contribute to differences in absorption of lutein compared to other species (other than the rat, which also lacks a gallbladder). In the horse, bile is secreted continuously from the liver. Bile secreted from a gallbladder is much more concentrated than that secreted by the liver due to reabsorption of water and inorganic salts by the mucosal cells of the gallbladder viscus (Ullrey, 1972). Differences in bile composition may affect the emulsification of dietary fats and fat-soluble vitamins, interactions with pancreatic lipase, and the formation of micelles. Because bile salts initiate the process of digestion and absorption of fats and carotenoids, alterations in composition could affect the absorption of carotenoids. Despite the differences in bile secretion and composition, equids are very adept at digesting and absorbing dietary fats (Kronfeld et al., 2004). In part, this may be due to the relatively high concentration of lipase secreted by the equine pancreas. Lorenzo-Figueras et al. (2007) reported that the cellular concentration of lipase was more than 20-fold greater than amylase and 500–1,000 times greater than elastase, trypsin, and chymotrypsin in pancreatic tissue harvested from horses immediately after euthanasia. In addition, the relative activity of each pancreatic enzyme closely followed the cellular concentrations. When the authors compared the pancreatic lipase activity in adult horses to tissue obtained from other species, they found this enzyme exhibited a similar level of activity to adult pigs, but was slightly higher than that found in rats.

Another factor that might distinguish lutein absorption kinetics in the horse is the consumption of rations much higher in fiber and lower in fat compared to those typically consumed by rats, humans, dogs, and cats. Dietary fiber has been shown to reduce lutein absorption in humans (Riedl et al., 1999). In contrast, the bioavailability of some carotenoids seems to be enhanced by higher levels of dietary fat. Fecal excretion of β-carotene was reduced by 20 percent when a diet of straw, oats, beet pulp, and grass meal (2.5 percent crude fat) was supplemented with plant oil (6.5 percent crude fat) in ponies, suggesting a positive benefit of a small amount of fat on β-carotene absorption (Kienzle et al., 2003). In humans, dietary fat has a limited affect on β-carotene absorption, but seems to have a greater role in facilitating the absorption of lutein. A certain quantity of dietary fat seems to be required for sufficient solubilization of lutein diesters in foods and/or secretion of esterases and lipases from the pancreas (Roodenburg et al., 2000). The hydrolysis of lutein esters is mediated by these enzymes and is regulated by the presence of fat in the duodenum (Roodenburg et al., 2000). The diester form of lutein is more hydrophobic, making it more difficult to solubilize. Adding oils and high-fat feedstuffs to the diet of horses is a common industry practice. Therefore, higher absorption of lutein might be anticipated when fat is added to the normal diet of horses.

Disease and Age on Disposition

Granado et al. (2003) reviewed serum lutein concentrations in a large number of human medical patients afflicted with various illnesses. The lowest concentration range reported (μmol/L) was less than 0.05 up to 0.25 (median 0.05) in patients with malabsorption and the highest ranged from 0.1 to 0.5 (median 0.25) in patients with myocardial infarction. In their review, Alves-Rodrigues and Shao (2004) noted that a number of factors, including age, body mass index, smoking, and alcohol, impact absorption of lutein. Diseases, including those associated with fat maldigestion or malabsorption, liver or renal disease, or endocrine abnormalities (including hyperthyroidism), also are associated with altered absorption.

SAFETY

Toxicity Studies

Target Species

To the committee's knowledge, no toxicity studies have been performed with lutein in horses, dogs, or cats.

Nontarget Species

Humans

Shao and Hathcock (2006), Alves-Rodrigues and Shao (2004), and the JECFA (2005) have reviewed in vivo toxicity data for lutein. The Joint Committee focused on xanthophylls in marigold (*Tagetes erecta*) and, with its most recent report, those preparations with high (> 80 percent) lutein content compared to previous reports that focused on low-content preparations. An assessment of lutein toxicity data led to the conclusion that free lutein and zeaxanthin are safe for human consumption as long as the daily human consumption is kept to 2 mg/kg BW or 145 mg lutein + zeaxanthin. Shao and Hathcock (2006) argued that excess lutein should not cause clinical signs consistent with vitamin A toxicity because lutein is not a substrate for 15,15-monoxygenase that cleaves β-carotene.

Rats

Purified (crystalline) lutein has been studied several times in Fisher rats. Inclusion of 35 mg (as an oil suspension) in the diet resulted in significantly lower lung and brain weights and in weight gain in animals receiving a high dose, although the latter was attributed to higher oil intake. Studies in rats receiving 208 mg (for 13 weeks) to 639 mg/kg BW (for 4 weeks) reached doses over 10,000-fold higher than the mean daily intake of 0.02 mg/kg BW in humans. Yet, no adverse events occurred, including changes in body or organ weight or hematological parameters (Kruger et al., 2002). The highest dose in rats associated with no observable adverse event was 639 mg/kg BW/day. Parameters assessed included complete blood counts, serum chemistry profiles, organ weights, and histologic examination of liver, spleen, skin, and mesenteric lymph nodes. In addition to these outcome measures, another study by the same authors (Kruger et al., 2002) also included assessment of coagulation tests and histological examination of over 40 organs, including the central nervous system.

Monkeys

Monkeys receiving 20 mg/kg BW/day for 52 weeks developed no adverse events despite a dose-dependent lutein increase in the plasma, liver, and retina (cited by JECFA, 2005). A more recent study in rhesus monkeys found that up to 9.34 mg/kg BW lutein (with 0.5 mg/kg BW) per day for 12 months resulted in no ocular toxicity or other evidence of adverse events (Khachik et al., 2006a).

Based on their review of data in the rat and monkey, the JECFA (2005) cites the oral median lethal dose of lutein as > 2,000 mg/kg BW.

Ex Vivo Studies

Target Species

Kim et al. (2000a,b) evaluated the effect of lutein on immunomodulatory function in dogs and cats and found positive, rather than negative, effects. Further, lutein (20 mg/day for 30 days) was found to increase plasma antioxidant activity in Alaskan sled dogs (Baskin et al., 2000). A number of ex vivo studies have focused on immunomodulatory or safety effects of lutein on DNA (Sujak et al., 1999; Haegele et al., 2000; Chew et al., 2000). Concentrations appear to inversely correlate with oxidative DNA damage (Haegele et al., 2000).

In Vitro Studies

Mutagenicity studies revealed no mutagenic effects; indeed, antimutagenic effects were demonstrated in *Salmonella typhimurium* (De Mejía, et al., 1997). The JECFA (2005) concluded in their review of lutein that studies focusing on genotoxicity were negative for significant findings.

Adverse Event Reporting Programs

The National Animal Supplement Council (NASC) has provided data related to adverse events reported for lutein products registered as part of their Compliance Plus® program (Chapter 3). The data provided to the committee regarding lutein use were limited to the number of products registered (types and strengths not provided), the level (mg/kg) of use, the number of units sold, and adverse events (including serious ones) during each reporting year. At the time of the committee report, lutein had been marketed for 8 years and six products were registered.

Horses: No data were provided for horses.

Dogs: No adverse events to lutein in dogs were reported to NASC during a 5-year reporting period. Approximately 415,000 lutein units were sold during this time. Lutein intake in dogs ranged from 0.35 to 0.87 mg/kg BW (most recent mean of 0.35 mg/kg).

Cats: No adverse events to lutein in cats were reported to NASC during a 9-year reporting period (1999–2007). During this time, approximately 1.65 million units of lutein were sold. Lutein intake cited for the six registered lutein products ranged from 0.53 to 1.76 mg/kg BW (most recent mean of 1.15 mg/kg).

Nonsafety Studies

Target Species

Horses

To the committee's knowledge, no clinical or field trials have been performed in horses with the intent of investigating the effects of dietary lutein supplementation on equids.

Dogs

In a randomized, controlled, clinical trial in experimental animals, the effects of lutein on immune function were studied in dogs (Kim et al., 2000b). Young adult (17–18 month) female Beagles (n = 56; 11 kg) were supplemented with 5 (0.45 mg/kg BW), 10 (0.9 mg/kg BW), or 20 mg (1.9 mg/kg BW) crystallized lutein suspended in soybean oil and administered orally for 12 weeks. The authors did not specifically address potential adverse events other than weight loss, which did not occur during the study period.

Cats

In a randomized, controlled, clinical trial in experimental animals, the effects of lutein on immune function were studied in cats (Kim et al., 2000b). Young adult (10-month) female Tabby cats (n = 56; 1.41 kg) were supplemented with 1 (0.71 mg/kg BW), 5 (3.6 mg/kg BW), or 10 mg (7.2 mg/kg BW) crystallized lutein incorporated into the basal diet for 12 weeks. It is not clear if the supplement was first mixed with oil. The authors did not specifically address potential adverse events other than weight loss, which did not occur during the study period. The highest plasma lutein concentration measured approximately 0.12 μmol/L. Plasma concentrations appeared to be close to steady state by the study end at 12 weeks (Kim et al., 2000b).

Nontarget Species

Humans

Elderly humans (n = 45) received 2.5, 5, or 10 mg of pure lutein a day for 6 months such that the pattern of lutein and metabolites could be described. The 10 mg/day (0.143 mg/kg BW) dose was several times higher than the average human dietary consumption in fruits and vegetables. No evidence of side effects emerged during a 6-month dosing period followed by a 6-month dose-free period. Serum concentrations of lutein reached 1,000 nmol/L (Khachik et al., 2006b). Granado et al. (2003) offered a range of safe concentrations in humans to be between 0.5 and 1.0 μmol/L.

Shao and Hathcock (2006) systematically reviewed safety data for lutein in humans receiving the pure product, for which lutein concentrations are most likely to be highest. They reviewed 30 peer-reviewed published clinical trials involving lutein in humans and focused on 11 of the most relevant. Each involved all-*trans* lutein as either the free or esterified compound. Their evaluation was based on risk assessment methods described by the Council for Responsible Nutrition's *Vitamin and Mineral Safety*, 2nd Edition, which in turn incorporates fundamental steps proposed by the U.S. Food and Nutrition Board in its Dietary Reference Intakes of 1997 (cited by Shao and Hathcock, 2006). The methods of assessment included: (1) a search for data that might identify a hazard related to excessive intake, (2) assessment of dose-response relationships for the hazard, and (3) assessment of uncertainty such that an uncertainty factor might be assigned. An Upper Level of Intake (UL) was determined by adjusting the NOAEL by the uncertainty factor. In the event that data do not exist upon which a NOAEL could be based, then the highest intake level with sufficient evidence of safety was identified as the Observed Safe Level (OSL).

The authors noted that no published human studies focused specifically on safety of lutein supplementation, and only a few of the studies assessing beneficial effects monitored adverse effects, with monitoring reflecting self-reporting. The doses used in the clinical trials generally were 5- to 20-fold higher than the 2 mg/day mean level lutein human consumption. The highest dose studied was 40 mg/day (0.57 mg/kg BW) for 9 weeks, followed by 20 mg/day (0.29 mg/kg BW) for 17 weeks. The next highest doses studied were 30 mg/day for 12 weeks and 20 mg/day for 24 weeks. The longest duration of supplementation identified was 12 months at 10 mg/day (0.143 mg/kg BW). The only adverse event associated with lutein was carotenodermia (yellowish discoloration of the skin), which occurred in 40 percent of humans in two studies involving 15 mg/day (0.21 mg/kg BW) for 4 to 5 months. However, this event has been classified by the Institute of Medicine as harmless (Shao and Hathcock, 2006). The authors noted in their review that only short-term lutein effects were considered, even with long-term studies. No adverse events (hazards) were identified in any clinical trial included in their review. As such, neither a NOAEL nor UL could be identified from the review of clinical trials. However, based on studies in rats, the authors reasoned that a dose of 639 mg/kg/day extrapolates to a human dose of 38,000 mg/day, and applied a 1,000-fold uncertainty factor to yield a NOAEL at > 40 mg/day (0.57 mg/kg BW) all-*trans* lutein. Further, the authors noted the absence of any pattern of adverse effects related to lutein consumption warranted a high level of confidence in lutein safety. For an OSL, the authors proposed 20 mg/day (0.29 mg/kg BW) based on the study with the most appropriate design (double blinded, placebo controlled, clinically relevant signals and minimal disease in study subjects) and no adverse events. Although not used in determination of OSL, serum lutein concentrations were recorded for several clinical trials reviewed by the authors. The highest serum lutein concentration documented in humans among these trials with no adverse effects was 1.73 μmol/L at 15 mg/day for 26 days (n = 20).

Ex Vivo Studies

Target Species

To the committee's knowledge, no ex vivo studies have been performed with lutein in horses, dogs, or cats.

In Vitro Studies

Target Species

To the committee's knowledge, no in vitro studies have been performed with lutein in horses, dogs, or cats.

Use, Risk, and Exposure as a Supplement

Target Species

Horses

Lutein supplementation of equine diets does not appear to be a common practice in North America. A cursory search for animal dietary supplements containing purified lutein that are marketed for use in horses yielded no results. Product information describing the contents of herbal dietary supplements infrequently listed marigold petals in their formula. Some supplements marketed as "hair coat color enhancers" for horses contain small amounts of paprika (< 1 percent) that may provide a source of supplemental lutein.

Dogs

No data could be found by the committee to indicate adverse events associated with lutein when added to the canine diet. Data provided by the Pet Food Institute (PFI) indicate that lutein was associated with no adverse effects in two groups of dogs.[1] The first group was comprised of predominantly neutered adults (n = 40 and 20 control, 4 ± 2 years, and three feeding periods) representing six breeds, fed 0.05 to 0.089 mg/kg BW lutein for 8 weeks. The

[1]These data and some other personal communications were provided by commercial companies with the understanding that for proprietary reasons full details would not be shared. These data do provide important information where very little other is available.

second group was growing puppies (approximately 6 weeks of age, n = 17 and 16 control). Six breeds were represented, with Labradors and Greyhounds represented by four dogs each in treatment and control groups. The remaining breeds spanned the size of most common breeds. Puppies were fed 0.5 mg/400 kcal (1.25 mg/1,000 kcal) during growth with no overt side effects. Based on the 2006 *Nutrient Requirements of Dogs and Cats*, which assumes that a puppy weighs 5.5 kg and consumes 1,000 kcal/day, this equates to 0.23 mg lutein/kg BW. Signals observed included changes in weight, food intake, and clinical pathology. Although no statistical differences in adverse events were noted in the report, methodology regarding statistical analysis, including power of the study, was not provided. In its accumulated adverse event reporting data, the NASC indicated a lutein dosing range of 0.35 to 0.87 mg/kg.

Cats

Lutein feeding data in cats provided by PFI were reviewed by the committee. The lutein was provided as marigold meal in each of these studies. The data indicate that lutein was associated with no adverse effects in three groups of cats. The first study was in adult cats (n = 5, 7 control, 4.1 ± 2.9 years) receiving 3.6 mg/kg BW for 2 months. The second was in older adults (n = 10, 10 control, 9.3 ± 1.2 years) fed 0.07 mg/kg BW lutein for 12 weeks. The third study followed 2 years of lutein supplementation in older adult cats (n = 14, 14 control, 8.7 ± 2 years) at a rate of 2.35 ± 0.57 mg lutein /1,000 kcal diet (0.94 mg/400 kcal diet or 10 mg/kg DM). Assuming an average 4 kg cat requires 250 kcal ME/day (NRC, 2006), this results in a daily lutein intake of approximately 0.15 mg/kg BW. No overt side effects were reported for lutein supplementation in cats in these studies. Signals evaluated for potential adversity appeared to include body weight, food intake, and clinical pathology. A fourth study provided for committee review by PFI was performed in young adult, first litter gestational queens (n = 10, 10 control, 1.2 ± 1.0 years) during 24 weeks of prebreeding (6 weeks), gestation, and lactation. Cats received 1.75 mg lutein/g canned kitten diet (0.7 mg lutein/400 mg diet; approximately 7 to 9 mg lutein/kg food on a dry basis, depending on the moisture content of the food). Using the same body weight and maintenance energy requirement assumptions discussed above and assuming that a cat at peak lactation increases her consumption 3-fold over maintenance, estimated lutein intake ranged from approximately 0.1 mg/kg BW/day during early gestation to 0.3 mg/kg BW/day during peak lactation. In the lutein group, one litter was resorbed late in gestation and another cat kittened early, although this cat subsequently produced a healthy litter while continuing to receive the same lutein-supplemented diet. A third cat rejected her kittens at birth, resulting in the loss of the litter, although this is not unusual in first-litter queens. No litters were lost in the control group. The total number of stillborn kittens in the lutein-supplemented group was five compared to two in the control group (average 0.6 and 0.2 per live litter for the lutein and control groups, respectively); postbirth kitten deaths were 2 in the lutein group compared to 3 in the control group. No abnormalities were reported in any of the dead kittens with the exception of a cleft-palate in one of the kittens whose mother had been fed the control diet. There were no statistically significant differences between the two diets in litter size, still birth rates, or postbirth death rates. However, analysis did not take into account assessment of in utero deaths. The concentration of lutein in the test food (7 to 9 mg/kg food, dry basis) is lower than the average lutein content of dry cat foods containing corn gluten meal (28 to 50 mg/kg food, dry basis) and is in line with the average lutein content of corn gluten meal-free dry foods (3–9 mg/kg food, dry basis) and canned cat foods (7–20 mg/kg food, dry basis) (Kemin Nutrisurance, 2007). Corn gluten meal has been a common ingredient in nutritionally complete dry cat foods for many years. Therefore, while the unexplained loss of two litters in the test group and none in the control group cannot be ignored, the committee considered that it was unlikely to be due to the lutein content of the test food.

Nontarget Species

Several general observations speak to the safety of lutein when added to the diet in humans. First, Khachik et al. (1995) noted in their study that animal toxicology data are not required by the FDA for short-term studies involving food source carotenoids such as lutein and zeaxanthin if the daily dose is within several-fold of the average daily dietary levels in humans (see the next section on Consumption as Part of Normal Diet). As such, safe consumption is implied for foods, even those containing high lutein content. Second, the FDA has responded to Kemin Food's assessment of lutein as GRAS with a letter of non-objection (GRAS Notice No. GRN 00140; http://www.cfsan.fda.gov/~rdb/opa-g140.html).

Third, ingestion of lutein as a dietary supplement has been occurring in humans since 1996 with no evidence of adverse events. Doses recommended for therapeutic indications vary. Vitamin preparations may contain as little as 0.25 mg lutein. The most common doses cited for specific therapeutic intent include 10 mg for prevention of macular degeneration and 6 to 7.5 mg for cancer protection. At the 63rd meeting of the FAO/WHO Joint Expert Committee on Food Additives (JECFA, 2005), average daily lutein intake from dietary supplements could not be predicted. Finally, lutein intake as supplements in participants of clinical trials reviewed as part of lutein risk assessment by Shao and Hathcock (2006) ranged from 8 to 40 mg/day, well above the average amount consumed in foods, and generally higher than that recommended for prevention of AMD.

Consumption as Part of Normal Diet

Target Species

A common level of intake apparently has not been recommended in the dog, cat, or horse, although content might be determined from normal diets. A dietary requirement for lutein has not been established in horses, dogs, and cats (NRC, 2006, 2007) nor has a specific level of lutein supplementation been recommended for these species.

Horses

Feedstuffs commonly fed to horses (i.e., roughages, cereal grains, and plant protein sources) will likely contain some level of naturally occurring lutein. Although available data specific to lutein are limited, lutein seems to be the predominant carotenoid in forages, constituting 40 to 75 percent of total carotenoid pigments (Prache et al., 2003; Reynoso et al., 2004; Calderón et al., 2006; Cardinault et al., 2006). The lutein content of forages reported in the literature range from just < 20 to > 600 mg/kg DM (NRC, 1994; Prache et al., 2003; Reynoso et al., 2004; Chauveau-Duriot et al., 2005; Calderón et al., 2006, 2007).

Because lutein has reportedly never been fed to horses intentionally as a dietary supplement, recommendations on its relative safety for horses are difficult. The horse's natural diet, particularly if high in fresh-growing forages, can be quite high in lutein. For example, utilizing the value of 415 mg lutein/kg DM reported by Prache et al. (2003) for mixed cool-season grass pasture in June, a 500 kg horse eating 10 kg (2 percent of BW) of this forage would have a lutein intake of 4.15 g/day (8.3 mg/kg BW). This is 14.5-times higher than the 38 mg/day (0.57 mg/kg BW) cited for humans when lutein is consumed as a dietary supplement (Shao and Hathcock, 2006) and 44-fold higher than the 90th percentile of human consumption of lutein from natural sources (13 mg/day; JECFA, 2005). However, the relative availability of lutein from feedstuffs typically found in equine rations has not been evaluated.

Dogs and Cats

Pet food ingredients that contain lutein include dried tomatoes, carrots, broccoli, spinach, corn, and corn gluten (Kemin Nutrisurance, 2007). The amount of lutein in canine and feline diets seems to be determined principally by the amount of corn gluten the diet contains (Table 6-1). Canned diets generally do not contain much corn gluten, resulting in a lower lutein content, compared to dried diets, which may contain low to high corn gluten and thus lutein content. In general, dry diets containing a high content of corn gluten contain 28–50 mg/kg DM lutein compared to dry diets without corn gluten, which contain 3–9 mg/kg DM lutein. In contrast, canned diets contain 1.5–4.5 mg/kg lutein "as fed" or 7–20 mg/kg DM (data provided by Kemin Nutrisurance, 2007). When normalized to body weight, the estimated daily intake of lutein in dogs ranges from 0.2–33 mg, or 0.18–0.45 mg/kg BW/day. Cats exhibit a more narrow range of caloric intake, resulting in a more narrow range of daily lutein intake approximated at 0.2–6.2 mg, or 0.11–0.85 mg/kg BW/day.

Nontarget Species

A plethora of data is available regarding the content of lutein in various natural foods. Assumptions can be made regarding safe use when lutein is part of the normal diet. This is supported by a study of humans in the Fiji Islands, where 25 mg lutein generally is normally consumed each day by part of the population. This equates to 0.37 mg/kg BW for a 70-kg person or greater than 10-fold higher than normal human consumption in the United States. The population is characterized by lower lung cancer rates, despite a greater content of tar and nicotine in local cigarettes, with the negative correlation greatest for dietary lutein and vitamin E. However, a positive correlation was also documented for increased cholesterol (Le Marchand et al., 1995). Other side potential effects were not addressed.

Humans

Government recommendations do not exist for daily intake of lutein in humans (Lienau et al., 2003). Further, the FDA has indicated than an optimum daily amount of lutein intake has not been determined in humans. However, lutein consumption as part of the daily diet in humans is associated with a substantial history of use, without evidence of adverse events. These include ingestion of diets naturally rich in lutein. For example, inhabitants of the Fiji Islands consume 200 g dark greens daily, resulting in an intake of approximately 25 mg (0.357 mg/kg BW) daily. Humans have been ingesting foods originating from animals for which diets have been manipulated to increase lutein content. Lutein has been used as a human food colorant (e.g., 0.4 percent marigold powder in butter; Sowbhagya et al., 2004) with no evidence of adversity.

Alves-Rodrigues and Shao (2004) suggested that the daily intake of lutein from dark green, leafy vegetables approximates 6 mg/day. However, absorption from unprocessed vegetables may be half that from supplemented materials. According to the USDA, current intake in the United States is about 1.7 mg (0.024 mg/kg BW), which is less than that associated with reduced risk of acute macular degeneration (Alves-Rodrigues and Shao, 2004). Based on this level of intake, the 90th percentile is 3 mg/day (0.043 mg/kg BW) with the mean intake of lutein in unsupplemented diets by Americans being less than 2 mg/day (0.028 mg/kg BW) (Shao and Hathcock, 2006). Intake may increase in states of disease, ranging from 5–30 mg/day (0.071 to 0.43 mg/kg BW).

The 63rd meeting of the FAO/WHO Joint Expert Committee on Food Additives (JECFA, 2005) indicated that North American and European intake of lutein from natural sources ranges from 1 to 2 mg (0.01 to 0.03 mg/kg BW) each day. Based on simulations, JECFA predicted the mean and 90th percentile intake of lutein with zeaxanthin to be 7 and 13 mg/day (0.1 mg/kg BW and 0.186 mg/kg BW), respectively. The JECFA committee could not predict intake from dietary supplements.

Safety of Similar Compounds

Concern has been expressed that very high doses of carotenoids may be harmful, possibly due to pro-oxidant activity. This concern might be supported by a study in smokers receiving β-carotene (Lienau et al., 2003). Beta-carotene and retinol supplementation has been associated with an increase in the incidence of lung cancer (Goodman et al., 2004); research in ferrets suggest this reflects its pro-vitamin A activity (decrease expression of retinoic acid receptor β and increase expression of AP-1 complex, altering regulation of cell differentiation and proliferation). However, because side effects to β-carotene reflect its pro-vitamin A status, lutein should not manifest similar effects. Cats fed 5 or 10 mg/day of β-carotene for 14 days showed no adverse events (Chew et al., 2000). However, longer studies would be necessary to adequately assess carcinogenicity of β-carotene.

CURRENT REGULATORY STATUS OF LUTEIN

Lutein is the subject of two GRAS (generally recognized as safe) Notifications for intended use in human food including crystalline lutein (Kemin, GRN 000140) and lutein esters (Cognis, GRN 000110). The FDA has not reached an independent conclusion in either case that lutein is GRAS, although the agency "has no questions" about the sponsors' determinations of GRAS status for these substances. FDA does advise both sponsors that use of lutein as a color additive would require premarket approval separate from the GRAS determination. The FDA does not currently accept GRAS notifications for animal feed ingredients, and there is not yet an FDA-recognized mechanism for self-determination of GRAS status for animal feed ingredients or "animal dietary supplements," as defined by this report (Box 1-3).

The marigold flower is the common commercial source of lutein (Kruger, 2002). *Tagetes* (Aztec marigold) meal and extract is an approved color additive under 21 CFR 73.295. The meal form consists of dried ground flower petals of *Tagetes erecta* L., while the extract form is a hexane extract of the petals mixed with a vegetable oil. Both forms may contain up to 0.3 percent lutein. The regulation restricts its use to inclusion in chicken feeds for the sole purpose of enhancing the yellow color of chicken skin and egg yolks. Use of marigold extract in other animal feeds, or as a nutritional source of lutein, is not allowed under current regulations. In the review of marigold extract as food colorant, Sowbhagya et al. (2004) noted that as long as toxicity data do not exist for lutein, it cannot be used as food colorant.

LIMITATIONS TO THE ASSESSMENT OF SAFETY

A number of limitations underlie the assessment of safety of lutein in target species. Pharmacokinetic studies, including dose-concentration relationships, have not been performed. The impact of processing, food matrix, concentration of lutein, and concentration of other carotenoids necessitates some basic level of information. Reaching consensus among studies in other species also is limited by differences in the proportion of free versus esterified lutein, the different sources, the impact of esterification on disposition and the relevance of data from one type of product (i.e., protein-bound or free lutein, mono- vs. diesterified lutein, or free (extracted) crystalline lutein). Formulation (e.g., suspended in oil versus directly applied to food) may profoundly impact results. Clear guidance on the impact of processing and, specifically, differences in products in regards to oral bioavailability is paramount. These differences include, but are not necessarily limited to, the impact of light on oxidation status, isomeric conversion to less biologically active forms, the appropriateness of standardization of lutein content based on color, and the risk of microbial, pesticide, herbicide, and heavy metal contamination. The lack of a standard, which limited previous studies, may have been rectified with the generation of a USP lutein monograph. However, analytical methods must be standardized and should include specifications to ensure that lutein and its metabolites are not detected together.

Although lutein seems to be safe (see next section on Risk Assessment), understanding species differences in the disposition of the compound are important not only to demonstrate safety, but also to establish a minimum recommended dose for efficacy. Scientific studies and reviews of lutein, particularly the earlier studies, tended to originate from countries in which lutein was often used empirically and in which the sources of lutein were not limited by patent rights. For example, a lutein palmitate preparation (Adaptinol; Helenien) seems to have been the most common preparation used in scientific studies outside the United States, whereas many U.S. studies involve crystalline lutein (Granado et al., 2003). Often, xanthophylls (including zeaxanthin) or metabolites are included as "lutein" in analytical methods and what actually is measured should be carefully determined. Exposure of tissue samples post-collection to light, oxygen, and temperature differences affect lutein measurements.

Recommendations regarding dose are complicated by the lack of consistency in analytical methods and interpretability of standards for measurement of concentrations in human serum. Intake of lutein seems to vary markedly among and within populations (Granado et al., 2003). Accurate determination of intake is also clouded by external factors such as dietary changes and seasons. Food factors that impact on reliability of data include failure to properly identify the food or the part of the plant consumed, its ripeness (which markedly influences xanthophyll content), and the impact of food processing that influences retention, stability, and bioavailability.

RISK ASSESSMENT

A number of considerations support the safety of lutein intake as a supplement. In humans, no consistent pattern of clinically relevant adverse events has emerged despite the following: (1) a long history of intake of foods naturally containing high lutein content, (2) approximately a decade of history of therapeutic intake of lutein as a dietary supplement, and (3) many clinical trials in which lutein supplementation was higher than that recommended therapeutically. Further, lutein extracted from *Tagetes erecta* L. has been a subject of review four times (31st, 55th, 57th, and 63rd) by the Joint Food and Agriculture Organization/World Health Organization Expert Committee on Food Additives. The most recent review incorporated preparations with high lutein content and included toxicologic assessment (JECFA, 2005). Likewise, in their review, Shao and Hathcock (2006) noted that a 2000 report of the Institute of Medicine found no clinically relevant adverse effects associated with consumption of lutein. The observations of these different reviews were based, in part, on toxicity data in rats receiving lutein at a rate of 638 mg/kg BW for 4 weeks and monkeys receiving lutein at a rate of 20 mg/kg BW for 52 weeks. Finally, although it is a carotenoid, multiple authors have noted that side effects typical of provitamin A or vitamin A compounds should not occur with lutein because mammals do not have the enzymatic capability of converting it to retinol. Even in populations at risk, higher than expected lutein tissue concentrations might reasonably be expected to result in no to minimal risk of adverse effects.

In the target species, history of safe use is supported by the lack of any apparent adverse effects in association with ingestion of diets containing lutein at a content that results in an approximate daily intake (mg/kg BW) of up to 8.3, 0.45, and 0.85 in horses, dogs, and cats, respectively (Table 6-2). Studies provided by PFI support safe use in cats at 3.6 mg/kg BW for 8 weeks and 0.94 mg/kg BW for 2 years, and in dogs at 0.89 mg/kg BW for 8 weeks. One study in gestational first-litter cats suggested the possibility of gestationally related adverse events. Although the perceived risk remains low, the possibility of gestationally related adverse events in cats warrants further consideration. Finally, studies focusing on the impact of lutein on immune function reported no adverse events in dogs or cats receiving lutein at a rate of 1.9 mg/kg BW and 7.0 mg/kg BW for 12 weeks, respectively. Accordingly, the following recommendations are offered.

Horses

Forage, whether in the form of pasture or hay, is an important part of the diet for horses in the United States. Forage is also likely to be the most abundant source of lutein in the equine diet. As discussed above, the lutein content of fresh and preserved forages reported in the literature ranges from > 20 to < 600 mg/kg DM (NRC, 1994; Prache et al., 2003; Reynoso et al., 2004; Chauveau-Duriot et al., 2005; Calderón et al., 2006, 2007). Fresh forage usually contains more lutein than hay, but not all horses have access to fresh forage. In addition, the lutein concentration in forage can change throughout the growing season and with feed storage conditions. Ultimately, the committee chose the lutein value of 415 mg/kg DM reported by Prache et al. (2003) for mixed cool-season grass pasture to represent a reasonable upper end of exposure of naturally occuring lutein in horses. On average, a horse can be expected to consume about 2 percent of BW per day as forage, resulting in a lutein intake of 8.3 mg/kg BW. This value was deemed by the committee as the upper end of historical safe intake (HSI) for the horse.

Despite the fact the horse's natural diet may contain reasonable levels of lutein, the absorption, metabolism, and utilization of lutein by the horse have never been reported and have presumably never been studied. Such a lack of information adds to the difficulty in evaluating the potential effects of lutein supplemented beyond that naturally occurring in typical feedstuffs.

Furthermore, despite reports that lutein is nontoxic, noncarcinogenic, and nonteratogenic in other species, available research does indicate there are significant differences in carotenoid metabolism between horses and other species. In addition, the composition of the typical equine ration is much different (higher in fiber, lower in fat) than the diet of species most commonly used for lutein supplementation testing and could potentially affect lutein absorption kinetics. Lutein may negatively affect the absorption of other carotenoids, in particular, beta-carotene (Kostic et al., 1995). Horses can derive their vitamin A naturally and entirely if sufficient levels of β-carotene are present in the diet. It is not clear if a negative effect of lutein supplementation on β-carotene absorption might lead to reductions in vitamin A status and vitamin A deficiency in horses, but the potential warrants consideration. Horses that would be most susceptible would be those with high vitamin A requirements (i.e., growing horses, pregnant and lactating mares, and horses with compromised immune status) and those maintained on hay for long periods without sufficient vitamin A supplementation (e.g., in the form of retinyl-palmitate or retinyl-acetate). Furthermore, β-carotene aids in the control of progesterone secretion by the corpus luteum; therefore, insufficient dietary β-carotene may impair reproductive performance in broodmares. This implies that horses likely have a physiological requirement for β-carotene beyond that needed as a provitamin A precursor. If supplemental lutein can impact the horse's β-carotene status, the biological functions relying on β-carotene may be negatively affected.

Based on the relatively high lutein content in forages consumed by horses, as well as the lack of adverse events reported in a wide variety of other species consuming lutein supplements, it seems likely that supplementary lutein is relatively safe for the horse. However, because of the complete lack of data on circulating and storage levels of lutein in the horse, as well as the lack of data directly applicable to lutein digestion, absorption, metabolism, and excretion in the horse, the committee believes basic testing is needed in the horse before recommendations can be provided on the presumed safe intake (PSI) of lutein when supplemented to the equine diet. Accordingly, the PSI for lutein is the same as the HSI in the horse and represents only the intake of lutein that is naturally occurring in common feedstuffs fed to horses (e.g., forage). The following summarize recommendations regarding lutein intake in horses (Table 6-3):

Historical safe intake of lutein: 8.3 mg/kg BW
Presumed safe intake of lutein: 8.3 mg/kg BW

Dogs

In dogs, history of safe use is supported by the lack of any apparent adverse effects in association with ingestion of diets containing lutein at a content that results in an approximate daily intake of up to 0.45 mg/kg (Table 6-3). Studies provided by PFI support safe use in dogs at 0.89 mg/kg BW for 8 weeks. Further, a study focusing on the impact of lutein on immune function reported no adverse events in dogs receiving lutein at a rate of 1.9 mg/kg BW for 12 weeks. Accordingly, the following recommendations are offered for lutein in dogs (Table 6-3):

Historical safe intake of lutein: 0.45 mg/kg BW
Presumed safe intake of lutein: 1.8 mg/kg BW

Cats

In cats, history of safe use is supported by the lack of any apparent adverse effects in association with ingestion of diets containing lutein at a content that results in an approximate daily intake of up to 0.85 mg/kg BW (Table 6-3). Studies provided by PFI support safe use in cats at 3.6 mg/kg BW for 8 weeks and 0.94 mg/kg BW for 2 years. One study in gestational first-litter cats suggests the possibility of gestationally related adverse events. Although the perceived risk remains low, the possibility of gestationally related adverse events in cats warrants further consideration. Finally, studies focusing on the impact of lutein on immune function reported no adverse events in cats receiving lutein at a rate of 7.2 mg/kg BW for 12 weeks, respectively. Accordingly, the following recommendations are offered regarding lutein in cats (Table 6-3):

TABLE 6-3 Historical Safe Intake (HSI) and Presumed Safe Intake (PSI) of Lutein in Horses, Dogs, and Cats (mg/kg BW per day)

Species	HSI	PSI
Horses[a]	8.30	8.30
Dogs	0.45	1.80
Cats	0.85	7.20

[a]When ingested as forage or other natural sources.

Historical safe intake of lutein: 0.85 mg/kg BW
Presumed safe intake of lutein: 7.2 mg/kg BW

OTHER RECOMMENDATIONS

Lutein seems to be safe when offered as a natural ingredient of food or, in dogs and cats, as a dietary supplement. Although target species toxicity data are not available, data in other species suggest that toxic concentrations far exceed concentrations likely to be achieved at recommended and beyond recommended doses. However, the absence of data in target species warrants further investigation, with the following recommendations:

- Analytical methods must be standardized and validated in each target population. Methods should distinguish between parent compound and metabolites. Methods should include directives that minimize lutein-containing solutions (whether "stock" analytical solutions or lutein-containing tissue samples) exposure to UV light or variations in temperature.
- General guidelines should be promulgated regarding the impact of processing and differential sources of lutein on lutein bioavailability and safety. Safety should include rate of exposure to lutein, but more importantly, risk of exposure to unintended contaminants.
- Recommendations should be offered regarding safe levels of intake when included as part of the food or as a supplement, with recommendations varying with the type of product offered (i.e., extracted versus nonextracted).
- Data should be promulgated to ensure maintenance of potency when stored according to labeled recommendations. Standards should be promulgated to define optimum storage conditions, with a focus on impact of UV light, environmental oxygen, and storage temperatures.
- Manufacturers should be directed to label ingredients as to total lutein in mg/weight of unit dose and to describe the preparation of lutein (e.g., crystalline or esters) being studied.
- Feline susceptibility to retinal toxicity with fluorquinolones suggests marked species differences in retinal physiology that predispose it to adversity. Special considerations should be made in assessing the role of lutein in feline vision.

REFERENCES

Alves-Rodrigues, A., and A. Shao. 2004. The science behind lutein. Toxicol. Lett. 150:57–83.

Aman, R., R. Carle, J. Conrad, U. Beifuss, and A. Schieber. 2005. Isolation of carotenoids from plant materials and dietary supplements by high-speed counter-current chromatography. J. Chromatogr. A. 1074:99–105.

Bailey, C. A., and B. H. Chen. 1988. Research note: Carotene and xanthophyll changes during growth and processing of turf bermudagrass. Poult. Sci. 67:1644–1646.

Baskin, C. R., K. W. Hinchcliff, R. A. Disilvestro, G. A. Reinhart, G. Hayek, B. P. Chew, J. R. Burr, and R. A. Swenson. 2000. Effects of dietary antioxidant supplementation on oxidative damage and resistance to oxidative damage during prolonged exercise in sled dogs. Am. J. Vet Res. 61:866–891.

Berardo, N., O. V. Brenna, A. Amato, P. Valoti, V. Pisacane, and M. Motto. 2004. Carotenoids concentration among maize genotypes measured by near infrared reflectance spectroscopy (NIRS). Innovative Food Science and Emerging Technol. 5:393–398.

Bhosale, P., D. Y. Zhao, and P. S. Bernstein. 2007a. HPLC measurement of ocular carotenoid levels in human donor eyes in the lutein supplementation era. Invest. Ophthalmol. & Visual Sci. 48:543–549.

Bhosale, P., B. Serban, D. Y. Zhao, and P. S. Bernstein. 2007b. Identification and metabolic transformations of carotenoids in ocular tissues of the Japanese quail *Coturnix japonica*. Biochemistry 46:9050–9057.

Blount, J. D. 2004. Carotenoids and life-history evolution in animals. Arch. Biochem. Biophys. 430:10–15.

Bowen, P. E., S. M. Herbst-Espinosa, E. A. Hussain, and M. Stacewicz-Sapuntzakis. 2002. Esterification does not impair lutein bioavailability in humans. J. Nutr. 132:3668–3673.

Bradbury, J. 2001. Lutein may help reduce atherosclerosis. The Lancet 357:2030.

Breithaupt, D. E. 2007. Modern application of xanthophylls in animal feeding—a review. Trends Food Sci. Technol. 18:501–506.

Burri, B. J., and A. J. Clifford. 2004. Carotenoid and retinoid metabolism: Insights from isotope studies. Arch. Biochem. Biophys. 430:110–119.

Burri, B. J., T. R. Neidlinger, and A. J. Clifford. 2001. Serum carotenoid depletion follows first-order kinetics in healthy adult women fed naturally low carotenoid diets. J. Nutr. 131:2096–2100.

Calderón, F., G. Tornambé, B. Martin, P. Pradel, B. Chauveau-Duriot, and P. Nozière. 2006. Effects of mountain grassland maturity stage and grazing management on carotenoids in sward and cow's milk. Anim. Res. 55:533–544.

Calderón, F., B. Chauveau-Duriot, B. Martin, B. Graulet, M. Doreau, and P. Nozière. 2007. Variations in carotenoids, vitamins A and E, and color in cow's plasma and milk during late pregnancy and the first three months of lactation. J. Dairy Sci. 90:2335–2346.

Cardinault, N., M. Doreau, and P. Nozière. 2004. Devenir des caroténoides dans le rumen. Renc. Rech. Ruminants 11:82 (abstr.).

Cardinault, N., M. Doreau, C. Poncet, and P. Nozière. 2006. Digestion and absorption of carotenoids in sheep given fresh red clover. Anim. Sci. 82:49–55.

Chauveau-Duriot, B., D. Thomas, J. Portelli, and M. Doreau. 2005. Carotenoids content in forages: Variation during conservation. Renc. Rech. Ruminants. 12:117.

Chew, B. P., J. S. Park, B. C. Weng, T. S. Wong, M. G. Hayek, and G. A. Reinhart. 2000. Dietary β-carotene absorption by blood plasma and leukocytes in domestic cats. J. Nutr. 130:2322–2325.

Cisneros, M., J. Benavides, C. H. Brenes, and M. Rito-Palomares. 2004. Recovery in aqueous two-phase systems of lutein produced by the green microalga *Chlorella protothecoides*. J. Chromatogr. B 807:105–110.

De Mejía, E. G., M. Ramos-Gómez, and G. Loarca-Piña. 1997. Antimutagenicity of natural xanthophylls against aflatoxin B_1 in *Salmonella typhimurium*. Environ. Mol. Mutagen. 30:346–353.

de Oliveira, G. P. R., and D. B. Rodriguez-Amaya. 2007. Processed and prepared corn products as sources of lutein and zeaxanthin: Compositional variation in the food chain. J. Food Sci. 72:S79–S85.

Delgado-Vargas, F., and O. Paredes-López. 1997. Effects of enzymatic treatments of marigold flowers on lutein isomeric profiles. J. Agric. Food Chem. 45:1097–1102.

Dwyer, J. H., M. Navab, K. M. Dwyer, K. Hassan, P. Sun, A. Shircore, S. Hama-Levy, G. Hough, X. Wang, T. Drake, C. N. Bairey Merz, and A. M. Fogelman. 2001. Oxygenated carotenoid lutein and progression of early atherosclerosis. The Los Angeles atherosclerosis study. Circulation 103:2922–2927.

Fonnesbeck, P. V., and L. D. Symons. 1967. Utilization of the carotene of hay by horses. J. Anim. Sci. 26:1030–1038.

Gartner, C., W. Stahl, and H. Sies. 1996. Preferential increase in chylomicron levels of the xanthophylls lutein and compared to β-carotene in the human. Int. J. Vitam. Nutr. Res. 66:119–125.

Gay, L. S., D. S. Kronfeld, A. Grimsley-Cook, J. J. Dascanio, A. O. Ordakowski-Burk, R. K. Splan, E. A. Dunnington, and D. J. Sklan. 2004. Retinol, β-carotene and β-tocopherol concentrations in mare and foal plasma and in colostrum. J. Equine Vet. Sci. 24:115–120.

Goodman, G. E., M. D. Thornquist, J. Balmes, M. R. Cullen, F. L. Meyskens, Jr., G. S. Omenn, B. Valanis, and J. H. Williams Jr. 2004. The Beta-Carotene and Retinol Efficacy Trial: Incidence of lung cancer and cardiovascular disease mortality during 6-year follow-up after stopping beta-carotene and retinol supplements. J. Nat. Cancer Inst. 96:1729–1731.

Gradelet, S., P. Astorg, J. Leclerc, J. Chevalier, M.-F. Vernevaut, and M. H. Siess. 1996. Effects of canthaxanthin, astaxanthin, lycopene and lutein on liver xenobiotic-metabolizing enzymes in the rat. Xenobiotica 26:49–63.

Granado, F., B. Olmedilla, and I. Blanco. 2003. Nutritional and clinical relevance of lutein in human health. Br. J. Nutr. 90:487–502.

Greiwe-Crandell, K. M., D. S. Kronfeld, L. S. Gay, D. Sklan, W. Tiegs, and P. A. Harris. 1997. Vitamin A repletion in Thoroughbred mares with retinyl palmitate or β-carotene. J. Anim. Sci. 75:2684–2690.

Gugliemelli, L. A., H. L. Mitchell, and R. E. Silker. 1954. The xanthophylls of alfalfa. Trans. Kans. Acad. Sci. 57:368–373.

Haegele, A. D., C. Gillette, C. O'Neill, P. Wolfe, J. Heimendinger, S. Sedlacek, and H. J. Thompson. 2000. Plasma xanthophyll carotenoids correlate inversely with indices of oxidative DNA damage and lipid peroxidation. Cancer Epidemiol. Biomark. Prev. 9:421–425.

Hinds, T. S., W. L. West, and E. M. Knight. 1997. Carotenoids and retinoids: A review of research, clinical, and public health applications. J. Clin. Pharmacol. 37:551–558.

Humphries, J. M., and F. Khachik. 2003. Distribution of lutein, zeaxanthin, and related geometrical isomers in fruit, vegetables, wheat, and pasta products. J. Agric. Food Chem. 51:1322–1327.

Humphries, J. M., R. D. Graham, and D. J. Mares. 2004. Application of reflectance colour measurement to the estimation of carotene and lutein content in wheat and triticale. J. Cereal Sci. 40:151–159.

Itagaki, S., W. Ogura, Y. Sato, T. Noda, T. Hirano, S. Mizuno, and K. Iseki. 2006. Characterization of the disposition of lutein after i.v. administration to rats. Biol. Pharm. Bull. 29:2123–2125.

Jaramillo-Flores, M. E., L. González-Cruz, M. Cornejo-Mazón, L. Dorantes-Alvarez, G. F. Gutiérrez-López, and H. Hernández-Sánchez. 2003. Effect of thermal treatment on the antioxidant activity and content of carotenoids and phenolic compounds of cactus pear cladodes (*Opuntia ficus-indica*). Food Sci. Technol. Int. 9:271–278.

JECFA (Joint Expert Committee on Food Additives). 2005. Evaluation of certain food additives. World Health Organization Technical Report Series 928:1–156. Rome: Food and Agriculture Organization of the United Nations; World Health Organization.

Jenkins, M. Y., G. V. Mitchell, and E. Grundel. 2000. Natural tocopherols in a dietary supplement of lutein affect tissue distribution of tocopherols in young rats. Nutr. Cancer 37:207–214.

Jewell, C., and N. M. O'Brien. 1999. Effect of dietary supplementation with carotenoids on xenobiotic metabolizing enzymes in the liver, lung, kidney and small intestine of the rat. Br. J. Nutr. 81:235–242.

Jiang, X. Y., L. S. Chen, and C. S. Zhou. 2005. Lutein and lutein esters in marigold flowers by high performance chromatography. J. Central South Univ. Technol. 12:306–308.

Johnson, E. 2004 A biological role for lutein (Review). Food Rev. Int. 20:1–16.

Johnson, J. D. 2007. Lutein and zeaxanthin. An introduction to the chemistry of dietary carotenoids. Online at: http://www.chm.bris.ac.uk/motm/carotenoids/ccarotenoids.htm. Accessed February 12, 2008.

Kemin Nutrisurance. 2007. Information Pertaining to the Safety of Lutein for Use as a Food Ingredient. Des Moines, IA: Kemin Nutrisurance.

Khachik, F., G. R. Beecher, and J. C. Smith, Jr. 1995. Lutein, lycopene and their oxidative metabolites in chemoprevention of cancer. J. Cell. Biochem. Suppl. 22:236–246.

Khachik, F., C. J. Spangler, J. C. Smith, Jr., L. M. Canfield, A. Steck, and H. Pfander. 1997a. Identification, quantification, and relative concentrations of carotenoids and their metabolites in human milk and serum. Anal. Chem. 69:1873–1881.

Khachik, F., A. Steck, and H. Pfander. 1997b. Bioavailability, metabolism, and possible mechanism of chemoprevention by lutein and lycopene in humans. Pp. 542–547 in Food Factors for Cancer Prevention, H. Unigash, T. Osawa, J. Terao, S. Wantanabe, and T. Yoshikawa, eds. Tokyo: Springer-Verlag.

Khachik, F., E. London, F. F. de Moura, M. Johnson, S. Steidl, L. Detolla, S. Shipley, R. Sanchez, X. Q. Chen, J. Flaws, G. Lutty, S. McLeod, and B. Fowler. 2006a. Chronic ingestion of (3R,3′R,6′R)-lutein and (3R,3′R)- in the female rhesus macaque. Invest. Ophthalmol. & Visual Sci. 47(12):5476–86.

Khachik, F., F. F., de Moura, E. Y. Chew, L. W. Douglass, F. L. Ferris, 3rd, J. Kim, and D. J. Thompson. 2006b. The effect of lutein and supplementation on metabolites of these carotenoids in the serum of persons aged 60 or older. Invest. Ophthalmol. & Visual Sci. 47:5234–5242.

Kienzle, E., C. Kaden, P. P. Hoppe, and B. Opitz. 2003. Serum β-carotene and α-tocopherol in horses fed β-carotene via grass-meal or a synthetic beadlet preparation with and without added dietary fat. J. Anim. Physiol. Anim. Nutr. 87:174–180.

Kim, H. W., B. P. Chew, T. S. Wong, J. S. Park, B. B. C. Weng, K. M. Byrne, M. G. Hayek, and G. A. Reinhart. 2000a. Modulation of humoral and cell-mediated immune responses by dietary lutein in cats. Vet. Immunol. Immunopathol. 73:331–341.

Kim, H. W., B. P. Chew, T. S. Wong, J. S. Park, B. B. C. Weng, K. M. Byrne, M. G. Hayek, and G. A. Reinhart. 2000b. Dietary lutein stimulates immune response in the canine. Vet. Immunol. Immunopathol. 74:315–327.

Kim, J., and D. DellaPenna. 2006. Defining the primary route for lutein synthesis in plants: The role of *Arabidopsis* carotenoid β-ring hydroxylase CYP97A3. Proc. Nat. Acad. Sci. U.S.A. 103:3474–3479.

Kim, J. M., S. Araki, D. J. Kim, C. B. Park, N. Takasuka, H. Baba-Toriyama, T. Ota, Z. Nir, F. Khachik, N. Shimidzu, Y. Tanaka, T. Osawa, T. Uraji, M. Murakoshi, H. Nishino, and H. Tsuda. 1998. Chemopreventive effects of carotenoids and curcumins on mouse colon carcinogenesis after 1,2-dimethylhydrazine initiation. Carcinogenesis 19:81–85.

Korytko, P. J., K. A. Rodvold, J. A. Crowell, M. Stacewicz-Sapuntzakis, V. Diwadkar-Navsariwala, P. E. Bowen, W. Schalch, and B. S. Levine. 2003. Pharmacokinetics and tissue distribution of orally administered lycopene in male dogs. J. Nutr. 133:2788–2792.

Kostic, D., W. S. White, and J. A. Olson. 1995. Intestinal absorption, serum clearance, and interactions between lutein and β-carotene when administered to human adults in separate or combined oral doses. Am. J. Clin. Nutr. 62:604–610.

Krinsky, N. I., J. T. Landrum, and R. A. Bone. 2003. Biologic mechanisms of the protective role of lutein and in the eye. Annu. Rev. Nutr. 23:171–201.

Kronfeld, D. S., J. L. Holland, G. A. Rich, T. N. Meacham, J. P. Fontenot, D. J. Sklan, and P. A. Harris. 2004. Fat digestibility in Equus caballus follows increasing first-order kinetics. J. Anim. Sci. 82:1773–1780.

Kruger, C. L., M. Murphy, Z. DeFreitas, F. Pfannkuch, and J. Heimbach. 2002. An innovative approach to the determination of safety for a dietary ingredient derived from a new source: Case study using a crystalline lutein product. Food Chem. Toxicol. 40:1535–1549.

Landrum, J. T., and R. A. Bone. 2000. Lutein and the macular pigment. Arch. Biochem. Biophys. 385:28–40.

Le Marchand, L., J. H. Hankin, F. Bach, L. N. Kolonel, L. R. Wilkens, M. Stacewicz-Sapuntzakis, P. E. Bowen, G. R. Beecher, F. Laudon, P. Baque, R. Daniel, L. Seruvatu, and B. E. Henderson. 1995. An ecological study of diet and lung cancer in the South Pacific. Int. J. Cancer 63:18–23.

Lee, E. H., D. Faulhaber, K. M. Hanson, W. Ding, S. Peters, S. Kodali, and R. D. Granstein. 2004. Dietary lutein reduces ultraviolet radiation-induced inflammation and immunosuppression. J. Investig. Dermatol. 1:510–517.

Lee, S., and L. Caston. 2004. Enrichment of eggs with lutein. Poult. Sci. 83:1709–1712.

Lienau, A., T. Glaser, G. Tang, G. G. Dolnikowski, M. A. Grusak, and K. Albert. 2003. Bioavailability of lutein in humans from intrinsically labeled vegetables determined by LC-APCI-MS. J. Nutr. Biochem. 11:663–670.

Livingston, A. L., D. Smith, H. L. Carnahan, R. E. Knowles, J. W. Nelson, and G. O. Kohler. 1968. Variation in the xanthophyll and carotene content of Lucerne, clovers and grasses. J. Sci. Food Agric. 19:632–636.

López-Hernández, E., E. Ponce-Alquicira, F. Cruz-Sosa, and I. Guerrero-Legarreta. 2001. Characterization and stability of pigments extracted from *Terminalia Catappa* leaves. J. Food Sci. 66:832–836.

Lorenzo-Figueras, M., S. M. Morisset, J. Morisset, J. Laine, and A. M. Merritt. 2007. Digestive enzyme concentrations and activities in healthy pancreatic tissue of horses. Am. J. Vet. Res. 68:1070–1072.

Lu, Y., H. Yaoa, Y. Gonga, and Q. Shenga. 2005. Effects of enzymatic treatment of corn gluten meal on lutein and extraction. Int. J. Food Prop. 8:161–169.

McDowell, L. R. 2000. Vitamins in Animal and Human Nutrition, second edition. Ames, IA: Iowa State University Press.

McEligot, A. J., C. L. Rock, T. G. Shanks, S. W. Flatt, V. Newman, S. Faerber, and J. P. Pierce. 1999. Comparison of serum carotenoid responses between women consuming vegetable juice and women consuming raw or cooked vegetables. Cancer Epidemiol. Biomarkers Prev. 8:227–231.

Molldrem, K. L., J. Li, P. W. Simon, and S. A. Tanumihardjo. 2004. Lutein and β-carotene from lutein-containing yellow carrots are bioavailable in humans. Am. J. Clin. Nutr. 80:131–136.

Mora, O., J. L. Romano, E. González, F. J. Ruiz, and A. Shimada. 1999. In vitro and in situ disappearance of β-carotene and lutein from lucerne (*Medicago sativa*) hay in bovine and caprine ruminal fluids. J. Sci. Food Agric. 79:273–276.

Moss, R. W. 2006. Should patients undergoing chemotherapy and radiotherapy be prescribed antioxidants? Integr. Cancer Ther. 5:63–82.

Nozière, P., B. Graulet, A. Lucas, B. Martin, P. Grolier, and M. Doreau. 2006. Carotenoids for ruminants: from forages to dairy products. Anim. Feed Sci. Tech. 131:418-450.

NRC (National Research Council). 1994. Nutrient Requirements of Poultry, 9th Ed. Washington, DC: National Academy Press.

NRC. 2006. Nutrient Requirements of Dogs and Cats. Washington, DC: The National Academies Press.

NRC. 2007. Nutrient Requirements of Horses, 6th Revised Ed. Washington, DC: The National Academies Press.

O'Neill, M. E., and D. I. Thurnham. 1998. Intestinal absorption of β-carotene, lycopene and lutein in men and women following a standard meal: response curves in the triacylglycerol-rich lipoprotein fraction. Br. J. Nutr. 79:149–159.

Park, Y. M., M. J. Anderson, J. L. Walters, and A. W. Mahoney. 1983. Effects of processing methods and agronomic variables on carotene contents in forages and predicting carotene in alfalfa hay with near-infrared reflectance spectroscopy. J. Dairy Sci. 66:235–245.

Philip, T., C. W. Weber, and J. W. Berry. 1976. Utilization of lutein and lutein-fatty acid esters by laying hens. J. Food Sci. 41:23–25.

Piccaglia, R., M. Marotti, and S. Grandi. 1998. Lutein and lutein ester content in different types of *Tagetes patula* and *T. erecta*. Ind. Crop. Prod. 8:45–51.

Prache, S., A. Priolo, and P. Grolier. 2003. Persistence of carotenoid pigments in the blood of concentrate-finished grazing sheep: Its significance for the traceability of grass-feeding. J. Anim. Sci. 81:360–367.

Pullakhandam, R., and M. L. Failla. 2007. Micellarization and intestinal cell uptake of β-carotene and lutein from drumstick (*Moringa oleifera*) leaves. J. Med. Food 10:252–257.

Reynoso, C. R., O. Mora, V. Nieves, A. Shimada, and G. de Mejía. 2004. β-carotene and lutein in forage and bovine adipose tissue in two tropical regions of Mexico. Anim. Feed Sci. Technol. 113:183–190.

Riedl, J., J. Linseisen, J. Hoffmann, and G. Wolfram. 1999. Some dietary fibers reduce the absorption of carotenoids in women. J. Nutr. 129:2170–2176.

Rock, C. L., M. E. Swendseid, R. A. Jacob, and R. W. McKee. 1992. Plasma carotenoid levels in human subjects fed a low carotenoid diet. J. Nutr. 122:96–100.

Roodenburg, A. J. C., R. Leenen, K. H. van het Hof, J. A. Weststrate, and L. B. M. Tijburg. 2000. Amount of fat in the diet affects bioavailability of lutein esters but not of α-carotene, β-carotene, and vitamin E in humans. Am. J. Clin. Nutr. 71:1187–1193.

Rosenthal, J. M., J. Kim, F. de Monasterio, D. J. Thompson, R. A. Bone, J. T. Landrum, F. F. de Moura, F. Khachik, H. Chen, R. L. Schleicher, F. L. Ferris, III, and E. Y. Chew. 2006. Dose-ranging study of lutein supplementation in persons aged 60 years or older. Invest. Ophthalmol. & Visual Sci. 47:5227–5233.

Schalch, W., W. Cohn, F. M. Barker, W. Köpcke, J. Mellerio, A. C. Bird, A. G. Robson, F. F. Fitzke, and F. J. G. M. van Kuijk. 2007. Xanthophyll accumulation in the human retina during supplementation with lutein or the LUXEA (LUtein Xanthophyll Eye Accumulation) study. Arch. Biochem. Biophys. 458:128–135.

Schieber, A., and R. Carle. 2005. Occurrence of carotenoids cis-isomers in food: Technological, analytical, and nutritional implications. Trends Food Sci. Technol. 16:416–422.

Schweigert, F. J., J. Raila, B. Wichert, and E. Kienzle. 2002. Cats absorb β-carotene, but it is not converted to vitamin A. J. Nutr. 132:1610S–1612S.

Shao, A., and J. N. Hathcock. 2006. Risk assessment for the carotenoids lutein and lycopene. Regul. Toxicol. Pharmacol. 45:289–298.

Snodderly, D. M., M. D. Russett, R. I. Land, and N. I. Krinsky. 1990. Plasma carotenoids of monkeys (*Macasa fascicularis* and *Saimiri sciureus*) fed a nonpurified diet. J. Nutr. 120:1663–1671.

Sowbhagya, H. B., S. R. Sampathu, and N. Krishnamurthy. 2004. Natural colorant from marigold-chemistry and technology. Food Rev. Int. 20:33–50.

Sturz, A. V., and J. Kimpinski. 2004. Endoroot bacteria derived from marigolds (*Tagetes* spp.) can decrease soil population densities of root-lesion nematodes in the potato root zone. Plant Soil 262(1-2):241–249.

Su, Q., K. G. Rowley, and K. O'Dea. 1999. Stability of individual carotenoids, retinol and tocopherols in human plasma during exposure to light and after extraction. J. Chromatogr. B: Biomed. Sci. Appl. 729(1–2):191–198.

Sujak, A., J. Gabrielska, W. Grudzinski, R. Borc, P. Mazurek, and W. I. Gruszecki. 1999. Lutein and zeaxanthin as protectors of lipid membranes against oxidative damage: The structural aspects. Arch. Biochem. Biophys. 371:301–307.

Tanumihardjo, S. A., J. Li, and M. P. Dosti. 2005. Lutein absorption is facilitated with cosupplementation of ascorbic acid in young adults. J. Am. Diet. Assoc. 105:114–118.

Thurmann, P. A., W. Schalch, J. C. Aebischer, U. Tenter, and W. Cohn. 2005. Plasma kinetics of lutein, and 3'-dehydro-lutein after multiple oral doses of a lutein supplement. Am. J. Clin. Nutr. 82:88–97.

Tsao, R., and R. Yang. 2006. Lutein in selected Canadian crops and agrifood processing byproducts and purification by high-speed counter-current chromatography. J. Chromatogr. A. 1112:202–208.

Tucker, R. E., G. E. Mitchell, and C. O. Little. 1967. Absorption of labeled carotene from the large intestine of sheep. J. Anim. Sci. 26:225 (abstr.).

Ullrey, D. E. 1972. Biological availability of fat-soluble vitamins: vitamin A and carotene. J. Anim. Sci. 35:648–657.

Updike, A. A., and S. J. Schwartz. 2003. Thermal processing of vegetables increases Cis Isomers of lutein and zeaxanthin. J. Agric. Food Chem. 51:6184–6190.

USDA (United States Department of Agriculture). 2006. Composition of Foods. Raw, Processed, Prepared. Agricultural Research Service, Nutrient Data Laboratory. USDA National Nutrient Database for Standard Reference, Release 13.

USP (United States Pharmacopeia). 2007. Dietary Supplements: Lutein. Rockville, MD: U.S. Pharmacopeia.

van den Berg, H., and T. van Vliet. 1998. Effect of simultaneous, single oral doses of β-carotene with lutein or lycopene on the β-carotene and retinyl ester responses in the triacylglycerol-rich lipoprotein fraction of men. Am. J. Clin. Nutr. 68:82–89.

van het Hof, K. H., I. A. Brouwer, C. E. West, E. Haddeman, R. P. M. Steegers-Theunissen, M. van Dusseldorp, J. A Weststrate, T. K. A. B. Eskes, and J. G. A. J. Hautvast. 1999a. Bioavailability of lutein from vegetables is 5 times higher than that of β-carotene. Am. J. Clin. Nutr. 70:261–268.

van het Hof, K. H., L. B. M Tijburg, K. Pietrzik, and J. A. Weststrate. 1999b. Influence of feeding different vegetables on plasma levels of carotenoids, folate and vitamin C. Effect of disruption of the vegetable matrix. Br. J. Nutr. 82:203–212.

Wang, M., R. Tsao, S. Zhang, Z. Dong, R. Yang, J. Gong, and Y. Pei. 2006. Antioxidant activity, mutagenicity/anti-mutagenicity, and clastogenicity/anti-clastogenicity of lutein from marigold flowers. Food Chem. Toxicol. 44:1522–1529.

Wei, Y., T. Zhang, G. Xu, and Y. Ito. 2003. Application of CCC for the separation of lutein from a crude extract of marigold flower petals. J. Liq. Chromatogr. Relat. Technol. 26:1659–1669.

Wells, C., W. Bertsch, and M. Perich. 1993. Insecticidal volatiles from the marigold plant (genus *tagetes*). Effect of species and sample manipulation. Chromatographia 35(3-4):209–205.

Yemelyanov, A. Y., N. B. Katz, and P. S. Bernstein. 2001. Ligand-binding characterization of xanthophylls carotenoids to solubilized membrane proteins derived from human retina. Exp. Eye Res. 72:381–392.

7

Evening Primrose Oil

DESCRIPTION

Common Names and Synonyms

The scientific name for evening primrose oil is *Oleum Oenothera biennis.* Common names used for the evening primrose plant include common evening primrose, scabish, king's cure-all, night-willow herb, German rampion, hog weed, and fever-plant.

Source and Botanical Characteristics

Evening primrose oil (EPO) is the oil obtained from the seeds of the evening primrose plant (*Oenothera* spp.) from the Onagraceae family. Common evening primrose (*Oenothera biennis* L.) is the economically more important species for the production of EPO, but oils obtained from other *Oenothera* species and hybrids, including *O. lamarckiana* and *O. parviflora*, are equally commercialized as EPO (Lapinskas, 1993; Clough, 2001; Yu-Cheng et al., 2001; Knorr and Hamburger, 2004).

Common evening primrose (*O. biennis* L.) is a biennial, herbaceous forb reaching 90–180 cm in height. The evening primrose derives its name from the slightly phosphorescent yellow color of its flowers, which partially to fully close during the day and open in the evening. Evening primrose is completely distinct from the true primroses (*Primula* spp.) and is more closely related to the willow herbs (*Epilobium* spp.). Evening primrose is native to North America, according to the USDA-NRCS Plant Database (USDA, undated), and is now widely distributed in the wild in Europe, Asia, and the southern hemisphere.

In the northern hemisphere, flowering begins in late June/early July, with each bloom only lasting one to two days (Clough, 2001). Seed formation and ripening generally occurs from September through November; thus, all seed does not mature at the same rate (Fieldsend, 1996; Yu-Cheng et al., 2001). Seed is formed in pods, which contain hundreds of small, sesame-sized seeds. Examination of wild-growing evening primrose has estimated that each plant may have 140 seed pods, each containing an average of 180 seeds, yielding 25,200 seeds per plant (Hall et al., 1988); however, Stephens (1932) estimated seed numbers of wild varieties to be around 118,500 per plant. This wide variation in seed yield may reflect differences in plant variety and stage of seed maturation at the time of sampling. Evening primrose seed is very fine, with the 1,000 seed weight averaging 0.33 g, but can range from 0.2 to 0.6 g (Yu-Cheng et al., 2001).

Domestication and cultivation of evening primrose for commercial oil production began in the early 1970s (Lapinskas, 1993). Early crops were grown from seed obtained from wild evening primrose, but they were found unsuitable for commercial production due to the splitting of seed capsules prior to harvest and the relatively low seed yields (Fieldsend, 1996). Subsequent breeding programs created closed-podded, high-yielding (1,000–1,200 kg/ha) evening primrose varieties that were more conducive to large-scale agricultural production (Fieldsend, 1996; Clough, 2001). In addition, *Oenothera* varieties with higher oil and/or γ-linolenic acid contents have been developed for commercial oil production (Clough, 2001).

Field-scale production of evening primrose started in the United Kingdom in 1970 (Clough, 2001). By the early 1980s, production had also been established in the Netherlands, the United States, New Zealand, and Hungary. However, by 1989, production had started to decline in these countries due to cheaper costs of production, first in Eastern Europe and then in China. Since 1993, China has been the major producer of evening primrose seed in the world, with an estimated 90 percent of total supply (Yu-Cheng et al., 2001). In 2001, Yu-Cheng et al. estimated that export demand from China was approximately 1 million kg EPO per year (7.2–8.6 million kg of seed-equivalent). Lapinskas (2000) estimated that the global annual consumption of EPO (humans and animals) is in the range of 1.1 to 1.3 million kg.

Chemical Composition

Nomenclature for Fatty Acids

Evening primrose oil is made up primarily of triacyglycerols containing a variety of fatty acids, to some of which the biological activity of EPO can be attributed. There are many systems of nomenclature commonly used for fatty acids. As a result, a brief description of the fatty acid nomenclature used in this chapter is warranted before further description of the composition of EPO.

Trivial names are routinely used in the scientific and popular press when describing fatty acids relevant to EPO (e.g., γ-linolenic acid). Therefore, the committee has retained the use of trivial fatty acid nomenclature throughout this chapter. To avoid potential ambiguity, however, systematic nomenclature supported by the International Union of Pure and Applied Chemists and the International Union of Biochemistry (IUPAC-IUBMB) will also be provided in parenthesis at the first mention of each fatty acid in this chapter (see IUPAC-IUB, 1976; Fahy et al., 2005). Briefly, the length of the fatty acid chain (representing the number of carbon atoms) and the number of double bonds will be provided via the official systematic name. This name will be preceded by the numerical position of each double bond using the delta (Δ) nomenclature system (i.e., the position of unsaturation will be numbered with reference to the first of the pair of carbon atoms between which the double bond occurs, and the numbering of carbon atoms in the fatty acid will begin with the carboxyl carbon of the acyl chain as number one). The double bond geometry will also precede the systematic name. Although IUPAC-IUBMB has encouraged the use of *Z/E* to describe the configuration of the double bond, the committee has retained the use of the more traditional and common *cis/trans* designations to describe the geometry of the double bond(s) within the fatty acid. For example, the systemic name for γ-linolenic acid is all-*cis*-6,9,12-octadecatrienoic acid, which denotes it as an 18-carbon fatty acid with three *cis*-configuration double bonds between positions 6–7, 9–10, and 12–13 as numbered from the carboxyl carbon (see Figure 7-1).

To facilitate faster recognition of specific fatty acids described in this chapter, a shorthand nomenclature system will also be used. The shorthand nomenclature will consist of two numbers separated by a colon. The number to the left of the colon indicates the number of carbon atoms in the fatty acid and the number to the right of the colon denotes the number of double bonds. To further distinguish the specific fatty acid described by the shorthand system, the specific omega family will also be noted, where appropriate. Although it is an older nomenclature system, the methyl carbon in the fatty acid chain furthest from the carboxyl end is commonly referred to as the omega carbon. The reference to the omega carbon is often made when describing essential fatty acids. For example, an omega-3 (often written as ω-3 or *n-3*) fatty acid describes a fatty acid with a double bond between carbon atoms 3 and 4 from the omega end of the fatty acid chain. Using the shorthand version of nomenclature, γ-linolenic acid is represented as C18:3*n-6*, which describes this fatty acid as an 18-carbon fatty acid with three double bonds that is a member of the omega-6 family (see Figure 7-1).

Chemical Analysis of Evening Primrose Oil

The seed of *Oenotherna biennis* was reported to contain 15 percent crude protein, 26 percent crude fat, and 43 percent cellulose plus lignin (Hudson, 1984). Stasiniewicz et al. (1998) reported that the seed of *Oenotherna paradoxa* contained 19 percent crude protein, 26 percent crude fat, 20 percent crude fiber, and 6 percent ash. The oil content of evening primrose seed can vary with the age of the seed, cultivar, and growth conditions. In a recent study, the oil content of evening primrose (*Oenotherna biennis*) seed ranged from 23.4 to 29.8 percent and the crude protein content ranged from 14.0 to 17.1 percent over varying harvest schedules (fall vs. spring) and harvest methods (Ghasemnezhad and Honermeier, 2007).

Over 98 percent of EPO is made up of triacyglycerols (Hudson, 1984). The predominant fatty acid components of EPO include linoleic acid (*cis,cis*-9,12-octadecadienoic

γ-Linolenic acid

18 17 16 15 14 13 12 11 10 9 8 7 6 5 4 3 2 1 Δ

$CH_3{\bullet}CH_2{\bullet}CH_2{\bullet}CH_2{\bullet}CH_2{\bullet}CH{=}CH{\bullet}CH_2{\bullet}CH{=}CH{\bullet}CH_2{\bullet}CH{=}CH{\bullet}CH_2{\bullet}CH_2{\bullet}CH_2{\bullet}CH_2{\bullet}COOH$

n or ω 1 2 3 4 5 6 7 8 9 10 11 12 13 14 15 16 17 18

$CH_3{\bullet}CH_2{\bullet}CH_2{\bullet}CH_2{\bullet}CH_2{\bullet}CH{=}CH{\bullet}CH_2{\bullet}CH{=}CH{\bullet}CH_2{\bullet}CH_2{\bullet}CH_2{\bullet}CH_2{\bullet}CH_2{\bullet}CH_2{\bullet}CH_2{\bullet}COOH$

18 17 16 15 14 13 12 11 10 9 8 7 6 5 4 3 2 1 Δ

Linoleic acid

FIGURE 7-1 Chemical structures of γ-linolenic and linoleic acids.

acid; C18:2*n-6*), γ-linolenic acid (GLA; all-*cis*-6,9,12-octadecatrienoic acid; C18:3*n-6*), oleic acid (*cis*-9-octadecaenoic acid; C18:1*n-9*), palmitic acid (hexadecanoic acid; C16:0), and stearic acid (octadecanoic acid; C18:0). These fatty acids are normally present in the relative proportions listed in Table 7-1 (Hudson, 1984), although there may be EPO samples that fall outside the ranges cited. In commercial production, early varieties of EPO typically had GLA in the range 8.0–9.0 percent, but more recently, 9 percent has been an accepted minimum for traded oils, with prices for those with GLA below this substantially discounted (Clough, 2001).

A number of fatty acids are also present in EPO at low concentrations, including myristic acid (C14:0), palmitoleic acid (C16:1*n-7*), vaccenic acid (C18:1*n-7*), α-linolenic acid (C18:3*n-3*), eicosanoic acid (C20:0), and eicosenoic acid (C20:1*n-9*). Court et al. (1993) reported a comprehensive fatty acid analysis of EPO, and data for a single oil sample in which minor fatty acids were also identified and quantified are listed in Table 7-2.

The triacylglycerol species in EPO have been eluted and identified (Redden et al., 1995a; Shimizu and Nakano, 2003). The triacylglycerol species containing two or more GLA molecules represent less than 1 percent of the total triacylglycerol mass. Most of the GLA-containing species consist of only one molecule of GLA per triacylglycerol molecule, accompanied primarily by two molecules of linoleic acid (~80 percent of total triacylglycerol mass) or by one molecule of linoleic acid and one molecule of either palmitic or oleic acid.

Stereospecific analysis to determine the fatty acid distribution over the three binding positions of the triacylglycerol molecule has also been performed on EPO. Researchers have found GLA to be concentrated in the *sn*-2 and *sn*-3 positions of triacylglycerols (Lawson and Hughes, 1988; Redden et al., 1995b). Of the triacylglycerols containing GLA, 13 percent had the fatty acid at the *sn*-1 position, 28 percent had GLA at the *sn*-2 position, and 49 percent had GLA at the *sn*-3 position (Lawson and Hughes, 1988). Within the total triacylglycerol mass of EPO, 10.3–10.7 percent contained GLA at the *sn*-2 position, and 10.3–10.7 percent contained GLA at the *sn*-3 position. By comparison, linoleic acid was nearly evenly distributed in all positions, with approximately 73 percent, 79 percent and 74 percent of total triacylglycerol mass in EPO containing linoleic acid at the *sn-1*, *sn-2*, or *sn-3* positions, respectively (Lawson and Hughes, 1988).

In addition to triacylglycerols, the remaining fraction of EPO consists of small amounts of other lipids (nonesterified fatty acids, diacylglycerols, phospholipids) and about 1–2 percent unsaponifiable matter, of which sterols and tocopherols are of some importance (Hudson, 1984; Christie, 1999). These minor components have been reviewed by Clough (2001). The average total sterol content of EPO is 1640 mg/100 g oil. The predominant (~80 percent) sterol fraction in EPO is β-sitosterol, with the remainder including campesterol (9 percent), 24-stigmastadienol (5 percent), and avenasterol (4 percent), as well as others (Clough, 2001). The natural tocopherol components include γ-tocopherol (161–758 mg/kg oil) and α-tocopherol (72–204 mg/kg oil) (Hudson, 1984; Clough, 2001). Small amounts of δ-tocopherol may also be present (Uzzan et al., 1992 as reported in Christie, 1999). Phospholipids comprise only about 0.05 percent of the oil and include phosphatidylcholine

TABLE 7-1 Select Fatty Acid Composition of Evening Primrose Oil

Fatty Acid	Symbol	Normal Range (g/100 g Fatty Acids)
Palmitic acid	C16:0	7–10
Stearic acid	C18:0	1.5–3.5
Oleic acid	C18:1*n-9*	6–11
Linoleic acid	C18:2*n-6*	65–80
γ-Linolenic acid	C18:3*n-6*	8–14

SOURCE: Based on data in Hudson (1984).

TABLE 7-2 Detailed Fatty Acid Composition of a Single Sample of Evening Primrose Oil

Saturated Fatty Acids	g/100 g Fatty Acids	Monounsaturated Fatty Acids	g/100 g Fatty Acids	Polyunsaturated Fatty Acids	g/100 g Fatty Acids
C12:0	0.04	C16:1*n-9*	0.04	C18:2*n-6*	71.20
C14:0	0.07	C16:1*n-7*	0.07	C18:3*n-6*	8.72
C15:0	0.03	C17:1*n-8*	0.04	C18:3*n-3*	0.18
C16:0	6.44	C18:1*n-7*	0.84	C20:2*n-6*	0.03
C17:0	0.06	C18:1*n-9*	9.76	—	—
C18:0	1.81	C20:1*n-9*	0.23	—	—
C20:0	0.31	—	—	—	—
C22:0	0.12	—	—	—	—
C24:0	0.04	—	—	—	—

SOURCE: Based on data in Court et al. (1993).

(31.9 percent), phosphatidylinositol (27.1 percent), phosphatidylethanolamine (17.6 percent), phosphatidylglycerol (16.7 percent), and phosphatidic acid (6.7 percent) (Lotti and Quartacci, 1990, as reported in Christie, 1999).

More recently, a detailed analysis of the non-triacylglycerol constituents of cold-pressed, unrefined EPO revealed three pentacyclic triterpenes identified as 3-*O*-*trans*-caffeoyl derivatives of betulinic, morolic, and oleanic acid (Hamburger et al., 2002). These lipophilic substances have been shown to have free radical scavenging and cyclooxygenase plus neutrophil elastase inhibitory activities in vitro (Hamburger et al., 2002). A quantitative survey of commercially available EPO products found that cold-pressed oils showed the highest non-triacylglyceride content (Knorr and Hamburger, 2004). Analysis of this fraction revealed that pentacyclic triterpenes were found only in cold-pressed oils. In contrast, refined oils or EPO obtained by supercritical carbon dioxide extraction had only trace amounts or were even below the limit of detection of the triterpenoidal esters (Knorr and Hamburger, 2004). These findings were confirmed by Puri (2004), who also recovered a pentacyclic triterpene ester in a commercially available cold-pressed, unrefined EPO preparation. Subsequently, the triterpenoidal esters were reported to be localized in the endosperm of the evening primrose seed, and the amount was approximately 72 percent greater than that found in cold-pressed unrefined EPO (Zuagg et al., 2006).

The composition of residues of evening primrose seeds remaining after cold-pressed oil extraction (referred to as seed meal or seed cake) have also been studied. Depending on the method and extent of oil extraction, evening primrose seed meal has been reported to contain 21–26 percent crude protein, 9–17 percent crude fat, and approximately 23 percent crude fiber (Hanczakowski et al., 1993; Stasiniewicz et al., 1998; Strzetelski et al., 1998a,b, 1999). The protein fraction of evening primrose seed meal is higher in methionine and cystine, but lower in lysine, compared to soybean meal (Stasiniewicz et al., 1998). High levels of tannins and anti-trypsin activity have also been identified in seed meal from evening primrose (Hanczakowski et al., 1993; Stasiniewicz et al., 1998), which has been suggested to limit the digestibility of protein in rats (Hanczakowski et al., 1993) and ruminants (Stasiniewicz et al., 1998; Strzetelski et al., 1998a,b, 1999). The fat in evening primrose seed meal was reported to contain approximately 73 percent linoleic acid, 9.0 percent GLA, and 6 percent oleic acid (Stasiniewicz et al., 1998), which closely mimics the relative proportions of these fatty acids found in EPO (see Table 7-1). Evening primrose seed meal has also been found to be a rich source of phenolic antioxidants, including catechin, epicatechin, and gallic acid (Balasinksa and Troszynska, 1998; Wettasinghe and Shahidi, 1999; Birch et al., 2001; Wettasinghe et al., 2002). Peschel et al. (2007) reported that crude extracts of evening primrose seed meal yielded a high total phenolic content similar to already commercialized antioxidants from rosemary, green tea, and grape seeds. Of several extracts tested, evening primrose seed meal exhibited the greatest potency for free radical scavenging activity and was very effective in scavenging superoxide anion radicals and inhibiting lipid oxidation (Peschel et al., 2007).

In addition to investigations on the composition of evening primrose seed oil and seed meal, the phytochemistry of the evening primrose plant itself has been studied. The fatty acid profile in the evening primrose plant differs from the oil in the seeds, with α-linolenic, linoleic, and palmitic acids dominant in the total fatty acid content of the plant. At all stages of growth, GLA (found in high amounts in the seed oil) was lacking in the evening primrose plant (Peiretti et al., 2004). Triterpenoids, gallic acid derivatives, and functionalized long-chain alcohols and acids were identified in the roots (Shukla et al., 1999). Numerous flavonol glycosides, gallic acid derivatives, phenylpropanoids, and anthocyanins have been reported in polar plant extracts (Abdullazhanova et al., 2000). In addition, the aerial parts of evening primrose contain a high content of phenolics and hydrolyzable tannins.

Variation in the Composition of Evening Primrose Oil

The relative fatty acid composition of EPO can vary according to factors such as the age of the seed, the cultivar, and growth conditions (Ghasemnezhad and Honermeier, 2007). Furthermore, as noted elsewhere in this chapter, the method of oil extraction from evening primrose seed may impact the non-triacylglycerol composition of EPO. Specifically, cold-pressed, unrefined EPO may contain a higher non-triacylglycerol content than refined EPO or that obtained by supercritical fluid/carbon dioxide extraction (Knorr and Hamburger, 2004). As a result, cold-pressed EPO can contain higher levels of triterpenoidal esters (Hamburger et al., 2002; Knorr and Hamburger, 2004) and plant sterols (Clough, 2001). In addition, subjecting the crude oil to heat during various phases of the refining process, especially high-heat deodorization, may reduce naturally occurring tocopherols, as well as result in some stereomutation (i.e., *cis* to *trans* conversion) of fatty acid double bonds (Wolff and Sebedio, 1994). In production systems where evening primrose seed is harvested from the wild and manually cleaned, separation of immature and mature seed can be incomplete, which can influence seed oil content (lowering to < 20 percent oil) and fatty acid composition (Clough, 2001). Manual cleaning and inefficient drying practices can also adversely affect seed and oil quality, due to a mixture of excess moisture, immature seed, and contamination with plant material and soil (Clough, 2001).

A study evaluating the amount of GLA in 16 different commercial preparations of EPO (and in most cases, 3 separate batches of each) found that most brands contained between 7 percent and 10 percent GLA, with a range of 1.9–10.5 percent (Gibson et al., 1992). The manufacturers had labeled the products as containing 5.2–10 percent GLA. With the exception of one brand, the actual amount of GLA agreed very closely with the labeled amount (on average, within ± 0.5 percent). However, the authors noted that a few of the products evaluated appeared to contain small amounts of borage oil (another GLA-rich oil) based on the recovery of low levels of the monoenes C22:1 and C24:1, which are usually not found in EPO. The authors further speculated that the addition of borage oil might be an attempt by manufacturers to supply oils with a standard GLA content, as most of the products thought to contain EPO/borage oil blends also contained GLA levels close to 10 percent.

While reviewing the literature in the preparation of this document, the committee noted relatively small variations in the amount of GLA and linoleic acid contained in the EPO supplements used in research trials. The fatty acid composition of EPO supplements employed in these studies usually fell within the ranges presented in Table 7-1. However, in some studies the fatty acid composition of the products used was not always well described (e.g., only the total amount of EPO fed was provided). In addition, several studies conducted in the target species used a blended oil product (usually EPO and fish oil), but did not report the composition of the individual oils nor the proportion of each oil supplied in the blend.

Putative Active Compounds and Proposed Biological Activity

Putative Active Compounds

The primary ingredients in EPO purported to have biological effects are GLA and linoleic acid. In this regard, EPO is unique compared to most oilseed oils in that it has a relatively high concentration of GLA and linoleic acid, but virtually no α-linolenic acid (Tables 7-1 to 7-3). A comparison of the chemical structures of linoleic acid and GLA is shown in Figure 7-1.

Proposed Biological Activity

The proposed biological activity of EPO has been elucidated primarily from studies conducted in vitro or in rodents, with either supplementation of EPO or specific fatty acids found in EPO. Although some aspects of the proposed biological activity have been confirmed in humans, the mechanics have not specifically been studied for their similarities or differences in horses, dogs, or cats. Therefore, the discussion on proposed biological activity that follows is considered general knowledge, and it is presumed it would be similar for all mammals. Specific information known about the target species as it relates to the discussion is provided.

In vivo, GLA is rapidly elongated by the addition of two carbons to dihomo-γ-linolenic acid (DGLA; all-*cis*-8,11,14-eicosatrienoic acid; C20:3*n-6*) (Gurr et al., 2002). Depending on the cell type, DGLA can be oxidized via cyclooxygenase isoenzymes (COX 1 or 2) to yield prostaglandins of the 1-series (e.g., PGE_1). Alternatively, DGLA can be oxidized by 15-lipoxygenase to 15-(S)-hydroxy-8,11,13-eicosatrienoic acid (15-HETrE) (Gurr et al., 2002).

Most of the biological effects ascribed to GLA can be attributed to PGE_1 and 15-HETrE. The PGE_1 is an eicosanoid with direct anti-inflammatory effects, showing clinical application in the suppression of chronic inflammation, vasodilation, and lowering of blood pressure in humans and laboratory animals (see reviews by Fan and Chapkin, 1998; Kapoor and Huang, 2006). In addition, DGLA competes with arachidonic acid (all-*cis*-5,8,11,14-eicosatetraenoic acid; 20:4*n-6*) for cycloxygenase isoenzymes to form PGE_1. As a result, fewer 2-series prostaglandins, which are more pro-inflammatory than the 1-series, are formed from oxidation of arachidonic acid. In comparison to PGE_1, 15-HETrE has indirect anti-inflammatory activity. In addition, 15-HETrE has been shown to inhibit the biosynthesis of the 4-series leukotrienes from arachidonic acid (Fan and

TABLE 7-3 A Comparison of the Composition of Select Fatty Acids Present in Evening Primrose, Borage, Black Currant, Hemp Seed, and Fungal Oils

		g/100 g Fatty Acids				
Fatty acid	Symbol	Evening Primrose Oil	Borage Oil	Black Currant Oil	Hemp Seed Oil	Fungal Oil
Saturated	—	7	14	8	9	17
Oleic acid	C18:1*n-9*	9	17	12	11	37
Linoleic acid	C18:2*n-6*	74	37	45	54	17
γ-Linolenic acid	C18:3*n-6*	9	23	17	2	25
α-Linolenic acid	C18:3*n-6*	< 1	< 1	13	21	2
Stearidonic acid	C18:4*n-3*	—	< 1	3	1	6
Erucic acid	C22:1*n-9*	< 1	3	—	—	—
Other	—	< 1	< 5	2	2	2

SOURCES: Based on data in Court et al. (1993); Dines et al. (1996); Barre (2001); Clough (2001); and Kriese et al. (2004).

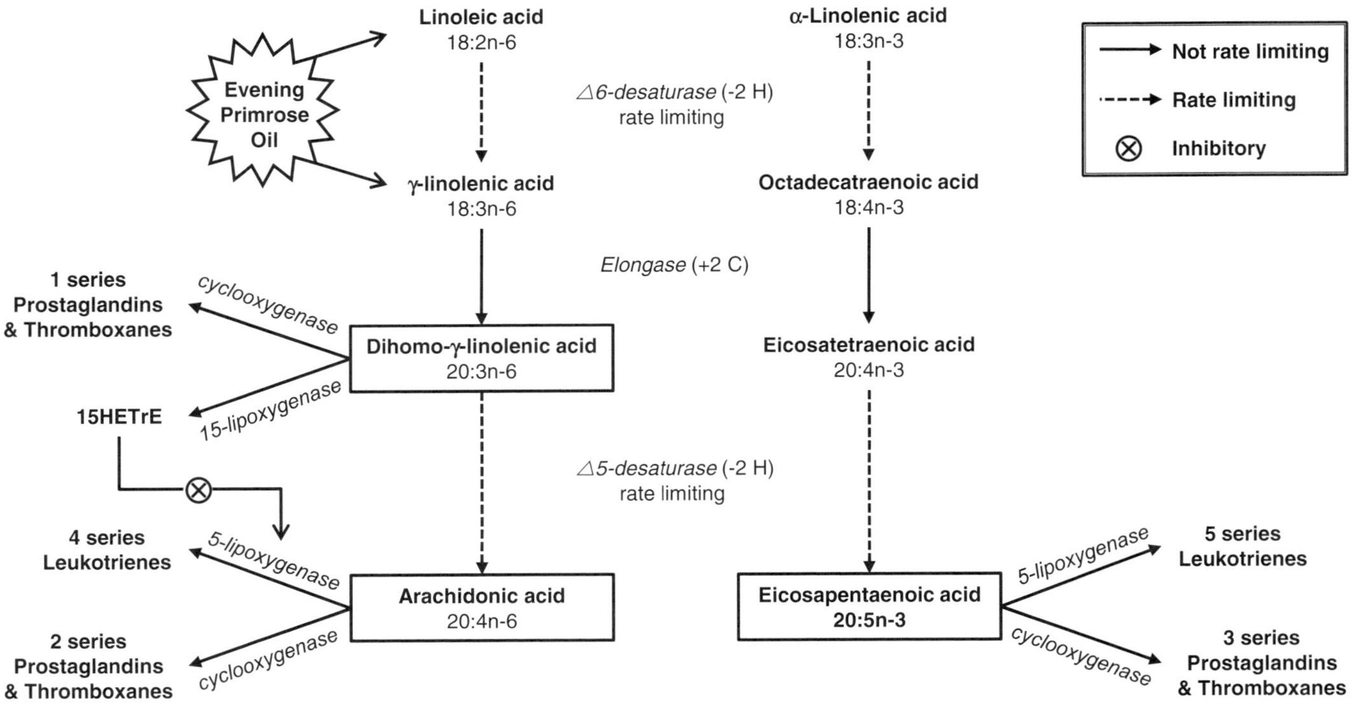

FIGURE 7-2 Elongation and desaturation of essential fatty acids and their metabolism to leukotrienes, prostaglandins, and thromboxanes. NOTE: The precursor fatty acids that come from dietary evening primrose oil supplementation are highlighted.

Chapkin, 1998; Kapoor and Huang, 2006). The 4-series leukotrienes exert greater pro-inflammatory effects than leukotrienes of other series. Collectively, DGLA and its metabolites, PGE_1 and 15-HETrE, produce a lesser inflammatory response compared to those metabolites formed from arachidonic acid. The formation of DGLA from GLA and its subsequent effects on arachidonic acid metabolism are illustrated in Figure 7-2.

As a member of the omega-6 fatty acid family, GLA is naturally formed from linoleic acid in the body. However, this reaction, which is catalyzed by the enzyme, Δ6-desaturase, usually proceeds very slowly (see Figure 7-2). It has been hypothesized that supplying GLA in EPO helps to bypass this rate-limiting step (Horrobin, 1992). In essence, the GLA in EPO is thought to be readily available for elongation to DGLA, a step that is not rate-limiting and proceeds rapidly. Subsequently, the increased supply of DGLA may facilitate the biosynthesis of desired anti-inflammatory eicosanoids and competitively inhibit the pro-inflammatory products generated from arachidonic acid (Horrobin, 1992).

A systemic decline in Δ6-desaturation, and the resulting decline in the capacity to convert linoleic acid to GLA (and subsequently arachidonic acid), has been associated with various physiologic and pathophysiologic states, including aging, diabetes, alcoholism, atopic dermatitis, premenstrual syndrome, rheumatoid arthritis, cancer, and cardiovascular disease (see reviews by Horrobin, 1993; Fan and Chapkin, 1998). It has been hypothesized that dietary supplementation with EPO may serve to alleviate a systemic decline in Δ6-desaturation by bypassing this rate-limiting step with its supply of GLA. As a result, GLA and oils rich in GLA have been prescribed and/or recommended with respect to alleviating some of the symptoms of these diseases.

A secondary component of EPO that may have biological importance is linoleic acid, which makes up 65–80 percent of EPO by weight. Linoleic acid cannot be synthesized de novo by mammals. Therefore, linoleic acid is recognized as an essential fatty acid and must be supplied in the diet. Further, linoleic acid is considered essential because of the roles it plays in the body: maintaining the integrity of cell membranes; the modulation of membrane-bound proteins such as receptors, transport proteins, and ion channels; the expression of certain genes; and as a precursor for biologically active metabolites, the eicosanoids (Gurr et al., 2002).

It is generally thought that all mammals (including humans) require 1 percent of total dietary energy intake as linoleic acid to prevent essential fatty acid deficiency (Gurr et al., 2002). In the horse, the NRC (2007) recommended a linoleic acid intake of 0.5 percent of total dietary energy; however, the Committee on the Nutrient Requirements of Horses did not provide justification for the lower linoleic acid requirement in horses compared to other animals. To the knowledge of the present committee, an essential fatty acid deficiency has not been described for the horse, even in those consuming diets almost devoid of fat. Sallmann et al. (1991) observed no clinical abnormalities in ponies fed diets containing 0.05 percent and 0.22 percent total fat containing 0.03 percent and 0.14 percent linoleic acid, respectively, for 7 months. The lack of clinical abnormalities in these ponies could have resulted from the mobilization of body fat stores, which may have been sufficient to meet the biological need for essential fatty acids during the prolonged period of low fat intake.

In dogs, the requirements for essential fatty acids have been recently reviewed (NRC, 2006). The Committee on the Nutrient Requirements of Dogs and Cats determined the adequate intake for linoleic acid in dogs to be 3, 2.8, and 2.4 g per 1,000 kcal of metabolizable energy for growing puppies, bitches during late gestation and peak lactation, and adult dogs at maintenance, respectively. This committee also set the adequate intake of α-linolenic acid at 0.18 g per 1,000 kcal of metabolizable energy for puppies and reproduction and 0.09 g for adult dogs at maintenance. This committee further stated that the α-linolenic acid requirement of dogs is dependent upon the linoleic acid content of the diet and that the ratio of linoleic acid to α-linolenic acid should be between 2.6:1 and 16:1. The NRC (2006) also lists a recommendation for eicosapentaenoic and docosahexaenoic acids in dogs: 0.13 g per 1,000 kcal of metabolizable energy for growth and reproduction and 0.11 g for adult maintenance, with 50–60 percent of the intake as eicosapentaenoic acid and 40–50 percent as docosahexaenoic acid. An adequate intake of 0.08 g of arachidonic acid per 1,000 kcal of metabolizable energy was also recommended for growing puppies. Although these requirements were formally listed (NRC, 2006), the committee noted that a lack of published studies made it difficult to define precise requirements for eicosapentaenoic, docosahexaenoic, and arachidonic acids for dogs.

Cats are unusual among mammals in that neither linoleic nor α-linolenic acid alone is sufficient to protect against the effects of fatty acid deficiency (Rivers et al., 1975). Presumably, this is because cats have limited Δ6-desaturase enzyme activity (Rivers et al., 1975; Hassam et al., 1977). It has also been suggested that cats lack the Δ5-desaturase enzyme (Hassam et al., 1977; Frankel and Rivers, 1978). More recently, it was reported that both Δ5- and Δ6-desaturases are active in cats, but the amount of activity does not appear to be adequate for maintaining tissue stores of long-chain polyunsaturated fatty acids (Pawloski et al., 1994). As a result, cats require preformed long-chain polyunsaturated fatty acids, such as arachidonic, eicosapentaenoic, and docosahexaenoic acids in their diet, in addition to the parent linoleic and α-linolenic acids. The NRC (2006) set the adequate daily intake of fatty acids for cats as follows: (1) linoleic acid: 1.4 g/1,000 kcal metabolizable energy for kittens, adult cats at maintenance, and queens in late gestation and peak lactation; (2) α-linolenic acid: 0.05 g/1,000 kcal metabolizable energy for kittens and queens in late gestation and peak lactation, with no recommendation set for adult cats at maintenance; (3) arachidonic acid: 0.05 g/1,000 kcal metabolizable energy for kittens and queens in late gestation and peak lactation and 0.005 g/1,000 kcal metabolizable energy for adult cats at maintenance; and (4) eicosapentaenoic and docosahexaenoic acids: 0.025 g/1,000 kcal metabolizable energy for kittens, adult cats at maintenance, and queens in late gestation and peak lactation. The NRC (2006) further recommends that the ratio of eicosapentaenoic acid to docosahexaenoic acid be less than 1.5:1 for kittens and gestating/lactating queens and less than 0.25:1 for adult cats at maintenance.

Recent research has demonstrated that EPO may also possess other moieties with potential biological activity. Triterpenoid caffeoyl esters have been isolated from the non-triacylglyercol fraction of cold-pressed, unrefined EPO. These pentacyclic triterpenes were identified as caffeoyl derivatives of beulinic, moralic, and oleanic acids (Hamburger et al., 2002). The catechol moieties in EPO were found to have free-radical scavenging properties (Hamburger et al., 2002) and likely act as natural antioxidants that protect the polyunsaturated fatty acids in unrefined EPO from autooxidation (Knorr and Hamburger, 2004). Caffeic acid derivatives in EPO were also shown to be strong inhibitors of leukocytic elastase in vitro (Hamburger et al., 2002), which is one of two main proteinases of neutrophils released as part of an inflammatory response. Elevated plasma levels of neutrophil elastase is a characteristic feature of active inflammation (Fischbach et al., 1987). The caffeoyl esters in EPO were also shown to inhibit cyclooxygenase 1 and 2 enzymes in vitro (Hamburger et al., 2002) and, as such, could possibly exert an anti-inflammatory effect. While these substances may contribute to the biological responses seen in humans and animals supplemented with EPO, their role (distinct from GLA and linoleic acid) has not been studied in vivo.

Methods of Analysis

Lipids are generally characterized by their ability to dissolve in water-immiscible organic solvents. Methods used for the extraction of lipids depend on the sample type. For example, extraction of lipids from biological samples is accomplished by homogenization with binary solvent mixtures, most commonly chloroform/methanol. In contrast, oils may be dissolved in hexane. In order to quantify the fatty acids in EPO, the fatty acid constituents must then be transmethylated (in the presence of an acidic or basic catalyst) to their methyl esters. There are numerous methods available for this purpose (Gurr et al., 2002), and, to the committee's knowledge, they have not been compared for their advantages and disadvantages in determining the fatty acid composition of EPO.

Extraction of lipids from samples is best accomplished as soon as possible to minimize the degradative changes that would otherwise take place. When storage has to take place, it is best done at as low a temperature as possible (–20°C or lower) and under an inert nitrogen atmosphere to minimize oxidation of the double bonds in polyunsaturated fatty acids (Gurr et al., 2002). In addition, before storage for any length of time, lipid extracts are best re-dissolved in a small amount of solvent containing an antioxidant such as 3,5-di-*t*-butyl-4-hydroxytolulene (BHT) before storage at –20°C or lower in the dark under nitrogen (Gurr et al., 2002).

Methods used to identify and quantify fatty acids, the fatty acid positional distribution on the triacylglycerol molecules, and the specific molecular species of triacylglycerols in EPO have been reviewed and described elsewhere (Christie, 1999). Briefly, capillary gas chromatography (GC) is the most widely used method for analysis of fatty acids in EPO. The GC heating and holding cycles may alter the sensitivity, possibly obscuring or incompletely separating the minor fatty acid components (Gurr et al., 2002). Fatty acid methyl esters should be identified by their retention times relative to authentic standards (Gurr et al., 2002). Identification of the fatty acid positional distribution on the triacylglycerol molecule and the specific molecular species of the triacylglycerols in EPO has been performed with silver-ion and reversed-phase chromatography, often used in conjunction with thin-layer chromatography or high-performance liquid chromatography (HPLC) (Christie, 1999). Reverse-phase HPLC has also been linked to mass spectrometry for triacylglycerol identification purposes. Identification of specific triacylglycerols and positional distribution of fatty acids is not routinely performed in clinical research trials nor is it generally included in the standard fatty analysis of commercial EPO products for labeling purposes.

Standardization

Although EPO contains several potential active ingredients, most preparations appear to be standardized or compared based on their GLA content. Nonetheless, product specifications for the amount of EPO and the proportion of GLA vary between manufacturers. According to the Longwood Task Force's monograph on EPO (Kemper, 1999), soft-gelatin capsule preparations for human use in the United States generally contain 500 to 1,000 mg of EPO per capsule, with many standardized to contain 8 percent GLA. Yu-Cheng et al. (2001) stated that EPO products originating from China generally fall into one of three specifications: 8–9 percent, 9–10 percent, or 10 percent GLA. Many encapsulated EPO products for companion animals contain a similar profile and are often produced by the same manufacturer as human EPO supplements. In addition, some animal owners may feed EPO products marketed for humans to their animals. However, EPO preparations can differ widely between manufacturers, both in chemical composition and the amount of oil present in capsules (Gibson et al., 1992). Various formulations also contain EPO blended with other oils (e.g., fish oils, linseed oil) or added vitamins, minerals, or herbal extracts (Clough, 2001). In addition to packaging in gel capsules, some EPO preparations come as bulk oils that must be measured out by the animal owner before feeding.

Related Compounds

Compounds that Provide Similar Active Ingredients

In addition to the Onagraceae family (which includes evening primrose), GLA can be found in other higher plants, mainly among species of the Boraginacae and Saxifragaceae. In the Boraginacae family, oil from the seeds of *Borago officianlis* L. and *Symphytum officianale* L. (both marketed as borage oil) contains higher levels of GLA (20–27 percent of total fatty acids), but only half the amount of linoleic acid (35–40 percent) compared to EPO (Miller et al., 1968; Dines et al., 1996). Borage oil also contains significant amounts of long-chain monounsaturated fatty acids (e.g., C20:1, C22:1, and C24:1). Borage oil, particularly in oil from *Symphytum officianale*, may also contain carcinogenic unsaturated pyrrolidizine alkaloids (Awang, 1990), although the prevalence of these toxic compounds in borage oils has been debated (see Clough, 2001). Other species within the Boraginacae family, such as *Echium vulgare*, *E. plantagineum*, *Onosmodium occidentale*, and *O. hipidissimum*, contain smaller quantities of GLA. Within the Saxifragaceae family, the seeds of the *Ribes* are used as a source of GLA-containing oils. Among them, seeds of black currant (*Ribes nigrum*) are the richest source of GLA (up to 19 percent) (Traitler et al., 1984, 1988). Black currant oil differs from EPO in that it also contains substantial amounts of omega-3 fatty acids (e.g., 12–14 percent α-linolenic acid and 2–4 percent stearidonic acid).

The seeds of other higher plants also contain significant quantities of GLA. For example, the seed oils of *Scruphularia marilandica*, *Acer negundo*, *Astelia trinerva*, *Humulus lupulus*, and *Anenome cylindrical* contain between 5 and 25 percent GLA (see review by Phillips and Huang, 1996). Oil extracted from the seeds of hemp (*Cannabis sativa* L.) contains 1–6 percent GLA (Deferne and Pate, 1996; Leizer et al., 2000; Oomah et al., 2002; Kriese et al., 2004).

Many species of microorganisms are rich in GLA (for reviews see Phillips and Huang, 1996; Certik and Shimizu, 1999). Fungal oils derived from species of mold in the order of Mucorales (especially *Mucor* and *Mortierella* spp.) can contain 7–26 percent GLA. Oils derived from *Spirulina* spp. (a blue-green algae) can contain 12–25 percent GLA. Many species of ciliated protozoa in the family Tetrahymenidae (e.g., *Tetrahymena pyriformis*) are rich in GLA (> 30 percent).

In addition to EPO, oils derived from borage, black currant, and hemp seeds, and fungal oils are currently the most common sources of GLA used in commercial dietary supplements. The relative proportions of the predominant fatty acids present in these oils are compared to the fatty acid profile of EPO in Table 7-3.

Several studies have compared EPO supplementation to that of other GLA sources, most often borage oil, to determine their relative effectiveness at eliciting a biological response. Some clinical work has shown the biological potency of EPO to be equivalent to borage oil when fed to provide similar amounts of GLA, suggesting that the absolute amount of GLA was more important than the source (Raederstorff and Moser, 1993). Other studies feeding equal amounts (by weight) of EPO and borage oil have demonstrated that borage oil produces lesser effects than would be predicted by its higher GLA content (Engler, 1993; Dines et al., 1996; Fan et al., 1996). Jenkins et al. (1988) showed higher levels of PGE_1 formation in rats fed EPO compared to those fed borage, black currant, or fungal oils in amounts that provided an equal quantity of GLA. Several authors have attributed differences in biological potency between EPO and other oils to differences in stereospecific distribution of fatty acids (i.e., GLA at position *sn*-1, *sn*-2, and/or *sn*-3 in triacylglycerols) and the nature of fatty acids adjacent to GLA in triacylglycerols (Lawson and Hughes, 1988; Redden et al., 1995a,b; Phillips and Huang, 1996; Shimizu and Nakano, 2003). Huang et al. (1995) demonstrated that the rate of in vitro hydrolysis of GLA by pancreatic lipase was greater when the triacylglycerol contained one GLA molecule (as occurs in > 99 percent of EPO) compared to two molecules GLA (as occurs in borage oil). The authors also found that the release of GLA from either outer position (*sn*-1 or *sn*-3) or the middle position (*sn*-2) was significantly slower when the other two stereospecific positions in the same triacylglycerol molecule were occupied by saturated or long-chain monounsaturated fatty acids (which are absent from EPO, but present in borage oil). In contrast, Høy and Christensen (1996) found no significant difference in the in vivo metabolism of GLA from borage, evening primrose, and black currant seed oils in rats. Ultimately, the relative importance of the position of GLA in the triacylglycerol structure remains unclear and requires further study.

In addition to the natural sources of GLA described above, new technologies have led to the development of purified GLA, enriched and "designer" oils, and genetically modified oilseeds that contain high levels of GLA. Concentration and/or purification of GLA are most commonly accomplished via selective lipase-catalyzed reactions that remove unwanted fatty acids within various oil sources. For example, the GLA content of EPO was enriched to 75 percent from an initial concentration of 9 percent using a fungal lipase preparation that preferentially discriminated against GLA in favor of other fatty acids (Syed-Rahmatullah et al., 1994). Use of enzymes for selective esterification has further permitted the creation of triacylglycerols with fatty acids in specific positions on the glycerol backbone. Advances in the cloning and manipulation of fatty acid desaturase genes have created a wide range of unusual fatty acids in transgenic oilseed crops. For example, the recombinant expression of fungal Δ12- and Δ6-desaturase genes in the canola plant has led to the development of a new canola strain capable of producing GLA at up to 43 percent of the fatty acids in the oil of the seed (Huang et al., 2001). Although this high GLA canola oil has not been compared to EPO in vivo, results from 6-week (Palombo et al., 2000) and 12-week (Liu et al., 2004) feeding studies in rats showed that supplementation with the modified canola oil had a similar biological effect on the growth and hepatic metabolism of *n-6* fatty acids as borage oil.

Compounds that Provide Similar Biological Activity

Eicosapentaenoic acid (all-*cis*-5,8,11,14,17-eicosapentaenoic; C20:5n-3; EPA) is a fatty acid that has been reported to have similar biological activity to the DGLA derivatives that originate from GLA. Eicosapentaenoic acid differs from GLA and DGLA in that it is an omega-3 (*n-3*) fatty acid, whereas the latter two are *n-6* fatty acids. As a result, eicosanoids derived from the oxidation of EPA by cyclooxygenase and lipoxygenase enzymes differ from those generated by the action of these same enzymes on DGLA (see Figure 7-2).

The anti-inflammatory effects of dietary EPA have been reviewed elsewhere (see Calder, 2006); thus, only a brief description as it relates to the active ingredients in EPO is provided here. Similar to DGLA, EPA reduces the generation of archidonic acid-derived mediators by competing with arachidonic acid for incorporation into cell membranes (thereby reducing the amount of arachidonic acid substrate available) and by competing for cyclooxygenase and lipoxygenase enzymes. Only EPA, DGLA, and arachidonic acid can serve as direct substrates for eicosanoid production. In general, those derived from EPA and DGLA have weaker inflammatory effects than those derived from arachidonic acid. Thus, EPA and DGLA have somewhat similar biological effects, although the derivatives that are actually responsible for these effects differ between these fatty acids (Figure 7-2).

Similar to other oils derived from the seeds of higher plants, EPO does not contain EPA. Rather, EPA-rich foods include marine oils derived from cold water fatty fishes (e.g., menhaden fish oil) and the algae they feed on. However, EPA can be synthesized by elongation and desaturation from the parent n-3 fatty acid, α-linolenic acid (18:3n-3) in most mammals via the same Δ6- and Δ5-desaturases used to synthesize GLA and arachidonic acid from linoleic acid. The exception, as described earlier, is the cat, which has limited ability to metabolize α-linolenic acid to the longer-chain polyunsaturated fatty acids due to limited desaturase activity. Only trace amounts of α-linolenic acid are found in EPO (see Table 7-2). The potential complementary actions of DGLA and EPA have resulted in the marketing of dietary supplements containing both EPO (and/or other sources of GLA) and fish oil (or other sources of EPA).

Effects of Manufacturing, Processing, and Storage on Composition

Manufacturing and Processing

Mechanical pressing and/or organic solvent extrusion are most commonly employed to extract the oil from evening primrose seed (Clough, 2001). Large-scale mechanical extraction of oil (expeller extrusion) is generally accomplished by pressing seeds in an hydraulic or screw press. Solvent extraction of oil is usually performed using volatile purified hydrocarbons, including hexane, heptanes, or petroleum ether. The organic solvent is percolated through the seed, dissolving the oil, which can then be recovered by evaporation of the solvent. More recently, supercritical fluid extraction with carbon dioxide as the extraction solvent has been employed to liberate the oil from evening primrose seed (Gawdzik et al., 1998), but a relatively small amount of seed is processed using this method (Clough, 2001). Supercritical fluid extraction involves pressurizing and heating carbon dioxide to the point that it has the properties of both a liquid and a gas. Flow of this "supercritical" carbon dioxide through the seeds acts as a solvent and extracts the oil from the seed. When the pressure is reduced, the carbon dioxide reverts to a gaseous state, leaving behind the solvent-free oil.

Solvent-based extraction commonly removes over 98 percent of the oil from evening primrose seed, whereas mechanical processing typically recovers only 50 to 60 percent of the oil (Clough, 2001). The relatively low oil content of evening primrose seed (≈ 20 percent) often renders mechanical extraction uneconomical. In China, it is common for seed (and the subsequent seed residue) to be pressed two or three times to maximize output (Clough, 2001). In other cases, the oil in evening primrose seed may be extracted by mechanical pressing first, followed by a second solvent extraction to recover the oil remaining in the seed meal residue. As a result, there is potential for some products to contain EPO that was mechanically extracted, solvent extracted, or a blend of both.

Evening primrose seed is comparatively small and the seed coat is hard. Therefore, in some cases, seed may be heat-treated or steamed prior to extraction to improve oil yield. In the case of mechanical oil extraction, some heat is usually generated due to friction, even if no external heat is applied. Oils that are truly "cold pressed" are those that have been mechanically extracted at temperatures less than 49°C with no external heat applied.

Once extracted, the extent of processing and refining applied to the crude oil can vary. "Virgin" oils are those that have been extracted by mechanical cold pressing and then filtered to clarify the oil, with no further processing. More commonly, crude oil obtained from either mechanical or solvent extraction will undergo further refining (also referred to as raffination) to remove colors, odors, and other undesirable components such as fatty acids, waxes, carotenoids, phospholipids, and other unsaponifiables. Refining of EPO usually follows conventional procedures for caustic refining of soft oils (Clough, 2001). Degumming and neutralizing is generally the first stage of refining, which involves a citric acid wash followed by treatment with alkali (sodium hydroxide and/or sodium carbonate) to neutralize and remove many of the undesirable components. The second stage is bleaching, whereby the oil is treated with bleaching earths, such as Fuller's earth, activated carbon, or activated clays, to improve color reduction and ensure removal of polyaromatic hydrocarbons (Clough, 2001). An alternative bleaching procedure involves heating the oil to more than 175°C (Christie, 1999). The last stage of refinement is deodorization to remove the taints and odors present in the oil at the beginning of the refining process, as well as those produced during the neutralizing and bleaching stages. Deodorization is carried out by passing high-pressure steam (at up to 240°C) through the oil under vacuum (Christie, 1999). However, in order to avoid thermal degradation and *trans* isomerization of GLA, it has been recommended that temperatures less than 200°C should be employed (Wolff and Sebedio, 1994). Following deodorization, the oils are either packaged and distributed as is or with the addition of an antioxidant. Antioxidants, if used, are either tocopherols (natural mixed tocopherols or di-α-tocopherol) at a level of 500 mg/kg or a blend of tocopherols and ascorbyl palmitate (Clough, 2001).

European oil extraction from evening primrose seed (either locally produced or imported) is almost exclusively done using solvent extraction (Clough, 2001). Apart from those users specifying that the oil be cold pressed and unrefined, most applications/end-users in Europe require that the oils be fully refined.

In China, where 90 percent of the world's EPO supply originates, it is common for oil to be extracted with a mechanical screw press. As described by Yu-Cheng et al. (2001), the Chinese first soften evening primrose seed using steam and extract the oil without additional heat using a spiral oil press. The oil is filtered and then refined by neutralizing with alkali, deodorizing with steam, and decoloring by charcoal filtration. It is then dried, filtered again, and vitamin E is added to the final product. Oil is also extracted in China using chemical solvents (usually hexane) and supercritical carbon dioxide extraction, although to a lesser extent than mechanical extraction (Yu-Cheng et al., 2001).

The method of extraction and the refining process can alter the composition and properties of the EPO. Cold-pressed, unrefined EPO has been shown to contain a higher non-triacylglycerol content than refined EPO or that obtained by supercritical carbon dioxide extraction (Knorr and Hamburger, 2004). As a result, cold-pressed EPO can contain higher levels of triterpenoidal esters (Hamburger et al., 2002; Knorr and Hamburger, 2004). Refining also reduces the plant sterol fraction of EPO (see review by Clough, 2001). Bleaching often reduces the resistance of the oil to rancidity, because some naturally occurring antioxidants are removed along with the impurities. In addition, each step of the refining process usually involves heating the oil to a certain extent, which can destroy endogenous antioxidants. High-heat deodorization has also been shown to alter the geometric configuration of double bonds in GLA and other unsaturated fatty acids (Wolff and Sebedio, 1994). The double bonds of polyunsaturated fatty acids in crude oil extracts of evening primrose seed are mostly of the *cis* geometrical configuration. Alteration to the *trans* configuration caused by excessive heating during oil extraction and refining can alter or destroy the biological function of the original fatty acid if consumed. In addition, intake of high concentrations of dietary *trans* fatty acids may adversely affect the metabolism of essential fatty acids (linoleic acid and α-linolenic acid) by inhibiting desaturase activity or by competing for desaturases (Gurr et al., 2002). *Trans* fatty acids may therefore cause abnormal eicosanoid metabolism, as well as a perturbance of cell membrane structure and function. Ingestion of large amounts of *trans* fatty acids has been shown to increase plasma biomarkers of inflammation (López-García et al., 2005).

Stability and Storage

As an oil with a high proportion of polyunsaturated fatty acids (> 80 percent of the oil by weight), the greatest threat to the stability of EPO is lipid peroxidation. The major pathway is attack at the double bonds of a polyunsaturated fatty acid by reactive oxygen radicals with the initial formation of a lipid peroxide. If left unchecked, each lipid peroxide can react with another unsaturated fatty acid, triggering a chain reaction. Lipid peroxidation is accelerated in the presence of catalysts (transitional metal ions or haem compounds) and by heating. If allowed to go too far, lipid peroxidation can significantly reduce the concentration of polyunsaturated fatty acids, such as linoleic acid and GLA, in EPO.

Unrefined plant oils tend to have some built-in resistance to oxidation (e.g., tocopherols, β-carotene, triterpenoidal esters, phosphorus component of phospholipids). Exogenous antioxidants are often (but not always) added to the final EPO product to increase resistance to prooxidants and improve shelf life (Clough, 2001).

The effects of seed harvesting, processing, and refining on the oxidative stability of EPO can be evaluated by several methods used for other food-grade oils, including the acid, peroxide, and anisidine values, the Oil Stability Index, the *trans* fatty acid content, and the moisture content. A typical specification for traded refined EPO provided by Clough (2001) lists the following maximum values: peroxide value < 5 meq/kg oil; acid value < 0.6 mg KOH/g oil; moisture < 0.1 percent; saponification value 175–196; and unsaponifiable matter < 2 percent. However, the author cautions that the actual purchase specifications can vary considerably in their stringency. A summary of values measured in refined and unrefined EPO by Christie (1999) is described in Table 7-4. With regard to seed quality, the hard coat of evening primrose seed makes it resistant to mechanical damage at harvest and in postharvest handling (Clough, 2001). As a result, the oil-containing cells are not generally exposed to moisture or oxygen and if dried efficiently soon after harvest, increases in seed free fatty acid levels are small. Good-quality evening primrose seed will typically have a free fatty acid content of less than 1 percent, although values have been reported in the range of 1.8–6.9 percent (Clough, 2001).

Packaging and postmarket handling of EPO can affect stability. Many commercially available EPO products are sold in encapsulated form, which reduces exposure to oxygen. In contrast, EPO products sold in bulk form (e.g.,

TABLE 7-4 Quality and Stability Characteristics of Evening Primrose Oil

Characteristic	Units	Typical Range	Absolute Range
Acid value	mg KOH/g oil	2.0–6.0	0.5–12.0
Peroxide value	$mEqO_2$	1.5–6.0	1.0–12.0
Anisidine value	—	4–8	2–48
Oil stability index (unrefined oil)	hours	4.5–5.5	—
Oil stability index (refined oil)	hours	2.5	—
Unsaponifiable matter	percent	1.3–2.0	1.0–3.0
Phosphorus (unrefined oil)	mg/kg	20–40	5–80
Phosphorus (refined oil)	mg/kg	0–5	—
β-Carotene	mg/kg	1–3	—
Moisture (unrefined oil)	mg/kg	500–900	—
Moisture (refined oil)	mg/kg	< 500	—

SOURCES: Based on data in Christie (1999) and Clough (2001).

bottled oils) may allow repeated exposure to oxygen and other prooxidants (e.g., a bottle that is open and closed at each feeding or bacteria introduced in the form of a spoon or syringe used to dispense the daily dosage), which could eventually overcome endogenous and exogenous antioxidant capacity and reduce shelf life. Storage of EPO at elevated ambient temperatures can also increase susceptibility to lipid peroxidation.

Oils with a sufficient degree of lipid peroxidation often exhibit off-taste and odors; however, this may not discourage voluntary intake in all animals. If ingested, lipid peroxides are rapidly metabolized in the mucosal cells of the small intestine to various oxyacids that are rapidly oxidized to carbon dioxide. High concentrations of lipid peroxides in the gut may damage the mucosa and potentiate the growth of tumors (Gurr et al., 2002). There is little evidence of the absorption of unchanged hydroperoxides or of their incorporation into tissue lipids. However, hydroperoxyalkenals (low molecular weight breakdown products of lipid hydroperoxides) are absorbed and may be toxic (Gurr et al., 2002).

Potential for Contamination or Adulteration

Potential for Contamination

Seed quality for evening primrose is primarily defined in terms of purity, moisture content, oil content, GLA content, and percentage free fatty acids. According to Clough (2001), 98 percent minimum purity and 9 percent maximum moisture would be typical contractual requirements. In some countries, seed may be harvested at an immature state in order to take advantage of high early season prices, which can affect both total oil and GLA content. Seed may also be cleaned manually. The lack of efficient mechanical cleaning and drying equipment can result in seed with a higher moisture content, incomplete separation of immature from mature seed, and seed with a high foreign matter content (Clough, 2001).

As with all vegetable oils, the possibility exists that EPO may be contaminated with herbicides and, particularly, pesticides that have been applied either to the crops or to the seeds postharvest or are simply residual in the soil/environment. According to Clough (2001), one or two insecticide applications may be required to achieve satisfactory control of insects and moth larvae and a fungicide may be applied to control mildew. In addition to being used to control weeds, herbicides may be applied when harvesting evening primrose seed by defoliation. In China, use of pesticides and herbicides is less likely, due to the unavailability and cost of agrochemicals (Clough, 2001). It is generally accepted that refining of edible oils largely removes residual pesticides, but the lower temperatures typically used to deodorize EPO (to protect the GLA) will be less efficient at their removal than normal (Clough, 2001). Limited data are available to assess the level of potential agrochemical contamination of EPO. Clough (2001) presented data from 15 crude and 35 refined EPO samples evaluated over several years and concluded that oils were generally free from most compounds or they were present at levels that should not cause concern. However, between 40 and 60 percent of all the oils did contain at least one residual compound at a detectable level. The refined oils contained significantly lower levels of pesticides than crude oils.

As an extract derived from a botanical, EPO also has the potential to be contaminated with heavy metals or transitional metal ions. Christie (1999) reported that "it is unheard of for samples of evening primrose oil to fail" routine quality control testing for lead, arsenic, iron, and copper. However, Stasiniewicz et al. (1998) reported that the level of zinc, cadmium, and lead in evening primrose seed meal exceeded the standards established in Poland. The level of heavy metals in evening primrose seed is heavily dependent on exposure to industrial and urban pollution (Lammer-Zarawska et al., 1992, as cited in Stasiniewicz et al., 1998). If the oil is mechanically extracted from metal contaminated seeds, there is potential for contamination of EPO with heavy metals. A typical specification for traded refined EPO provided by Clough (2001) indicated levels for lead, mercury, and arsenic were less than 0.1 mg/kg and cadmium less than 0.01 mg/kg. The specification also placed the following limits on microbiological contamination: yeast < 100/g, mold < 100/g, negative coliform count, and negative *Salmonella*. Again, it must be noted that actual purchase specifications adopted by various EPO dietary supplement manufacturers can vary considerably in their stringency.

As a rich source of polyunsaturated fatty acids, EPO is at risk for oxidation during processing and refining. The formation of lipid hydroperoxides, as well as the stereomutation of unsaturated fatty acids from *cis* to *trans* configuration can take place, thereby altering the composition and biological properties of the oil (see earlier discussion).

In several commercially available preparations, EPO is blended with other oils. Some of these oils may themselves contain contaminants (e.g., high levels of mercury in some fish oils or toxic unsaturated pyrrolidizine alkaloids reported in some borage oils). Therefore, potential exists for contaminants to be introduced via the oils added (intentionally or unintentionally) to an EPO product.

Potential for Adulteration

Borage, black currant, and fungal oils contains higher level of GLA than EPO (see earlier section on Related Compounds). In an effort to elevate the GLA content of their EPO product, some manufacturers may add these oils to EPO. The blending of various types of oil may not always be disclosed on the product labeling (Gibson et al., 1992). In the case of borage oil, there may be a safety concern.

Borage plant parts, including the leaf, flower, and seed, have been reported to contain unsaturated pyrrolizidine alkaloids, especially amabiline (Larson et al., 1984; Awang, 1990). These alkaloids can be hepatotoxic, carcinogenic, mutagenic, and teratogenic (Roeder, 1995). However, whether these alkaloids are present in borage oil or only in borage plant tissue has been debated (see Clough, 2001).

BIOLOGY

Absorption, Distribution, Metabolism, and Elimination

General

Much of what we know about the absorption, distribution, metabolism, and excretion (ADME) of fatty acids—from EPO or other dietary oil sources—stems from research conducted in rodents. Relatively less is known about fatty acid ADME in horses, dogs, and cats and, perhaps more importantly, ADME specifically in response to EPO supplementation has not been studied in these species. As a result, the bulk of the discussion on ADME of EPO that follows is derived from information gathered in nontarget species, unless otherwise noted. Although effects in horses, dogs, and cats are likely to be similar to those in humans and other animals, some known species differences exist and will be highlighted where appropriate. In addition, although most aspects of ADME have been studied in response to dietary EPO supplementation, some gaps in knowledge remain.

Absorption

In general, the triacylglycerols in EPO are digested and absorbed similar to other dietary lipids. Hydrolysis of triacylglycerols begins in the stomach, where gastric lipase and physical churning form lipid droplets. In the small intestine, the fat emulsion is mixed with bile salts and pancreatic juice, which include enzymes that catalyze the hydrolysis of fatty acids from triacylglycerols. Among these enzymes, pancreatic lipase is responsible for the hydrolysis of fatty acids from the outer positions (*sn*-1 and *sn*-3) of triacylglycerols, yielding two fatty acids and one monoglycerol (a fatty acid attached to the *sn*-2 position). The products formed from lipid hydrolysis in the small intestine disperse and form mixed micelles, which contain a monolayer of bile salts (or bile acids), monoglycerols, and lysophospholipids that surround a core of fatty acids, cholesterol, and fat-soluble vitamins.

Micelles deliver the lipids to the brush border of the small intestine. Once inside the enterocyte, the monoglycerol molecules and fatty acids are re-esterified to triacylglycerols. Fatty acids can also be re-esterified to the *sn*-1 position of lysophospholipids. Once formed, these phospholipids, along with an apolipoprotein skeleton, are packaged to form the outer monolayer of a chylomicron, with a core of triacylglycerols, cholesterol, fat-soluble vitamins, and some carbohydrates. Chylomicrons fuse with the basolateral membrane of the enterocyte and enter into tiny lymph vessels (lacteals). After transversing the lymphatic system, chylomicrons pass via the thoracic duct into circulation. The exceptions to the above are short- and medium-chained fatty acids (2 to 12 carbons), which are rapidly absorbed via the portal vein and transverse the liver before entering system circulation. However, EPO contains no short-chained fatty acids and virtually no medium-chained fatty acids (Court et al., 1993); therefore, uptake of the purported active components of EPO likely take the pathway of the chylomicrons described above. It is also worth noting that a true chylomicron fraction has never been isolated in adult horses (see review by Watson et al., 1993 and discussion in Chapter 4). Although horses are very capable of absorbing dietary fat (see Kronfeld et al., 2004), the exact mechanism has not been elucidated.

Absorption of triacylglycerols specifically from EPO has not been studied in horses, dogs, or cats, but evidence of EPO absorption has been reported by Høy and Christensen (1996) in rats. Male albino Wistar rats were cannulated in the main mesenteric lymph duct and lymph was collected before and for 24 hours after a single bolus injection of EPO (0.5 mL) into the stomach. The molar percentage of linoleic acid and GLA in lymph increased to maximum levels during the first 3 to 4 hours after administration of EPO and then declined after 7 hours, demonstrating the absorption of fatty acids associated with EPO. The proportion of fatty acids in the lymph was reflective of the composition of the supplemental EPO.

Only one study, performed in humans, has described the serum concentration versus time curve in response to the ingestion of EPO (Martens-Lobenhoffer and Meyer, 1998). Six healthy adult volunteers were orally administered six capsules of a commercially available EPO product at 0700 hours and a further six capsules at 1900 hours. Each capsule contained 466–536 mg EPO, adjusted to provide a total content of 40 mg GLA per capsule. In all volunteers, the fatty acid levels in serum were profiled for two, 24-hour periods: one with EPO supplementation and one without. On the days of investigation, subjects were fed low-fat meals. Following the 0700 hour EPO dose, serum GLA concentration remained at baseline until approximately 1.5 hours postdosing and then sharply increased, reaching a peak about 4 hours postdosing. Serum GLA then declined slowly and was near baseline at 12 hours postdosing. Following the 1900 hours EPO dosing, serum GLA concentration began to increase within 30 minutes of EPO administration, reaching a peak approximately 3 hours later. Again, serum GLA concentration slowly declined thereafter, reaching baseline approximately 12 hours postdosing (see Figure 7-3). The authors concluded GLA showed an absorption-elimination pattern in response to EPO administration, with an AUC_{24} and C_{max} significantly increased over

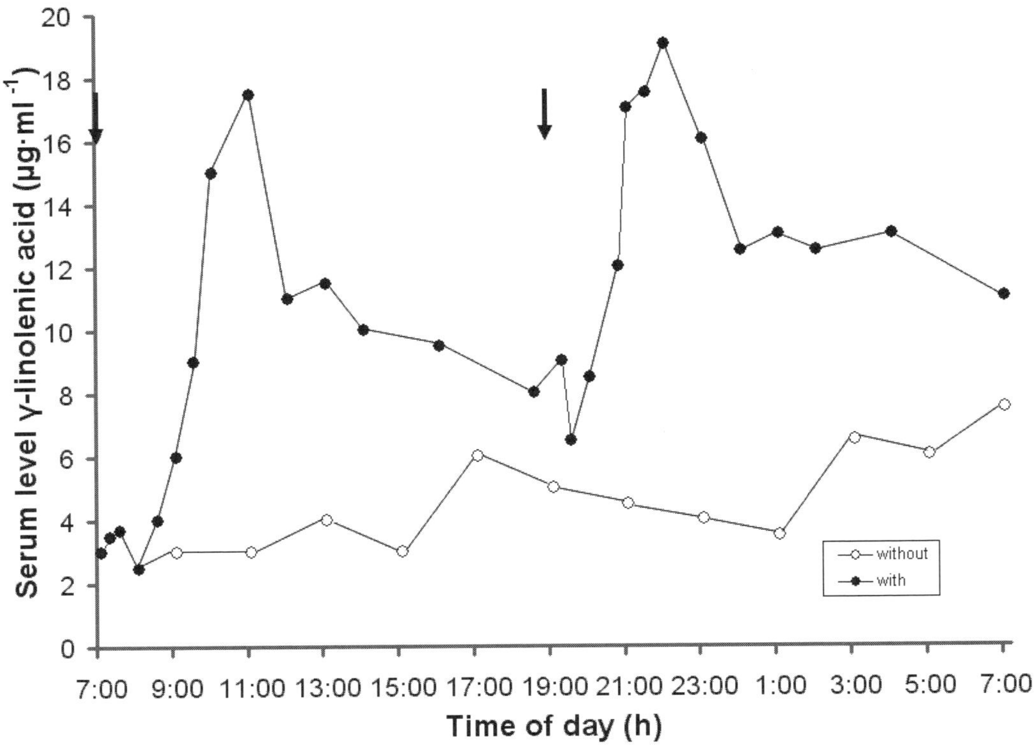

FIGURE 7-3 Pharmokinetics of γ-linolenic acid in serum in response to oral ingestion of evening primrose oil in humans.
NOTE: Average serum concentration of γ-linolenic acid over 24 hours without (○) and with (●) administration of six capsules of Epogam at 7:00 and 19:00 (indicated by arrows).
SOURCE: Redrawn from Martens-Lobenhoffer and Meyer (1998). Copyright 1998 by International Journal of Clinical Pharmacology and Therapeutics. Used with permission.

baseline values. The T_{max} after the 0700 hours EPO administration (4.4 ± 1.9 hours) was longer than after the 1900 hours EPO administration (2.7 ± 1.2 hours). The high standard deviations in specific serum fatty acid content demonstrated a high-level individual subject variation. The other seven fatty acids measured, in particular DGLA and arachidonic acid (both metabolites of GLA), did not increase in serum in response to acute EPO administration.

Distribution

After digestion, triacylglycerol-rich chylomicrons transport lipids of dietary origin and deliver them to tissues in need of fatty acids. Lipoprotein lipase, anchored to the luminal aspect of endothelial cells lining the capillaries of tissues and organs, binds to chylomicrons and rapidly hydrolyzes triacylglycerols in the core of the chylomicron. This releases fatty acids, which can diffuse across the cell membrane of tissues, either by simple diffusion or by facilitated diffusion using fatty acid transport proteins. Similar to pancreatic lipase, lipoprotein lipase more readily hydrolyzes the fatty acids at the *sn*-1 and *sn*-3 positions of the triacylglycerol. Once inside a tissue cell, the fatty acids can be oxidized for energy, re-esterified to triacylglycerols and stored (in adipose tissue and muscle), or re-esterified to phospholipids where they may become part of the cell membrane. Lipoprotein lipase reduces the triacylglycerol content of chylomicrons by about 75 percent and yields a chylomicron remnant that circulates to the liver where it is decomposed. Some of the lipid components will be repackaged into very low density lipoproteins (VLDL) that are synthesized by hepatocytes and secreted back into the blood. Presumably, dietary fatty acids originating from EPO or those previously stored in adipose tissue could be components of the VLDL synthesized by the liver. Once in circulation, lipoprotein lipase can again catalyze the removal of fatty acids (this time from VLDL), distributing them to tissues. The average turnover time for chylomicron triacyglycerols in the blood is about 7 minutes, whereas that for VLDL triacylglycerols is about 20 minutes (Olson, 1999).

The formation and clearance of chylomicrons in response to EPO supplementation has been studied in rats. Høy and Christensen (1996) administered an emulsion made of 0.3 mL EPO, 20 µCi [^{14}C]-oleic acid, 40 µCi [^{3}H]-cholesterol, and 10 ng di-pentadecanoyl-phosphatidylcholine through a feeding tube to male Wistar rats. They observed that the fatty acid profile of chylomicrons varied with time, reflecting the absorption of fat and the release of triacylglycerols into the lymph. By 8 hours, the chylomicron fatty acid composition reflected the composition of dietary EPO. The GLA was nearly evenly distributed among the three positions of the triacylglycerols within the chylomicrons. Further, the clearance of chylomicrons from circulation was rapid as indicated by the disappearance of labeled oleic acid (half-life ≈ 12 minutes) and cholesterol (half-life ≈ 5 minutes). Therefore, at least in the rat, the distribution of absorbed EPO appears to proceed in a similar manner to other dietary lipids.

Beyond the chylomicron, studies documenting the distribution of fatty acids originating specifically from EPO have not been reported. However, tracer studies using radio-labeled fatty acids, as well as tissue analysis following EPO or GLA supplementation, can be used to elucidate the distribution of specific fatty acids within the body. In vivo distribution of [1-^{14}C]-linoleic acid and [1-^{14}C]-GLA were compared following their administration by gavage to rats (Huang et al., 1996). After 24 hours, most of the radioactivity was recovered in phospholipids (mainly phosphatidycholine) and, to a lesser extent, in triacyglycerol fractions. Using [3-^{13}C]-GLA, Cunnane et al. (1996) observed that only low amounts (if any) of intact GLA reach the suckling rat or pig brain. Based on their results, the authors speculated that the low levels of GLA in the mammalian brain are due to relatively low access of GLA to the brain and are less likely due to rapid conversion of GLA to arachidonic acid. In rats fed diets with 10 percent (w/w) EPO for 11 weeks, significant incorporation of GLA into liver and adipose tissue triacylglycerols was observed; however, EPO did not appear to alter phospholipid omega-6 fatty acid concentrations in liver, heart, brain, kidney, or testes (Høy et al., 1983). In bulls fed 10 or 30 percent of the diet as evening primrose seed meal (containing 12.2 percent crude fat), the linoleic acid content of subcutaneous and kidney fat increased significantly, whereas the GLA content did not change (Strzetelski et al., 1998b). Only small amounts of GLA have been reported to accumulate in animal tissues, even after large quantities of GLA have been administered (see review by Phillips and Huang, 1996). This is likely due to the rapid elongation of GLA to DGLA, which is discussed further below.

Metabolism

Studies documenting the metabolism of fatty acids originating specifically from EPO have not been reported. However, tracer techniques have been used to elucidate the metabolism of specific long chain fatty acids, including linoleic acid and GLA.

Both linoleic acid and GLA are in the omega-6 fatty acid family and share some similar metabolic fates. Both fatty acids can be catabolized for energy via β-oxidation, resulting in the liberation of multiple acetyl-CoA molecules. These 2-carbon fragments can feed into the tricarboxylic acid cycle and subsequently undergo oxidative phosphorylation to generate adenosine tri-phosphate (ATP). However, there appears to be a preference for linoleic acid over GLA for energy production. Leyton et al. (1987) examined whole-body oxidation rates of omega-6 fatty acids in rats by measuring the radio-labeled carbon from the fatty acids in expired carbon dioxide over 24 hours. Seven hours after administration, the rate of oxidation of GLA, DGLA, and arachidonic acid was 27, 14, and 14 percent, respectively, of that observed for linoleic acid. Thus, the greater the degree of unsaturation and the longer the chain length, the slower the rate of fatty acid oxidation. Whole-body fatty acid balance studies in laboratory animals have shown that at the commonly accepted minimally adequate level for linoleic acid intake (2 percent of energy intake), complete oxidation accounts for about 75 percent of whole-body utilization of dietary linoleic acid. Only 6 percent is converted to longer chain omega-6 polyunsaturated fatty acids, while the rest is stored as linoleic acid itself, mostly in adipose tissue (as reviewed by Cunnane et al., 1996). At 0.3 percent of energy intake, at least 50 percent of dietary linoleic acid is still completely oxidized. With repeated cycles of 24-hour fasting followed by 72 hours refeeding, complete oxidation of linoleic acid exceeds 85 percent in male rats and can reach 100 percent in pregnancy (Cunnane et al., 1996).

Linoleic acid and GLA can also be used to synthesize longer-chain polyunsaturated fatty acids that play integral roles in cell membranes and maintenance of normal health. The process involves alternating steps of desaturation (the removal of two hydrogen atoms to create a double bond, via specific desaturase enzymes) and elongation of the fatty acid (by 2-carbon increments via elongase enzymes), thereby forming other fatty acids in the omega-6 family. Linoleic acid (C18:2) can be desaturated in a variety of tissues by Δ6-desaturase to form GLA (C18:3), which is rapidly elongated by two carbons to DGLA (C20:3). The cycle of desaturation and elongation continues when Δ5-desaturase acts on DGLA to form arachidonic acid (C20:4), which can be further elongated to adrenic acid (C22:4). The omega-6 fatty acid metabolic cascade is shown in Figure 7-2. In most mammals, linoleic acid is (or is presumed to be) metabolized by alternating desaturation and chain elongation reactions described above. In cats, an alternative pathway has been proposed, which bypasses the Δ6-desaturase step by first elongating linoleic acid (C18:2) to C20:2 and then desaturating this fatty acid with Δ8-desaturase to form DGLA (C20:3) (Frankel and Rivers, 1978; Sinclair et al., 1979). More recent evidence suggests that, at least in the liver, the cat possesses limited Δ6-desaturase, whereby linoleic acid can be directly desaturated to GLA and elongated to DGLA, as occurs in other mammals (Pawloski et al. 1994). Therefore, it is possible that both Δ6- and Δ8-desaturase function in the feline as routes of arachidonic acid and EPA synthesis. The synthesis of long-chain polyunsaturated fatty acids and their subsequent incorporation into membrane lipids are processes that are both localized primarily in the endoplasmic reticulum of the cell.

The enzymes involved in the desaturation of fatty acids (e.g., Δ6- and Δ5-desaturase) generally have limited activity. In addition, all long-chain fatty acids compete for the same desaturase enzymes. Members of the omega-3 fatty acid family (e.g., α-linolenic acid) have a greater affinity for desaturase enzymes, followed by omega-6 fatty acids (e.g., linoleic acid, GLA). The omega-9 fatty acids (e.g., oleic acid) have the lowest affinity (Gurr et al., 2002). However, omega-6 and omega-9 fatty acids are generally more prevalent in cell membranes; therefore, under normal conditions these fatty acid families are capable of securing a significant portion of the desaturase enzymes. Nonetheless, because the activities of Δ6- and Δ5-desaturase are limited, the desaturation steps are considered to be rate-limiting in the metabolism of long-chain fatty acids.

The activities of Δ6- and Δ5-desaturase, and thus the rate and amount of desaturation products (e.g., GLA, DGLA, and arachidonic acid) produced, can differ between species. In rats administered [1-^{14}C]-linoleic acid by oral gavage, most of the radioactivity remained as linoleic acid, whereas in rats given [1-^{14}C]-GLA up to two-thirds of the labeled fatty acid was elongated to DGLA and further metabolized to arachidonic acid (Huang et al., 1996). In the hamster, GLA feeding doubled the levels of DGLA in liver phospholipids, but only slightly increased the levels of arachidonic acid, demonstrating that the Δ5-desaturase activity in hamsters is very low (Ide et al., 1987). Similar to hamsters, rabbits have lower Δ5-desaturase activity. Administration of DGLA to rabbits had little effect on plasma arachidonic acid (Stone et al., 1979). In humans, excess linoleic acid intake has been shown to have no significant impact on circulating and tissue levels of GLA, DGLA, or arachidonic acid (Manku et al., 1988; Horrobin et al., 1991). In contrast, dietary supplementation with GLA significantly increased the levels of DGLA, and to a lesser extent, arachidonic acid in plasma phospholipids of humans (Manku et al., 1988; Richard et al., 1990). Therefore, both the Δ6- and Δ5-desaturase activities are slower in humans than rats (Ide et al., 1987). In the dog, the maximal velocity (V_{max}) for Δ6-desaturase was almost 10 times higher for α-linolenic acid than for linoleic acid in liver microsomes, compared to only a 3-fold difference in Δ6-desaturase V_{max} between these fatty acids in rats (Dunbar and Bauer, 2002). In contrast, the authors observed that the K_m for Δ6-desaturase was twice as high when using linoleic acid as a substrate than when using α-linolenic acid as a substrate. In addition, the concentrations of total free fatty acids and free linoleic acid were significantly higher and triacylglycerols significantly lower in dog liver microsomes than in rat liver microsomes. Both dogs and rats had very low concentrations of α-linolenic acid in liver microsomes. As a result, while α-linolenic acid is a preferential substrate for Δ6-desaturase, Dunbar and Bauer (2002) hypothesized that high dietary levels would probably be needed to effect physiological changes in omega-3 fatty acid metabolism in dogs. As mentioned earlier, both Δ5- and Δ6-desaturases appear to be active in cats, but the amount of activity does not appear to be adequate for maintaining tissue stores of long-chain polyunsaturated fatty acids (Pawloski et al., 1994). To the committee's knowledge, the relative activities of Δ6- and Δ5-desaturase in horses have not been established. Horses apparently have the ability to synthesize the longer-chain polyunsaturated fatty acids from the parent linoleic and α-linolenic acids, as evinced by the presence of archidonic acid, EPA, and docosahexaenoic acid (DHA) in cell membranes, despite not having consumed these fatty acids in the diet (Warren and Kivipelto, 2008).

In addition to species differences in fatty acid metabolism, there are differences between tissues, as not all cell types possess the ability to desaturate and elongate fatty acids. As reviewed by Huang et al. (1996), hepatocytes, human endothelial cells, fibroblasts, and lymphocytes can all desaturate and chain-elongate polyunsaturated fatty acids. Tissues other than liver do not sustain significant Δ6-desaturase activity. Kidney tissue cannot Δ6-desaturate linoleic acid to GLA, but can elongate GLA to DGLA, and to a smaller extent Δ5-desaturate DGLA to arachidonic acid. Platelets cannot desaturate linoleic acid to GLA, but can chain-elongate 18-carbon and 20-carbon unsaturated fatty acids. Mouse peritoneal macrophages possess an active elongase capable of converting GLA to DGLA, but possess only modest Δ5-desaturase activities. Feline brain appears to be able to desaturate C22:5*n-3* and C22:4*n-6* to C22:6*n-3* and C22:6*n-6*, respectively, whereas the same cannot happen in the cat's liver (Pawloski et al., 1994).

The longer-chain fatty acids can serve as replacements for oxidized fatty acids in the phospholipid bilayer of the cell membrane. Once incorporated into phospholipids, the fatty acids exert influence over cell membrane fluidity, protein receptor functioning, and gene transcription. The fatty acids can also be cleaved from the phospholipid by phospholipase A2 and transformed into eicosanoids, which serve as local mediators of inflammation, platelet aggregation, and blood pressure. Both DGLA and arachidonic acid can serve as precursors to eicosanoids, but they each yield a different series of these potent biological mediators. Eicosanoids generated from DGLA include the 1-series prostaglandins (e.g., PGE_1), prostacyclins (e.g., 6-keto-$PGF_{1\alpha}$), and thromboxanes (e.g., TxB_1) via cyclooxygenase and the 3-series leukotrienes via lipoxygenases. Eicosanoids generated from arachidonic acid include the 2-series prostaglandins (e.g., PGE_2), prostacyclins, and thromboxanes (e.g., TxB_2) via cyclooxygenase and the 4-series leukotrienes Figure 7-2. Eicosanoid formation represents a very small proportion of fatty acid turnover in the body (Gurr et al., 2002).

Excretion

Although not studied specifically, the excretion of fatty acids originating from EPO is likely no different than that of other oil products. Eicosanoids are metabolized very rapidly and their metabolites are excreted in the urine or bile (Gurr et al., 2002). Similarly, lipid hydroperoxides generated from fatty acid oxidation by free radicals and other reactive oxygen species will be catabolized. Fatty acids utilized for energy (ATP) production will result in carbon dioxide and water formation, which will be excreted via the lungs, urine, and sweat.

Purported Role in Health and Disease

The scientific and popular literature is replete with claims for the health benefits of GLA and EPO. Disorders for which the efficacy of EPO has been evaluated in controlled clinical trials in a variety of species include:

- Atopic dermatitis
- Rheumatoid arthritis
- Diabetic neuropathy
- Platelet aggregation
- Hypertension
- Multiple sclerosis
- Ulcerative colitis
- Premenstrual syndrome
- Hyperactivity
- Several cancers.

The available data on EPO supplementation in horses, dogs, and cats pale in comparison to the hundreds of studies performed in rodents and humans. Regardless of the animal model, results have been equivocal in almost all categories listed above. It is beyond the scope of the statement of task to address the efficacy of EPO (see Chapter 1). Therefore, the reader is directed towards published reviews and meta-analyses that discuss the efficacy of dietary EPO supplementation on various diseases and medical conditions (Horrobin, 1992, 1993; Kemper, 1999; Belch and Hill, 2000; Barre, 2001; Morse and Clough, 2006).

Regardless of their dietary origin, GLA and linoleic acid are widely recognized for their contributions to the maintenance of normal health and metabolism. The biological roles of these fatty acids are described in earlier sections of this chapter.

Drug Interactions

Early reports implied that EPO could cause or exacerbate epilepsy or seizures, particularly in schizophrenic patients or patients taking epileptogenic drugs such as phenothiazines (Vaddadi, 1981; Holman, 1983). A letter to the editor describing the possible exacerbation of epilepsy in a dog being fed a supplement containing EPO was also reported in the Veterinary Record (Arundel, 1992). As a result, many EPO monographs and herbal physician desk references have recommended that EPO be used cautiously in schizophrenic and epileptic patients or those treated with phenothiazines. However, the validity of these claims has recently been called into question by Puri (2007). The author highlighted that all five human patients being treated for schizophrenia were taking phenothiazines at the time of their alleged EPO-induced epileptic seizures, which are capable of lowering the threshold for seizures. Similarly, the dog that experienced a seizure while receiving an EPO-containing supplement (Arundel, 1992) had a history of epilepsy and seizures as evinced by maintenance of the dog on primidone, an antiseizure medication. In addition, Puri (2007) cited evidence of a strong link between schizophrenia and epilepsy, irrespective of the epileptogenic potential of phenothiazine treatment. Because of these factors, the author encouraged formularies to remove seizures and epilepsy as side effects of EPO, as well as removal of historical seizures or epilepsy as a contraindication to taking EPO. Despite the arguments presented by Puri (2007), new evidence that EPO does not induce seizures in schizophrenic or epileptic patients has not been introduced. Although linoleic and α-linolenic acid supplementation have shown no effect on seizure latency, duration, average severity, or incidence in rats (Taha et al., 2006), well-controlled clinical trials are still needed to elucidate potential complications of EPO and/or GLA supplementation in schizophrenic and epileptic patients. Phenothiazines are also commonly used as sedatives in animals; therefore, potential interactions should be investigated in EPO-supplemented animals given these drugs.

Theoretically, the biologically active drugs that affect prostaglandin metabolism, such as nonsteroidal anti-inflammatory drugs (NSAID) and corticosteroids, could alter the biological activity of GLA in EPO. Many NSAIDs reversibly (e.g., ibuprofen) or irreversibly (e.g., aspirin) block cyclooxygenase 1 and 2 enzymes from binding with arachidonic acid, thereby reducing 2-series prostaglandin release. The NSAID meclofenamate was shown to block changes in lung resistance and dynamic compliance induced by intravenous DGLA injection in mechanically ventilated paralyzed cats, presumably due to inhibition of prostaglandin production from DGLA (Levin et al., 1982).

Evening primrose oil has been shown to inhibit platelet aggregation in rats (Schölkens et al., 1982) and rabbits (De La Cruz, 1997) and to inhibit platelet-activating factor in humans (van Doormaal et al., 1988). Potentially, animals treated with anticoagulant drugs in conjunction with EPO should be monitored, as EPO supplementation may enhance the effects of these drugs.

Intragastric administration of EPO to rats was shown to enhance the hypotensive effects of dihydralazine, clonidine, and captopril (Hoffmann et al., 1984). Prostaglandin E_2 is the main arachidonic acid metabolite in the kidneys where it reduces antidiuretic hormone-induced water reabsorption and may help to control renin release (Gurr et al., 2002). The GLA in EPO, through its transformation to DGLA, competes with arachidonic acid for cyclooxygenase, resulting in greater production of the 1-series prostaglandins and less PGE_2 production.

Diet Interactions

The effects other components in the diet have on the bioavailability of EPO have not been well studied. The absorption of various oils and other dietary lipids has been shown to be reduced by high levels of dietary fiber in humans (Gurr et al., 2002). Similarly, it is unknown if the biological activity of GLA in EPO is altered with the manner in which it is given (e.g., whether EPO is given with food or not, or in single or multiple daily doses).

It is also unknown if EPO alters the absorption of other nutrients provided in the diet. In general, high levels of dietary fat have been shown to reduce fiber, protein, and calcium digestion in some species, which could ultimately affect dietary nutrient requirements. Dietary fat also facilitates the absorption of fat-soluble vitamins. In most cases this is beneficial for meeting the animal's vitamin requirements, but conditions may also exist to produce fat-soluble vitamin toxicity. None of these factors, however, is likely to be unique to EPO.

Evening primrose oil has the potential to affect vitamin E requirements if supplemented in large quantities. As a free radical scavenger, vitamin E protects cells from the potentially damaging effects of toxic oxygen radicals, whose major source is lipid metabolism. The dietary requirement of vitamin E, therefore, is linked to the dietary intake of polyunsaturated fatty acids (such as the linoleic acid and GLA in EPO). In particular, high-fat diets can induce a relative vitamin E deficiency. Typically, the expense of EPO would limit its use as the sole source of fat in a high-fat diet for horses, dogs, or cats. Nonetheless, EPO used in combination with other polyunsaturated fatty acids to create a high-fat diet would still impact vitamin E requirements.

The activities of the various enzymes involved in fatty acid metabolism have been shown to be affected by the carbohydrate, protein, minerals, and vitamins in the diet. Dietary protein quantity and quality have been shown to influence the activity of $\Delta5$- and $\Delta6$-desaturase enzymes. Feeding a low-protein diet to lactating rats strongly decreased the activity of $\Delta5$- and $\Delta6$-desaturase enzymes (Chanussot et al., 1988), whereas feeding diets high in casein were shown to increase these enzymes in rats (Peluffo et al., 1984). Although the activity of desaturase enzymes was not directly measured, higher concentrations of arachidonic acid and DHA (i.e., the desaturase products of linoleic and α-linolenic acids, respectively) were detected in liver and adipose tissue of cats fed casein compared to corn gluten (Szabo et al., 2003). Zinc and magnesium are cofactors for the desaturase enzymes, and zinc, calcium, and pyridoxine promote elongase activity (Bettger et al., 1979; Cunnane et al., 1984; Huang et al., 1988). Ultimately, the nutritional adequacy of the animal's basal diet may alter the metabolism of linoleic acid and GLA in supplemented EPO.

The sudden addition of large quantities of oil to the diet of an animal unaccustomed to a high level of dietary fat can result in side effects (e.g., diarrhea) or potentially more serious adverse events. As recommended for any dietary fat source, the animal should be adapted to EPO feeding by gradually increasing the amount fed over a sufficient period of time. In the committee's experience, the amount of time needed for adaptation to dietary fats and oils varies between species and between individual animals.

Impact of Disease

In disease conditions where lipid metabolism may be altered (e.g., hyperlipemia, hepatic dysfunction, renal failure, diabetes, or gastrointestinal disease), supplementation with any oil, including EPO, should be done with caution, unless the supplementation level is very low or the EPO is substituted for other fats in the diet while keeping the total level of fat in the diet constant.

Vulnerable Populations

Eicosanoids, particularly the various prostaglandins, are intimately involved in reproduction, including follicular development, ovulation, luteolysis and maternal recognition of pregnancy, and parturition (Allen and Harris, 2001; Weems et al., 2004). The 2-series prostaglandins (especially $PGF_{2\alpha}$ and PGE_2) derived from arachidonic acid dominate among the prostaglandins generated, likely because of the prevalence of arachidonic acid in cell membranes compared to other fatty acid precursors. As a source of linoleic acid and GLA, both of which are precursors to arachidonic acid, EPO has the potential to provide substrate for $PGF_{2\alpha}$ production. Furthermore, due to the rapid elongation of GLA to DGLA, EPO has the potential to shift the prostaglandin produced from a 2-series (derived from arachidonic acid) to a 1-series (derived from DGLA). The 2-series prostaglandins exhibit more potent biological activity than the 1- series (or 3-series) (Allen and Harris, 2001; Weems et al., 2006). Ultimately, by altering the types and ratios of the various prostaglandin series present through dietary fatty acid supplementation, reproductive function could be altered.

The effects of EPO on reproductive function have been investigated in only a few research studies. A retrospective analysis of records of healthy pregnant women found that EPO supplementation (0.5–1.5 g EPO/day) from week 37 of gestation to birth did not alter length of gestation or decrease overall length of labor (Dove and Johnson, 1999). However, there was a trend for a more protracted active phase of labor, prolonged rupture of membranes, and arrest of fetal descent in women receiving EPO supplementation (Dove and Johnson, 1999). Although the study design limits the establishment of a causal relationship, this study indicates that EPO supplementation may affect events associated with parturition. Frankel and Rivers (1988) fed cats a food containing EPO as the sole source of fat. The cats were successfully maintained on this diet for 10 months prior to breeding. While two of the three cats carried their kittens to term, only one live kitten was born. Because the EPO-added food was deficient in arachidonic acid and omega-3 fatty acids, the reproductive failure was most likely due to essential fatty acid deficiency. Tauson and Forsberg (1991) supplemented the diets of blue fox with EPO (4.5 mL EPO/day) during the breeding season through gestation and observed a lower incidence of barren females, but an increased rate of abortions compared to fox receiving the control diet. A study by the same researchers in mink found no effect of daily EPO supplementation (approximately 0.75 g/kg BW during gestation and 1.5 g/kg BW during lactation) on female reproductive performance, kit live weight, or kit growth rate (Tauson et al., 1991). Huang et al. (1992) supplemented rats with 5 percent EPO (resulting in an estimated daily intake of 1.5 g EPO/kg BW and 135 mg GLA/kg BW) and observed no differences in conception rates or litter size over four consecutive gestation/lactation cycles compared to rats fed an equal amount of safflower oil. The available data indicate there may be some species differences in the overall effects of EPO supplementation on reproductive function. While EPO supplementation likely contributes to the prostaglandin pool, predicting the changes in the pattern of prostaglandin synthesis following dietary modulation of fatty acids is difficult (Abayasekara and Wathes, 1999). In general, EPO appears to be unlikely to significantly alter the prostaglandin population and negatively affect reproductive performance unless fed in significant quantities or unless the female has altered essential fatty acid status or metabolism.

In one report (Levin et al., 1982) intrapulmonic arterial infusion of DGLA in cats resulted in increased airway resistance and constriction of the large and small airways. It is not possible to relate this dose or route of administration to oral intake in cats. While these data could suggest concern for use of high levels of DGLA or its precursors (i.e., EPO or GLA) in cats with asthma, GLA and its metabolite, PGE_1, are known to have the opposite effect in cats (bronchodilation, decreased lung resistance, and increased compliance) and would be considered beneficial in this same population.

SAFETY

Safety Studies

Target Species

Horses

To the committee's knowledge, acute toxicity studies designed to establish the mean lethal dose (LD_{50}) of orally administered EPO have not been performed in horses or other equids. Similarly, there appear to be no studies evaluating a dose response or chronic intake of EPO to establish the potential for subchronic or chronic toxicity in the horse.

Dogs

To the committee's knowledge, acute toxicity studies designed to establish the LD_{50} of orally administered EPO have not been performed in dogs or other canids.

Only one study investigating the potential for chronic EPO toxicity in the canine has been published. Everett et al. (1988a) supplemented 20 male and 20 female Beagle dogs with either 0, 1, 3, or 5 mL EPO/kg BW/day (corresponding to approximately 0, 1,000, 3,000, or 5,000 mg EPO/kg BW). Corn oil was used to balance each treatment so that all dogs received 5 percent total oil in the diet (w/w). The dogs weighed approximately 7 kg resulting in EPO doses of 0, 7, 21, or 35 mL/day. The EPO was a commercially available supplement (Efamol, Scotia Pharmaceuticals, Inc.) and contained 8.5–9 percent GLA and 70–73 percent linoleic acid. Therefore, dogs supplemented with EPO received between 0.6 and 3.1 mL GLA per day (approximately 88–438 mg/kg BW). Oils were administered by gavage and the dogs were supplemented for a total of 52 weeks. Food intake and body weight were monitored throughout the trial. Evaluations of blood hematology, blood chemistry, clotting time, reticulocyte count, and urinalysis were conducted at 0, 12, 26, and 50 weeks, and ophthalmoscopic examinations were conducted at 0, 25, and 52 weeks. At the termination of the study, dogs were euthanized and a postmortem analysis was conducted, including external and internal examination, description of gross lesions, and histopathological analysis of tissues. The authors reported the death of one dog fed an intermediate dose of evening primrose oil at week 46; the cause of death was not disclosed, but the authors stated it was not related to EPO intake. Upon necropsy, all groups (including corn oil-supplemented controls) had accumulation of oil droplets in the lungs and proliferation of lung alveolar macrophages. The authors stated that this finding was typical of animals given high doses of oil by gavage, but cited no supporting evidence from other researchers. The authors also stated that there were no consistent statistically significant differences in hematology, blood chemistry, body weight, organ weight, and organ histopathology between EPO and corn oil treatments; however, these data were not presented. The authors concluded that EPO appeared to be as safe as an equivalent weight of corn oil. This study used an appropriate control group, ample indicators of toxicity, and adequate trial length to assess chronic toxicity. However, the actual data collected from the dogs, while alluded to in the text, were not presented in the publication. As a result, critical evaluation of the data is not possible.

Cats

To the committee's knowledge, acute toxicity studies designed to establish the LD_{50} of orally administered EPO have not been performed in cats or other felids. In addition, there appear to be no studies evaluating chronic intake or varying doses of EPO to ascertain the potential for subchronic or chronic toxicity in the cat.

Nontarget Species

To the committee's knowledge, acute toxicity studies designed to establish the LD_{50} of orally administered EPO have not been performed in rodents or other nontarget species.

One study designed to investigate the potential for EPO to elicit chronic toxicity has been published using rats. Everett et al. (1988a) supplemented 100 male and 100 female Sprague-Dawley rats with 0, 0.3, 1.0, or 2.5 mL EPO/kg BW/day. Corn oil was used to balance each treatment so that all rats received 2.5 percent total oil in the diet (w/w). Rats entered the study at 5–6 weeks of age. The weight of the rats during the trial was not provided. Assuming male and female Sprague-Dawley rats weighed 120 g at the start of the trial, this would result in a daily EPO dose of 0, 0.036, 0.120, and 0.300 mL. Assuming male rats weighed 400 g and female rats weighed 250 g at the end of the trial, the daily EPO dose would be 0, 0.12, 0.4, and 1.0 mL for male rats and 0, 0.075, 0.250, and 0.625 mL for female rats by the end of the trial. The EPO was a commercially available supplement (Efamol, Scotia Pharmaceuticals, Inc.) and contained 8.5–9 percent GLA and 70–73 percent linoleic acid. Therefore, EPO-supplemented rats were receiving 3–26 μL GLA per day at the beginning of the trial and 7–88 μL GLA per day at the end of the trial (25–220 mg/kg BW). Oils were administered by gavage and rats were supplemented for 50 weeks. Food intake and body weight, blood hematology, blood chemistry, clotting time, urinalysis, and ophthalmoscopic examinations were performed at regular intervals. At the termination of the study, rats were euthanized and postmortem analysis, including external and internal examination and description of gross lesions was conducted. In addition, histopathological analysis of tissues was performed on 10 male and 10 female control and high EPO-dose rats. The authors reported the premature death of 11 rats, five in the control group (corn oil only) and six in the EPO-treated groups. The cause of the deaths was not disclosed; rather the authors stated "none of the deaths could be attributed to Efamol treatment." There were no significant differences between the different oil-treated groups in clinical signs, food consumption, or body weight changes. In addition, no consistent differences were seen in blood hematology, urinalysis, or clinical chemistry. Six EPO-treated rats were described as exhibiting areas of necrosis in the abdominal fat, which was not observed in control rats. The researchers stated the abdominal fat necrosis was likely a "chance occurrence" because the condition had been seen previously in their laboratory in control-fed rats; however, no supporting evidence from other researchers was cited. Male EPO-treated rats showed modestly reduced liver weights, but no histological abnormalities, which was also seen in controls. Six out of the 25 high-dose EPO-treated rats and 2 out of the 25 controls showed testicular shrinkage or softening. The researchers concluded that EPO appeared to be as safe as an equivalent weight of corn oil. Similar to the chronic toxicity study performed in dogs (which was conducted by the same authors), this study used an appropriate control group, ample indicators of toxicity, and adequate trial length to assess chronic toxicity. However, most, but not all, data were provided in the publication. Furthermore, potential signals of chronic toxicity (i.e., necrosis of abdominal fat and testicular shrinkage) were either superficially addressed or explanations simply not provided. In particular, the "necrosis" observed in abdominal fat tissue may have relevance to the safety of EPO in cats, if it was associated with pansteatitis; however, the similarity between the fat necrosis and pansteatitis could not be determined with the information provided by the authors.

Another study conducted by the same group (Everett et al., 1988b) investigated the potential carcinogenicity of EPO using rats and mice. In this study, 250 male and 250 female Sprague-Dawley rats were supplemented with 0, 0.3, 1.0, or 2.5 mL EPO/kg BW/day. The EPO was a commercially available supplement (Efamol, Scotia Pharmaceuticals, Inc.) and contained 8.5–9 percent GLA and 70–73 percent linoleic acid. Corn oil was used to balance the fat-added treatments so that they received 2.5 percent total oil in the diet (w/w). Fifty male and 50 female rats were not fed any oil (non-fat added diet) and were just maintained on a basal diet of standard laboratory chow. Rats entered the study at 5–6 weeks of age. The weight of the rats during the trial was not provided, but using the same assumptions described above, daily GLA intake can be estimated to range from 25–220 mg/kg BW over the course of the trial. Oils were administered by gavage and rats were supplemented for 104 weeks. All animals that died prior to the end of the study and all remaining animals at 104 weeks were subjected to complete postmortem examination with histopathological analysis of organs. An additional 250 male and 250 female CD-1 mice were also entered into a similar study at 5–6 weeks of age. Because the mice have a shorter lifespan than rats, the mouse study was terminated at 78 weeks; otherwise, the study design and objectives were similar to the study in rats. No biologically or statistically significant differences in tumor incidence existed between the EPO-supplemented diets and either the corn-oil control diet or the basal diet control animals. This study was well designed, but briefly described. In addition, not all data were presented for inspection.

In Vitro

To the committee's knowledge, no cytotoxicity studies using EPO have been performed in cell cultures in vitro.

Nonsafety Studies

Target Species

Horses

Two clinical research trials have been conducted in which horses were supplemented with EPO. In a double-blind, placebo-controlled trial, Craig et al. (1997) investigated the effects of EPO on adult horses and ponies (3–15 years of age) that had a history of recurrent seasonal pruritis. A commercially available mixed oil (Efamol Vet, Scotia Pharmaceuticals, Inc.) consisting of 80 percent EPO (containing 7.9 percent GLA) and 20 percent cold-water marine fish oil was provided to 16 horses/ponies. Another 17 horses/ponies received hydrogenated coconut oil and served as a control group. The oils were top-dressed on the evening feed by the individual horse owners at a rate of 0.1 g oil/kg BW. Thus, the horses treated with the mixed EPO received approximately 80 mg EPO/kg BW and 7.9 mg GLA/kg BW. Beyond the oils supplemented to the horses, the rest of the diet composition was not described. Horses were supplemented with the mixed EPO oil for 12 weeks. After 12 weeks, all horses/ponies were placed on the mixed EPO treatment for an additional 12 weeks. Blood samples were obtained from all horses at the start of the trial and at 12 and 24 weeks after supplementation commenced and analyzed for plasma phospholipid fatty acid concentrations. At week 12, horses receiving the mixed EPO had reduced linoleic acid concentrations in plasma phospholipids, and at 24 weeks EPO-treated horses had elevated levels of DGLA and α-linolenic acid in plasma phospholipids. Compared to the placebo, horses supplemented with mixed EPO had greater DGLA in plasma phospholipids after 12 weeks of supplementation. At 24 weeks, no differences in plasma phospholipid fatty acid concentration existed, as all horses had continued on the same mixed EPO from week 12 to 24. Finding measurable DGLA in the plasma phospholipids, as well as a rise in DGLA without a concurrent increase in GLA, suggests the horse is capable of rapidly elongating GLA originating from EPO to DGLA. In addition, the lack of change in the arachidonic acid concentration in plasma phospholipids indicates that Δ5-desaturase (and Δ6-desaturase) are rate-limiting steps in the metabolism of omega-6 fatty acids in the horse, similar to that observed in other species. Two horses receiving the mixed EPO were eliminated from the study prior to completion at 24 weeks. One horse was withdrawn after 4 weeks because it had developed "loose droppings," but the authors provided no information about whether this was due to EPO supplementation or some other cause. None of the other horses were described as having loose feces. The second horse was withdrawn due to owner noncompliance with the supplement protocol. Besides skin scrapings and clinical and owner evaluation of skin and pruritis severity (all related to the objectives of the study), no other data were reported. The authors provided no comments about the horses' general health or acceptance of the oil.

In a randomized, controlled (but not blinded) trial, Reilly et al. (1998) supplemented mature Irish draft–Thoroughbred cross horses with an oil mixture containing EPO in an effort to determine its effects on hoof growth and hoof lipid fractions. Six horses were supplemented with 30 mL/day of an oil mixture containing 18.75 mL EPO, 8.15 mL maize oil, and 3 mL cod liver oil. Body weights of EPO-treated horses ranged from 574–675 kg. The GLA content of the EPO or oil mixture was not provided by the authors. Assuming the EPO portion of the oil mixture contained 9 percent GLA (Court et al., 1993), 18.75 mL EPO per day would result in an estimated daily intake of 25–33 mg EPO/kg BW and 2.5–2.95 mg GLA/kg BW. An additional six horses received no oil supplementation and served as controls. The diet of the horses was described as follows: 6.8 kg of hay or haylage, split into two feedings daily; an additional 1.4 kg of roughage-based ingredients (> 18 percent crude fiber), and 1.4 kg of a grain mix concentrate. Feeds were reported to contain 2–3 percent crude fat, indicating that none of the feeds contained exogenous oil sources. Horses were supplemented with the mixed EPO for 164 days (≈ 23.4 weeks). With the exception of hoof measurements and sampling of hoof horn, no other data were reported. Supplementation with the mixed EPO did not alter hoof growth. One horse receiving the mixed EPO was removed from the study after 60 days due to "work commitments." The authors provided no comments about the horses' general health or acceptance of the oil.

Dogs

Lloyd and co-workers (Bond and Lloyd, 1992a,b; Scarff and Lloyd, 1992; Bond et al., 1993; Sture and Lloyd, 1995) published a number of studies evaluating the effect of EPO on skin health in adult dogs with atopy and/or pruritis (see summary in Table 7-5). Many of these studies used a combination of EPO and fish oil. The majority of the studies were blinded to treatment and placebo-controlled. The typical therapeutic dosage was lower than most of the dosages used by Everett et al. (1988a) to assess chronic toxicity. In many of these studies, however, it is difficult to determine the daily EPO intake because dosages were reported on a per kilogram body weight basis and body weight was not reported. For studies where a dosage calculation was possible, daily EPO intake ranged from 42 to 424 mg/kg BW, whereas it ranged from 1,000 to 5,000 mg/kg BW in the study by Everett et al. (1988a). Daily GLA intake ranged from 4 to

TABLE 7-5 Summary of Published Studies Investigating the Use of Evening Primrose Oil as a Dietary Supplement in Canids

Source of EPO	Species or Breed	No./ Diet	EPO dosage (mg/kg BW/ day)	GLA intake (mg/kg BW/day)	Duration	Design	Effects	Source
Evening Primrose Oil	Dog (Beagle)	10	0, 1,000, 3,000, 5,000	87.5–437.5	52 weeks	Substituted for corn oil; terminal study	No differences food intake, body weight, hematology, blood chemistry, ophthalmoscopic exams, histology	Everett et al. (1988a)
Evening Primrose Oil	Dog, variety of breeds, chronic pruritis	30	300	—	Placebo (olive oil) 3 weeks then placebo or EPO for 9 weeks, then opposite treatment for 9 weeks	Double blind, placebo-controlled crossover; placebo = olive oil	Improved erythema. Trend for improved pruritis, edema, and overall severity of skin symptoms. Increased plasma linoleic acid, arachidonic acid	Scarff and Lloyd (1992)
Efa Vet Regular (combo of EPO and fish oil)	Dog, variety of breeds, atopic dogs that had done well on Efa Vet (length of treatment unreported)	11	60–424 (mean 164)	5–36 (mean 14.1)	8 weeks	Double-blind, placebo-controlled; placebo = olive oil	Increased DGLA in blood of EPO dogs; no difference in blood linoleic, eicosapentaenoic and arachidonic acid	Bond and Lloyd (1992a)
Efa Vet (combo of EPO and fish oil) vs. HGF (concentrated source of fatty acids, but composition not described)	Dog, variety of breeds, atopic dogs previously responded well to Efa Vet	14	60–400 (mean 180) while on Efa Vet	5–34 (mean 15.5)	16 weeks (but had previously been on it for an unspecified period of time)	Randomized, single blind	Comparable efficacy; no negative effects reported	Bond and Lloyd (1992b)
HGF	Dog, atopic, previously responded poorly to EPO/fish oil combination	11	Pretest (4 months) 140–244 (mean 164)	12–21 (mean 15.5) pretest; 14 test	12 weeks	Case report	Diarrhea in one dog fed HGF; 8 of 11 dogs could decrease their prednisone intake; no negative effects of supplementation	Bond and Lloyd (1994)
Efa Vet or HGF capsules	Dog, atopic	—	Unknown	11–30 (mean 19.5)	8–18 weeks	Clinical trial	Decreased intradermal test response to allergens in some dogs	Bond et al. (1993)
Evening primrose oil compared to Efa Vet, DVM Derm Caps and fish oil	Dog, allergic pruritis	20	42	4.4	2 weeks	Double blind clinical trial, crossover (all dogs received all supplements)	Loose stools in one dog when fed any of the oil supplements	Scott et al. (1992)

continued

TABLE 7-5 Continued

Source of EPO	Species or Breed	No./ Diet	EPO dosage (mg/kg BW/ day)	GLA intake (mg/kg BW/day)	Duration	Design	Effects	Source
EPO/fish oil vs. olive oil placebo	Dog, atopic	15	Phase One 129; Phase Two 181	—	9 weeks per phase	3 weeks on olive oil, then Phase 1 = EPO/fish oil or olive oil; after 9 weeks crossover then continue 9 weeks	Some dogs appeared better, but no statistically significant differences	Sture and Lloyd (1995)
Efa-Vet 1 followed by Efa-Vet Regular	Dog, onychomadesis, Giant Schnauzer	1	Unknown	6–7	52 months	Case report	Claws returned to normal, no adverse effects reported	Bergvall (1998)
Efa-Vet 1 followed by Efa-Vet Regular	Dog with sudden loss of 8 claws, German Shepherd	1	Unknown	5	42 months	Case report	Claws markedly improved, no adverse effects reported	Bergvall (1998)
Efa-Vet 1 followed by Efa-Vet Regular	Dog with history of claw problems, Wirehaired Standard Dachshund	1	Unknown	3–3.4	34 months	Case report	Claws markedly improved, no adverse effects reported	Bergvall (1998)
Efa-Vet 1 followed by Efa-Vet Regular	Dog, onychomadesis and onycho-dystrophy, Giant Schnauzer	1	Unknown	6–7	31 months	Case report	Claws returned to normal, no adverse effects reported	Bergvall (1998)
Efa-Vet 1	Dog, acute claw loss, Standard Schnauzer	1	Unknown	3	30 months	Case report	Claws returned to normal, no adverse effects reported	Bergvall (1998)

36 mg/kg BW, whereas it ranged from 88 to 438 mg/kg BW in the study by Everett et al. (1988a). Plasma linoleic and arachidonic acids increased in dogs supplemented daily with 300 mg EPO/kg BW for 9 weeks (Scarff and Lloyd, 1992). Plasma linoleic acid, arachidonic acid, and EPA were similar in control dogs and dogs fed an EPO/fish oil supplement (Bond and Lloyd, 1992a), whereas plasma DGLA was lower in the control dogs. The GLA consumption in this study was estimated to be lower (approximately half) than the GLA consumption reported by Scarff and Lloyd (1992). Despite long-term use (up to 118 weeks in one study), the only side effect observed was loose stools in a small percentage of dogs (Scott et al., 1992; Bond and Lloyd, 1994). Although the dogs had dermatological conditions, there is no reason to believe that they would be more tolerant to excess primrose oil than clinically healthy dogs.

Cats

Four clinical studies have examined the use of EPO supplementation in the treatment of feline skin disorders. Only one of these studies was double-blinded and controlled (Logas and Kunkle, 1993). In that study, adult cats diagnosed with pruritic dermatitis received 0.5 mL EPO/day (which provided 37 mg GLA/day) and a control group of cats received an equivalent amount of olive oil. Ages and body weights of the cats were not provided by the investigators, but they indicated the EPO dose level was chosen for an average 4.54 kg adult cat; thus, the daily amount of EPO supplementation can be estimated at 110 mg/kg BW and daily GLA at 8.15 mg/kg BW. Cats were housed with their respective owners during the course of the study, and the owner of each cat administered the daily allowance of EPO or olive oil. Of the 15 cats that started the study, 11 finished all 8 weeks of supplementation. Reasons for removal from the study included owner noncompliance (n = 1), illness requiring prednisone therapy (n=1), and worsening of skin condition (n = 2). Of the remaining 11 cats, 7 received EPO treatment and 4 received olive oil. The authors stated that "no side effects attributable to the supplements were noted by the owners or the investigator for either group." However, it is worth noting that only external clinical symptoms were monitored by the investigators, as blood and tissue samples were not obtained during the study.

An open, controlled clinical trial randomly assigned 11 adult cats (≥ 3 years) diagnosed with papulocrustous dermatitis to either EPO or sunflower oil (which served as the isocaloric control group) supplementation for 12 weeks (supplementation occurred from week 7 to week 19) (Harvey, 1993b). Cats were entered into the study over a period of 2 months. Cats received 0.25 mL of EPO (n = 6) or sunflower oil (n = 5) per day. Based on this amount, and assuming an average body weight of 4 kg (NRC, 2006), daily EPO intake can be estimated at 62.5 mg/kg BW. Supplements were withdrawn from weeks 19–24. The cats were maintained on their original diets and were owner-fed during the trial. Blood samples were taken at the start of the trial and after 6, 12, 18, and 24 weeks, and the fatty acid composition of plasma and the phospholipid fraction of red blood cells were determined. Cats were examined clinically at 3-week intervals and scored for coat condition. No significant changes in plasma fatty acid concentrations were found. Analysis of the fatty acid composition of erythrocyte phospholipids showed an increase in oleic and linoleic acids in response to supplementation (at week 18), but no change in GLA, DGLA, or arachidonic acid. Two additional clinical trials, although open and uncontrolled, have also reported on EPO supplementation in cats with skin disorders. Harvey (1993a) supplemented 14 adult cats (≥ 1 year) diagnosed with miliary dermatitis with varying proportions of EPO and fish oil, totaling 0.5 mL/day for 24 weeks. The dosing schedule for all cats was reported as follows: weeks 1–6, 100 percent EPO; weeks 7–12, 80 percent EPO + 20 percent fish oil; weeks 13–18, 100 percent fish oil; weeks 19–24, 80 percent EPO + 20 percent fish oil. From these figures, and assuming an average BW of 4 kg (NRC, 2006), daily EPO intake can be estimated at 125 mg/kg BW when EPO was 100 percent of the supplement and 100 mg/kg BW when EPO was 80 percent of the supplement. The EPO was administered from a dropper. The fish oil and EPO/fish oil mixture were administered in 0.5-mL gelatin capsules. The cats were maintained on their original diets (owner-fed). The animals were examined at 3-week intervals and the presence or absence of crusted papules and other cutaneous lesions was determined. Blood samples were obtained at 6-week intervals and analyzed for changes in serum fatty acid content. Of the 14 cats, seven completed the entire 24-week protocol. Three cats withdrew after 12 weeks, two because of lack of response and one for noncompliance. A further four cats were withdrawn after 18 weeks because of their clinical deterioration. The author commented that "no side effects were observed in any of the cats during the period of study." No changes in serum linoleic acid, GLA, DGLA, or arachidonic acid were observed during the 24-week period. Serum EPA concentrations increased with the onset of the inclusion of fish oil in the supplement from weeks 6 through 24. In an earlier clinical trial, Harvey (1991) reported feeding a commercial preparation containing essential fatty acids (Efavet No. 2, Efamol Vet) to a group of 10 cats with miliary dermatitis for 3 months. The author reported that the supplement consisted of a blend of EPO and fish oil; however, the fatty acid composition of the supplement, the quantity of oil fed (it was simply stated that two capsules of the product were fed), and the body weights of the cats were not provided. Although the manufacturer of this product is still in existence, it is difficult to determine if the current Efavet product contains a similar fatty acid profile as the product used by Harvey (1991). Unfortunately, despite the author stating that ". . . the cats tolerated the capsules well," no other useful information can be gleaned from this study to evaluate safety.

While looking at the effects of various fatty acids on platelet aggregation, Davidson and Haggan (1990) supplemented the diets of adult and juvenile cats with EPO at a rate of 25 g/kg diet for 270 days. The EPO contained 8.5 percent GLA. The body weights of cats and DM intake were not presented; however, assuming an average body weight of 4 kg, daily caloric intake of 250 kcal and a diet energy content of 4 kcal/g (NRC, 2006), it can be estimated that the cats consumed an average of 391 mg EPO/kg BW and 33 mg GLA/kg BW per day. Cats fed the high EPO diet had similar aggregation profiles to cats fed the control food. The authors did not report the health status of the cats.

In an early study investigating the fatty acid requirements of cats, Frankel and Rivers (1978) included EPO at a rate of 125 g/kg diet in a semipurified complete food. The GLA made up 2.9 percent of the total fatty acids in the diet. The EPO source added to the food contained 7 percent GLA (as described in Rivers and Frankel, 1980); therefore, not all of the GLA in the diet originated from EPO. Six adult cats were used in a crossover design. All cats had previously been maintained on diets that provided only linoleic and α-linolenic acids and were thus deficient in long-chain polyunsaturated fatty acids (e.g., arachidonic acid) for 18 months prior to the start of the study. Half the cats remained on the fatty acid deficient (control) diet and the other three cats received the EPO-supplemented diet for 5 days. The EPO-supplemented cats were then returned to the fatty acid deficient (control) diet for 7 weeks and the opposite three cats were given the EPO-supplemented diet for 5 days. The body weights of cats were not provided by the authors and cats were allowed to eat ad libitum. Assuming an average body weight of 4 kg, daily caloric intake of 250 kcal, and diet energy content of 4 kcal/g (NRC, 2006), daily intake by cats can be estimated at 1,953 mg EPO/kg BW and 227 mg GLA/kg BW (136.5 mg GLA/kg BW directly from EPO). Evidence of GLA and DGLA in plasma phospholipids indicated the cats absorbed the fatty acids in EPO and that it was elongated to DGLA. Plasma arachidonic acid in EPO-supplemented cats was not different than that observed when cats received the fatty acid deficient diet. Some general signs of improvement in skin condition and estrus cycling were noted, compared to fatty acid deficient cats, but the authors commented that GLA alone could not be used to meet the fatty acid requirements of the cat.

In an effort to investigate the effects of omega-3 fatty acids on reproduction and fetal development in cats, Frankel and Rivers (1988) formulated an omega-3 deficient diet using soybean oil and EPO as the primary fat sources and compared the response to that of cats fed a fatty acid-sufficient diet. Actual diet composition was not provided in this study, but had been reported in an earlier report by Rivers and Frankel (1980) in which EPO was included at 125 g/kg diet. Thus, the EPO-added diet was similar to the study described above (Frankel and Rivers, 1978). The cats (three on each treatment) were successfully maintained on this diet for 10 months prior to breeding and through gestation. While two of the three cats on the EPO-added diet carried their kittens to term, only one live kitten out of six was born. Because the EPO-added food was deficient in arachidonic acid and omega-3 fatty acids, the reproductive failure was most likely due to essential fatty acid deficiency and not EPO per se.

Nontarget Species

Clinical research trials investigating the effect of EPO or GLA supplementation on various aspects of health and disease in humans and rodents are extensive (see the section in this chapter on Purported Role in Health and Disease). In humans, general adverse reactions, including headaches, nausea, loose stools, and diarrhea following treatment with EPO, have been reported (Briggs, 1986). It is worth noting that symptoms such as headaches would not be detectable in horses, dogs, or cats.

Three research studies have reported the feeding of cattle with evening primrose oilseed residues and/or full fat evening primrose seed (Strzetelski et al., 1998a,b, 1999). If only the amount of oil in these EPO-containing products is examined, average intake in cattle ranged from 31–1,090 mg EPO/kg BW. Enrichment of the diets of dairy cattle with EPO-containing products (providing approximately 31–142 mg EPO/kg BW) had no significant effects on milk production or the percentage of fat, protein, or lactose in milk (Strzetelski et al., 1998a, 1999). In addition, supplementation with evening primrose oilseed residue had no effect on prolactin, thyroid hormones, or bovine somatotropin concentrations in dairy cattle; however, a higher level of urea and creatinine in the blood was observed in cows fed evening primrose oilseed residue compared to control cows fed a non-fat-added diet, possibly indicating a lower efficiency of microbial protein synthesis (Strzetelski et al., 1998a). This finding is not atypical of fat-added diets, regardless of the source of fat, when fed to ruminants. High levels of EPO-containing seed residues fed to fattening bulls (providing approximately 1,090 mg EPO/kg BW) reduced dry matter, organic matter, crude protein, and crude fiber digestibility compared to bulls fed lower levels of EPO-containing seed residues (providing approximately 360 mg EPO/kg BW) or no seed residues (Strzetelski et al., 1998b). This finding further supports that the alterations to microbial digestion observed in ruminants can likely be attributed to high dietary fat concentrations, rather than to EPO specifically. Additional confirmation was provided recently by Jalc et al. (2005), who reported that in vitro fermentation of a hay:barley (60:40) diet with 5 percent w/w EPO did not alter any basal parameters of rumen fermentation (pH, ammonia-nitrogen, degradation of dry matter, organic matter, neutral detergent fiber, and acid detergent fiber).

Use, Risk, and Exposure as a Supplement

Target Species

Horses

Widespread use of dietary EPO supplements in horses appears to be uncommon in the United States. Because horses are not routinely supplemented with EPO, common levels of supplementation are difficult to establish. An intensive search by the committee for dietary supplements containing EPO that are marketed specifically for horses yielded no results. A short report of the clinical application of EPO to treat horses with *Culicoides* hypersensitivity in the United Kingdom was given by Craig (1992) as part of a veterinary dermatology workshop. The author reported providing horses with 20 g/day of a mixture of 80 percent EPO and 20 percent fish oil (thus, daily EPO intake can be estimated at 16 g/day). Body weights and GLA content were not provided. Assuming horses weighed an average of 500 kg, daily intake can be estimated at 32 mg EPO/kg BW. In a later study, Craig et al. (1997) investigated the effects of EPO on adult horses and ponies with a history of recurrent seasonal pruritis. Animals were fed a commercially available mixed oil (Efamol Vet) consisting of 80 percent EPO (containing 7.9 percent GLA) and 20 percent cold-water marine fish oil at a rate of 100 mg mixed oil/kg BW, resulting in an estimated 80 mg EPO/kg BW. Potential side effects of EPO supplementation were not addressed by either Craig (1992) or Craig et al. (1997).

Dogs

Dietary EPO supplements are commonly used to treat dogs with dermatological problems. Typical EPO dosages in published studies range from 42 to 424 mg/kg BW/day, with an average of approximately 170 mg/kg BW (see Table 7-5). This results in a typical daily intake of 4 to 36 mg GLA/kg BW.

Arundel (1992), in a letter to the editor in *Veterinary Journal*, reported that a 7-year-old Rottweiler that was described as being epileptic, had four epileptiform seizures within 48 hours after receiving a "compound containing evening primrose oil." The owner subsequently stopped administering the EPO compound. The dose of EPO, the other ingredients in the supplement, and the manufacturer were not reported. The author stated the dog was receiving primidone, which is an antiseizure medication and suggested the dog had a history of seizures. Additional medical history was not reported. A follow-up of the case was not published; therefore, it is unknown whether the dog had subsequent seizures. In a reply letter (Dobbin, 1992), Efamol Vet, the manufacturer of the EPO supplements EfaVet, Efa Vet Regular and EfaCoat, stated that they had not received any reports of epileptic seizures in dogs immediately after consumption of their EPO supplements. Taken in isolation, this case report is not adequate to raise a concern about a link between EPO and seizures in dogs, particularly when the incident occurred in a dog that appeared to have enough of a history of seizures to warrant antiseizure medication. To determine whether further investigation is necessary, the previous and subsequent seizure history of the dog is needed. In studies evaluating the tumorcidal action of GLA for gliomas (Das et al., 1995), intracerebral injections of GLA were conducted in three dogs and into the tumor bed of 19 affected humans. Dogs were injected intracerebrally with GLA (0.25 mg/dog) daily for 6 days. Computed tomography and histopathological examination of the brain of each dog revealed that GLA is not cytotoxic to normal dog brain cells. If epilepsy were a significant feature of GLA administration, direct central nervous system application might be expected to result in such clinical signs. An examination of adverse event reports, consumer comments, and consumer complaints is necessary to substantiate the history of safe use of the EPO product.

Bergvall (1998) summarized five case reports concerning the use of EPO in dogs with claw abnormalities. Daily intake of GLA ranged from 3 to 7 mg/kg BW for up to 52 weeks. Although the GLA content of the supplements was reported, the exact composition of the supplements was not. Therefore, the exact EPO intake is unknown. No adverse effects were reported in any of the patients. Bond and Lloyd (1994) reported successful use of EPO in 11 dogs fed 14 mg GLA/kg BW/day for 12 weeks. No adverse effects were reported. One of the dogs was reported to have diarrhea on two occasions during the 4-month pretrial period; dogs were reported to be consuming 12–21 mg GLA/kg BW during this pretrial period. There is no reason to believe that this tolerance data could not be extrapolated to clinically normal dogs.

The National Animal Supplement Council (NASC) monitored three EPO supplements used in dogs for adverse events (NASC, 2007, personal communication). While over 1.6 million administrations were sold, no serious adverse events were reported to the NASC from 2004 to 2007. During this 3-year time span, one adverse event was reported (but not described), resulting in an estimated 0.61 adverse events per 1 million administrations sold between 2004 and 2007, as reported by NASC. The EPO supplements monitored by NASC were reported to provide an average of 3 mg EPO/kg BW. This amount is substantially less than the dosage administered in the clinical trials described above.

Cats

Fatty acid supplements, including those containing EPO, have been used in the management of feline allergic skin diseases with mixed success. Daily EPO supplementation levels from published studies ranges from 62 to 125 mg/kg BW/day (Harvey 1993a,b; Logas and Kunkle, 1993). The addition of EPO to the diet was also used to investigate platelet function in cats at levels estimated to provide 391 mg EPO/kg BW/day (Davidson and Haggan, 1990). Not all studies reported the GLA content of the supplements used, but levels reported by Logas and Kunkle (1993) and Davidson and Haggan (1990) ranged from 8.15–33 mg GLA/kg BW/day.

Commercial EPO supplements for cats are readily available. The formulation of such products is often proprietary, so the actual EPO content and dosage is not generally available. Nonetheless, one EPO capsule product recommended providing cats with 22.5–45 mg GLA/day (or 5–10 mg/kg BW for a 4.5 kg cat). Another product containing a blend of EPO, fish oil, vitamins, and minerals recommended supplying cats with one capsule per 5 kg BW containing 15 mg GLA per capsule (i.e., 3 mg/kg BW). Assuming these commercial products utilize EPO containing 9 percent GLA, the daily intake of EPO can be estimated at 33–111 mg EPO/kg BW.

Between 2003 and 2007 the National Animal Supplement Council (NASC, 2007, personal communication) received no reports of adverse or serious adverse events for cats consuming EPO. The mean dosage was 2.71 mg/kg BW and over 127,000 administrations were sold during this time period. Similar to that observed in the dog, the average EPO dosage reported by the NASC for cats is substantially lower than that found in the literature.

Nontarget Species

Evening primrose oil was the first seed oil containing GLA to become commercially available and is the most used source of GLA for clinical and pharmaceutical applications (Horrobin, 1992). It is currently available in over 30 countries as a human nutritional supplement or as a constituent of specialty foods (Phillips and Huang, 1996). According to Horrobin (1992), "around 4,000 patients have been involved in trials of GLA, mainly in the form of primrose oil, given for 3 months or more in research studies in a hospital context. In the placebo-controlled studies, not a single adverse event has occurred significantly more frequently in the active GLA group as compared to the placebo group. In addition about half a million prescriptions of one month's supply of primrose oil as Epogam and Efamast [Scotia Pharmaceuticals, Ltd.] have been dispensed in the [United Kingdom] for atopic eczema or breast pain. The incidence of reported adverse events has been far lower than with most drugs, and no pattern has emerged suggesting that any adverse event is causally related to GLA consumption."

Daily doses of 1 g to over 20 g EPO (providing a few hundred milligrams up to 1.7 g of GLA/day) have been administered in human intervention studies (see review by Barre, 2001). Assuming this intake applies to a 70-kg man, this range of intake equates to approximately 14–286 mg EPO/kg BW (approximately 2.4–25 mg GLA/kg BW).

Recommended or suggested daily intake of EPO varies. Horrobin (1992) suggested GLA intakes range from 25–50 mg/day for nutritional purposes, 100–500 mg/day for therapeutic use, and 500–2,000 mg/day to provide a pharmacological effect. Assuming a GLA content of 9 percent, this equates to 0.28–0.56, 1.1–5.6, and 5.6–22.2 g EPO/day for nutritional, therapeutic and, pharmacological effects, respectively. The EPO monograph generated by the Longwood Herbal Task Force (Kemper, 1999) lists the following EPO doses: in adults, between 4–8 g/day are recommended, depending on the condition being treated; doses as high as 10–30 g EPO/day have been used in the treatment of rheumatoid arthritis. For children, 2–4 g EPO/day is suggested for eczema (Kemper, 1999). As indicated by health food supplement manufacturers, the typical daily intake of EPO as a source of GLA is two to six 500 mg capsules of EPO (approximately 1–3 g EPO/day) (Clough, 2001). Assuming a GLA content of 9 percent, this equates to between 90 and 270 mg GLA per day. In most cases, it appears that EPO supplementation is applied to conditions of poor health, as opposed to being used for preventative health maintenance.

Consumption as Part of Normal Diet

Target Species

Horses

Evening primrose plant tissue, evening primrose seed, and EPO are not routinely fed to horses as a source of nutrients. In addition, the committee is not aware of any evidence to suggest these materials have been a part of the evolutionary or voluntary diet of horses.

Linoleic acid can be found in a variety of feedstuffs consumed by horses, including cereal grains, grain byproducts, and soybean meal (NRC, 2007), with smaller amounts present in forages (Boufaïed et al., 2003; Warren and Kivipelto, 2007a,b). Vegetable oils (e.g., corn oil, soybean oil, and canola oil) and rice bran that are commonly added to equine diets are particularly rich sources of linoleic acid (NRC, 2007).

In contrast, available data on the GLA content of commonly used feeds indicate that this fatty acid does not appear to be found in significant quantities in traditional diets used for horses. Occurrence of significant levels of GLA in plants is rare; therefore, it is not surprising that GLA does not appear to be present in common forages consumed by horses (Warren and Kivipelto, 2007a,b).

Depending on the species of animal and the dam's diet, GLA appears to be a minor fatty acid in milk. Reviews on the lipid content of human breast milk have reported trace amounts of GLA (median 0.09 mol percent, range 0–0.33 mol percent) (Jensen, 1999; German and Dillard, 2006). A review of the lipid composition of bovine milk suggest that GLA is either absent or below the limits of detection in cow milk (Jensen, 2002), although the concentration of GLA in cow milk can be increased by feeding evening primrose seed meal (Strzetelski et al., 1999). Similarly, in mares fed bahiagrass pasture and grain concentrates, GLA was not detected in colostrum or milk samples obtained at 2-week intervals from parturition through the fourth month of lactation (Stelzleni, 2006). The lack of detectable quantities of GLA in the milk of cattle and horses may be due in part to the heavy reliance of forages in the diets of these animals.

Although data on all feed ingredients commonly used in the diets of horses are lacking, it can be concluded that the GLA content of common feeds is likely to be far lower than that provided in EPO supplements.

Dogs and Cats

Currently, evening primrose plant tissue and evening primrose seed are not routinely fed to dogs and cats as a source of nutrients, nor is there evidence to suggest these materials have been consumed voluntarily by free-foraging dogs and cats. On the other hand, EPO has been included as a source of dietary fatty acids in research diets and commercial pet foods. For example, in their studies on phosphorus requirements of cats, Kienzle et al. (1998) included 0.2 percent EPO in their basal cat diet. Based on the DM intake of the basal diet and the body weight of the cats in their study, daily consumption ranged from 20 to 24.6 mg EPO/kg BW. Evening primrose oil has also been added to some commercial dog foods. A patent was filed by Shields and Bennett (2000) describing seven dog foods that contained a guaranteed minimum of 0.1–0.4 percent EPO and a minimum of 0.02–0.05 percent GLA. Assuming EPO contains 8–14 percent GLA and a 15-kg dog requires 1,000 kcal/day (NRC, 2006), these foods would have provided approximately 40–105 mg EPO/kg BW/day. A statement was made in the patent for each of these dog foods that said, "animal feeding tests using the procedures of the Association of American Feed Control Officials substantiate [the formula] provides complete and balanced nutrition for all stages of life." Hence, the foods would have been fed throughout gestation, lactation, and growth and would have had to meet standards for blood parameters, growth, and reproductive performance (AAFCO, 2007). One of the criteria for passing an AAFCO protocol is that no animal can show "clinical or pathological signs of nutritional deficiency or excess" (AAFCO, 2007). Thus, dog foods containing 0.02–0.05 percent GLA (0.1–0.4 percent EPO) were able to maintain normal reproductive performance and growth with no overt signs of toxicity. Chapter 2 of this publication includes a more complete description of AAFCO Nutrition Claim Substantiation trials.

Linoleic acid can be found in a variety of feedstuffs consumed by dogs and cats (see NRC, 2006). By comparison, the GLA content of pet foods is substantially less and varies according to the types and amounts of animal-based products included in each product. Beef, pork, and poultry products such as meat, tallow/lard, and egg yolks have measurable GLA (Horrobin, 1992) (Table 7-6). Animal fat contains higher levels of GLA than meat; organ meats tend to be higher than skeletal muscle. Watson (1998) estimated that daily intake of canned dog food and dry dog food would provide approximately 60 mg and 25 mg GLA, respectively, for a 20-kg dog (or 1.25–3.0 mg/kg BW). The author also estimated that daily intake of canned cat food and dry cat food would provide approximately 18 mg and 8 mg GLA, respectively, for a 5-kg cat (or 1.6–3.6 mg/kg BW).

TABLE 7-6 γ-Linolenic Acid (GLA) Content of Select Animal and Poultry Products

Source	Lipid, Percent (Wet Weight)	Percent GLA in Lipid	mg GLA/100 g Source
Beef			
Lean, raw	2.0	0.11	2.2
Fat, raw	60.4	0.10	60.4
Liver, raw	4.6	0.22	10.1
Kidney, raw	3.1	0.16	5.0
Pork			
Lean, raw	3.3	trace	trace
Fat, raw	69.7	0.03	20.9
Chicken			
Lean, raw	2.9	0.13	3.8
Fat, raw	59.7	0.13	77.6
Egg yolk			
Free range hens	29.8	0.07	20.9
Commercial hens	31.5	0.06	18.9

SOURCE: Based on data in Horrobin (1992).

The GLA concentration in queen milk was reported to be approximately 0.12 percent of the total milk fat (Jacobsen et al., 2004). The fatty acid composition (as a percentage of milk fat) of cat milk was not affected by stage of lactation, litter size, or teat position (Jacobsen et al., 2004). Although the GLA content of canine milk was not presented in studies evaluating milk fatty acid composition (Bauer et al., 2004, 2006; Heinemann et al., 2005), small quantities of GLA (0.2–0.4 percent of milk fat) have been detected in canine milk (J. E. Bauer, 2007, personal communication).

Safety of Similar Compounds

Target Species

Horses

One study was performed in horses using oil from purple viper's bugloss (*Echium plantagineum*) seed (Bergero et al., 2002). As an *Echium*, purple viper's bugloss (PVB) is a member of the borage family of *Boraginaceae*. Four mature horses (426 kg) were used in a crossover design. In the first 30-day period, two of the horses were given 20 g PVB/day (4.7 g/100 kg BW) top-dressed on barley. The PVB was reported to contain 10.4 percent GLA, resulting in a daily intake of 2.1 g GLA (5 mg GLA/kg BW). The other two horses received only the basal diet. The basal diet consisted of 5.6 kg first-cut meadow hay and 3.1 kg barley per day. After 30 days of supplementation, horses were switched to the opposite treatment for an additional 30 days. Blood and skin were sampled on day 30 and 60 for determination of fatty acid composition. Supplementation with GLA in the form of PVB oil had no effect on plasma or skin fatty acid composition. The authors reported no other data related to the monitoring of the horse's health or the acceptability of the PVB oil.

Dogs

A study was performed to determine the effect of fatty acid supplementation on the need for steroid use in dogs with atopic dermatitis (Saevik et al., 2004). Dogs were fed either a placebo (medium chain triacylglycerol oil) or a borage/fish oil blend added at a rate of approximately one pump stroke per 10 kg BW/day for 84 days. One pump stroke was reported to contain 190 mg linoleic acid, 105 mg GLA, 9.9 mg EPA, and 6.6 mg docosahexaenoic acid. Therefore, daily consumption of GLA was approximately 10 mg/kg BW. Owners were able to decrease prednisone supplementation in dogs fed the borage/fish oil supplement. No adverse effects were reported. Harvey (1999) fed atopic dogs either placebo (olive oil), 88 mg borage/fish oil per kg BW, or 176 mg borage/fish oil per kg BW for 8 weeks in a blinded study. An 8:1 ratio of borage oil to fish oil was maintained in the two borage oil-treated groups. Olive oil was added to the borage/fish oil supplements in varied amounts so that the total supplemental oil intake was the same across the three groups of dogs. Corresponding daily GLA intakes were 0, 21, and 42 mg/kg BW, respectively. The higher dosage of borage/fish oil was reported to be more efficacious in treating atopy than the lower dosage. Two dogs were removed from the borage oil-supplemented groups because they failed to respond and one dog from the placebo group because it contracted scabies. No adverse effects were reported in any of the dogs.

Cats

Borage oil supplementation of cats with pruritic skin disorders has been the subject of investigation in a small number of clinical studies. In an open, uncontrolled trial, Miller et al. (1993) supplemented 28 cats with 110 mg/kg BW of a commercial fatty acid supplement (DVM Derm Cap Liquid, DVM Pharmaceutical, Inc.) containing borage oil and fish oil for 30 days and, in some cases, up to 10 months. Unfortunately, the composition of the oil was not provided. The authors reported that one cat vomited each time the supplement was given and three cats found the product unpalatable.

Similar to EPO, borage oil has been included as a source of essential fatty acids in feline research diets and commercial food products. For example, Szabo et al. (2003) included 0.15 percent borage oil to help meet the fatty acid requirements of overweight adult cats that were being fed to undergo rapid weight loss. Morris (1998) included 0.5 percent borage oil (containing 23 percent GLA) in the basal diet to help meet the fatty acid requirements of adult cats or kittens in his studies on vitamin D synthesis in cats. While indicators of safety were not specifically evaluated by these investigators, there were no indications that this concentration of borage oil was unsafe.

A controlled clinical trial where cats with miliary dermatitis were supplemented with a GLA-containing oil of undisclosed origin was reported by Lechowski et al. (1998). In this study, healthy cats and cats with miliary dermatitis received either no oil supplementation or were supplemented with 1 mL of an oil preparation that contained 9.1 percent GLA top-dressed on their daily food by the individual cat owner. Body weights of the animals were not provided, but for an average 4 kg cat, this level of oil would result in a daily intake of 22.8 mg GLA/kg BW. Cats were supplemented for 6 weeks and cats were clinically evaluated at 2-week intervals. Serum total cholesterol and high-density lipoprotein were lowered and serum triacylglycerols were elevated in oil-supplemented cats with miliary dermatitis compared to unsupplemented cats with miliary dermatitis, making values similar to healthy cats receiving diets with or without oil. Oil supplementation had no effect on these variables in healthy cats.

CURRENT REGULATORY STATUS

Evening primrose oil is not codified as GRAS (generally recognized as safe), an approved food additive, or prior-sanctioned for use in human food or animal feed. Further, it is not an AAFCO-defined animal feed ingredient. While there is some reference to ingestion of the leaves or roots of the plant by humans for food purposes, the prevailing intended use of evening primrose appears to be that of a medicinal herb, according to one online alternative health website (http://altnature.com/gallery/Evening_Primrose.htm). Documented evidence of use of the oil, the seeds from which the oil is derived, or the plant in general as an animal feed ingredient does not appear to be sufficient to establish a safe history of use. As such, its regulatory status would appear to be that of an unapproved food additive.

LIMITATIONS TO THE ASSESSMENT OF SAFETY

The following factors were limitations in the assessment of the safety of EPO in horses, dogs, and cats:

- As a botanically derived supplement, the composition of EPO can vary. In addition, variations in oil extraction and refining, packaging, and storage may affect the active ingredients present.
- The majority of studies conducted on EPO supplementation utilized products from a single manufacturer, which may have minimized the committee's ability to determine the impact that variable oil composition, as well as variable manufacturing and processing practices, can have on EPO supplement safety.
- Evening primrose oil contains multiple ingredients that have potential biological activity. The two fatty acids most commonly associated with the biological activity of EPO (i.e., linoleic acid and GLA) could have multiple effects on biological systems and these effects may be confounded by other fatty acids and dietary components, thus making them difficult to separate.
- A variety of fatty acids are consumed in the diets of target species, which can inhibit, augment, or have no effect on the fatty acids consumed in an EPO supplement. Therefore, careful consideration of the background fatty acid profile of the animal's diet is important. These data were rarely available in the studies utilized by the committee for the assessment of safety of EPO in horses, dogs, and cats.
- Animals have the ability to store fatty acids as phospholipids in cell membranes and as triacylglycerols in adipose tissue for long periods of time. Therefore, short-term feeding trials are not representative of the potential biological effects that may be seen with long-term (or even lifetime) EPO supplementation. Similarly, plasma and tissue fatty acid levels may take several weeks to achieve a plateau following dietary supplementation and short-term studies may not evaluate biological response at the period

of maximal tissue accretion. Few studies were available that documented the long-term safety of EPO supplementation.

- Inadequate data describing dose response or long-term feeding of EPO were available for the target species to establish the potential for subchronic or chronic toxicity. In the case of horses and cats, these data do not seem to exist. In dogs, only one study has reported on the dose response of EPO supplementation (Everett et al., 1988a), but the actual data were not presented and statistically significant data were not well described.
- The majority of data describing EPO supplementation in dogs and cats were generated from studies using adult animals with skin disorders.
- More clinical research data (not necessarily designed to assess safety) were available for the committee to evaluate safety based on a history of EPO use as a supplement in dogs than in horses or cats.
- Many clinical and experimental research trials investigating the application of EPO in the target species do not provide adequate information to assess safety (e.g., not placebo-controlled or blinded, do not provide body weight of animals, do not provide adequate description of the amount of EPO fed or the composition of the EPO product, fail to describe the composition of basal diet, and fail to report on measures of overall animal health).
- Many research trials investigating the application of EPO in the target species utilize other oils (e.g., fish oil) blended with EPO, which may confound results of EPO-specific biological effects.
- Some studies reported the use of a commercially available EPO product, but failed to provide the composition. The composition of commercial EPO products may change over time or may no longer be available, making the data useless for determining the level of safety.
- Data describing EPO supplementation during pregnancy, lactation, growth, and strenuous exercise in the target species have not been published. In addition, EPO supplementation of these vulnerable populations in non-target species has not been widely reported in the scientific literature.
- Studies examining the effects of species and breed on the absorption and response to essential fatty acid supplementation are needed.

RISK ASSESSMENT

Horses

To the committee's knowledge, comprehensive study on the safety of EPO supplementation in horses has never been completed. Evidence of use of EPO in horses has been demonstrated in only two research trials (Craig et al., 1997; Reilly et al., 1998) and one clinical report in the literature (Craig, 1992), and these trials supplied lower amounts of EPO (25–80 mg/kg BW) than is commonly reported for therapeutic use in humans and other animals (50–400 mg/kg BW). The longest period of EPO supplementation in horses documented in the literature is 24 weeks; therefore, effects of chronic supplementation in the horse are unknown.

The committee's consensus is that EPO supplementation at levels in common use in other species (50–400 mg/kg BW) is likely to be relatively safe in horses. This decision is based primarily on the relative safety of the fatty acids in EPO, as well as its reported use in other species without significant adverse events. Linoleic acid, found in the highest quantities in EPO, is found in almost all feedstuffs that are routinely included in equine diets (NRC, 2007). In addition, this fatty acid predominates in vegetable oils (e.g., corn oil, soybean oil) that may be added to the equine diet. Horses have been reported to tolerate up to 23 percent of the diet by weight as corn oil or soybean oil without adverse effects on digestion (as reviewed by Kronfeld et al., 2004). In contrast to linoleic acid, GLA does not appear to be found in measurable quantities in common feedstuffs fed to horses (see the section in this chapter on Consumption as Part of Normal Diet). Nonetheless, this fatty acid is an intermediate compound in the metabolism of omega-6 fatty acids and can presumably be synthesized in the horse from linoleic acid. The fate of GLA as DGLA is quite different than as arachidonic acid; however, this may only be a realistic concern when large quantities of EPO (in excess of 400 mg/kg BW) are supplied in the diet. The committee has set the Presumed Safe Intake (PSI) in horses at 400 mg EPO/kg BW (see Table 7-7). When adding EPO to the equine diet, other sources of dietary fat must be adjusted to accommodate the upper level of dietary fat tolerated by the individual horse.

Dogs

Based on history of safe use and long-term clinical efficacy trials, the committee concluded that the dosage of EPO typically administered in clinical trials (i.e., 42–424 mg EPO/kg BW or 4–36 mg GLA/kg BW) is well tolerated when fed long term to dogs. All of these trials were conducted with dogs that had skin disorders; however, the

TABLE 7-7 Historical Safe Intake (HSI) and Presumed Safe Intake (PSI) of Evening Primrose Oil in Horses, Dogs, and Cats (mg/kg BW per day)

Species	HSI	PSI
Horses[a]	25–80	400
Dogs	42–424	424
Cats[b]	20–391	391

[a]Presumes daily total fat intake by horses will not exceed 23% of the diet by weight, including any EPO added to the diet.

[b]Presumes dietary recommendations for arachidonic acid, α-linolenic acid, EPA, and DHA will be met by other dietary sources of fatty acids.

committee believes that similar levels of supplementation would be not harmful to normal, healthy dogs. One study reported on the dose response of EPO supplementation in healthy dogs (Everett et al., 1988a), but the actual data were not presented and statistically significant data were not well described. Therefore, despite the fact that the authors did not report any overt signs of toxicity at up to 5,000 mg EPO/kg BW, the data of Everett et al. (1988a) were not used in determination of the PSI. The committee has set the PSI for dogs at 424 mg/kg BW, which is the upper level used in clinical trials (Table 7-7). Most likely the upper safe intake for EPO is quite a bit higher than this in dogs.

Cats

The amount of daily EPO supplemented for the purposes of managing feline allergic skin diseases ranged from 62–110 mg/kg BW in published studies (Harvey 1993a,b; Logas and Kunkle, 1993). In their investigations of the effects of EPO on blood platelet function, Davidson and Haggan (1990) supplemented cats with EPO at 391 mg/kg BW for 270 days. While the safety of EPO was not specifically evaluated in this study, there was no indication of intolerance to EPO in cats at this level. Short-term (Frankel and Rivers, 1978) and long-term (Rivers and Frankel, 1980; Frankel and Rivers, 1988) feeding studies have included EPO as a source of fatty acids in cat foods at levels up to 125 g/kg diet, which result in an estimated intake of 1,953 mg/kg BW for an average 4-kg cat. Although no ill effects were noted that could be attributed to the high level of EPO inclusion in the diet, the diets were reported to be deficient in other fatty acids. In addition, because the cats were given ad libitum access to feed in the Rivers and Frankel studies, assumptions had to be made to estimate EPO intake. These factors reduce the committee's confidence in using these data to set the PSI for EPO in cats. Therefore, the committee has set the PSI for cats at 391 mg/kg BW (Table 7-7); however, it is likely that cats could tolerate higher levels of EPO. Because EPO does not contain adequate amounts of all the essential fatty acids (particularly arachidonic acid, α-linolenic acid, EPA, and DHA) and the cat has limited Δ5- and Δ6-desaturase activities (Rivers et al., 1975; Hassam et al., 1977; Frankel and Rivers, 1978; Pawloski et al., 1994), the main concern when feeding high concentrations of EPO (particularly above the PSI level) is a deficiency of essential fatty acids. Therefore, EPO intake should be limited to accommodate other dietary fat sources that will permit the essential fatty acid requirements of the cat to be met (NRC, 2006). In addition, EPO should not be used to replace all dietary fat sources in the cat (Frankel and Rivers, 1978, 1988). Finally, more vitamin E may be needed in the diets of cats, particularly those fed large amounts of EPO or EPO/fish oil blends, because of the potential risk of pansteatitis in this species.

OTHER RECOMMENDATIONS

Although available data are less than optimal for assessing potential toxicity in the target species, EPO seems to be relatively safe when offered at the low dosage often used in clinical applications, when the addition of EPO does not exceed the fat intake tolerance of the animal, and, in cats, when EPO is not included as the sole source of dietary fat. Nonetheless, the absence of toxicity or dose-response data in the target species warrants further investigation, with the following recommendations.

- There is a need for research to assess the effects of EPO on the fatty acid profile of phospholipids of cell membranes and tissues in horses, dogs, and cats. It is the fatty acids in the phospholipids of cells that are involved in cellular signaling through pathways such as eicosanoids. Fatty acid, triacylglycerol, and phospholipid concentrations in plasma are more commonly measured, but are not direct measures of this signaling potential. Much of the biological activity ascribed to EPO is rooted in specific eicosanoid synthesis, which is also where potential concerns for safety could arise (e.g., prostaglandins and pregnancy, thromboxanes and blood clotting, and leukotrienes and inflammation).
- Most research conducted with EPO in the target species was performed on mature animals. Research is needed to address the safety of EPO supplementation in the target species during pregnancy, growth, and, in the case of horses and dogs, athletic training.
- Most studies in the target species involved relatively short-term EPO supplementation. Because fatty acid turnover in the body can be slow, the safety of dietary EPO supplementation should be evaluated in response to long-term feeding trials in the target species. Furthermore, animals should be evaluated for a period of time once EPO supplementation has been discontinued to determine whether specific withdrawal strategies need to be implemented to maintain adequate biological function and health.
- To facilitate future evaluation of safety across studies, research manuscripts describing EPO supplementation should publish the fatty acid composition of the EPO supplement, the dosage fed (and/or the dose of EPO along with the body weight of the animals so dosage can be calculated), and the fatty acid composition of the animals' basal diet.
- Studies evaluating the efficacy of dietary EPO supplementation are to be encouraged to include some measures of safety (e.g., hematology and blood chemistry) in addition to their evaluations of EPO utility for specific health benefits. In addition, animals used in efficacy studies should be monitored for adverse health events during the period of supplementation, and detailed comments should be included in the publication to indicate what was monitored, the frequency of monitoring, and the specific outcome.

Finally, the committee recommends that a robust adverse event reporting program be instituted to capture common EPO usage data and a detailed record of adverse events (see Chapter 3).

REFERENCES

AAFCO (Association of American Feed Control Officials). 2007. Pp. 147–156 in Official Publication. Oxford, IN: Association of American Feed Control Officials.

Abayasekara, D. R. E., and D. C. Wathes. 1999. Effects of altering dietary fatty acid composition on prostaglandin synthesis and fertility. Prostaglandins Leukot. Essent. Fatty Acids. 61:275–287.

Abdullazhanova, N. G., S. M. Mavlyanov, and S. V. Abdullaev. 2000. Phenolic compounds from *Oenothera gigas*. Chem. Nat. Compd. 36:97–98.

Allen, K. G. D., and M. A. Harris. 2001. The role of n-3 fatty acids in gestation and parturition. Exp. Biol. Med. 226:498–506.

Arundel, B. L. 1992. Evening primrose oil and epilepsy. Vet. Rec. 131:543.

Awang, D. V. C. 1990. Herbal medicine: Borage. Can. Pharm. J. 123:121–126.

Balasinksa, B., and A. Troszynska. 1998. Total antioxidative activity of evening primrose (*Oenothera paradoxa*) cake extract measured in vitro by liposome model and murine L1210 cells. J. Agric. Food Chem. 46:3358–3563.

Barre, D. E. 2001. Potential of evening primrose, borage, black currant, and fungal oils in human health. Ann. Nutr. Metab. 45:47–57.

Bauer, J. E., K. M. Heinemann, K. E. Bigley, G. E. Lees, and M. K. Waldron. 2004. Maternal diet alpha-linolenic acid during gestation and lactation does not increase docosahexaenoic acid in canine milk. J. Nutr. 134(8 Suppl.):2035S–2038S.

Bauer, J. E., K. M. Heinemann, G. E. Lees, and M. K. Waldron. 2006. Docosahexaenoic acid accumulates in plasma of canine puppies raised on α-linolenic acid-rich milk during suckling but not when fed α-linolenic acid-rich diets after weaning. J. Nutr. 136:2087S–2089S.

Belch, J. J. F., and A. Hill. 2000. Evening primrose oil and borage oil in rheumatologic conditions. Am. J. Clin. Nutr. 71(Suppl.):252S–256S.

Bergero, D., N. Miraglia, M. Polidori, M. Ziino, and D. Gagliardi. 2002. Blood serum and skin fatty acid levels in horses and the use of dietary polyunsaturated fatty acids. Anim. Res. 51:157–163.

Bergvall, K. 1998. Case report. Treatment of symmetrical onychomadesis and onchodystrophy in five dogs with omega-3 and omega-6 fatty acids. Vet. Dermatol. 9:263–268.

Bettger, W. J., P. G. Reeves, E. A. Moscatelli, G. Reynolds, and B. L. O'Dell. 1979. Interaction of zinc and essential fatty acids in the rat. J. Nutr. 109:480–488.

Birch, A. E., G. P. Fenner, R. Watkins, and L. C. Boyd. 2001. Antioxidant properties of evening primrose seed extracts. J. Agric. Food Chem. 49:4502–4507.

Bond, R., and D. H. Lloyd. 1992a. A double-blind comparison of olive oil and a combination of evening primrose oil and fish oil in the management of canine atopy. Vet. Rec. 131:558–560.

Bond, R., and D. H. Lloyd. 1992b. Randomized single-blind comparison of an evening primrose oil and fish oil combination and concentrates of these oils in the management of canine atopy. Vet. Dermatol. 3:215–219.

Bond, R., and D. H. Lloyd. 1994. Combined treatment with concentrated essential fatty acids and prednisolone in the management of canine atopy. Vet. Rec. 134:30–32.

Bond, R., D. H. Lloyd, and J. M. Craig. 1993. The effects of essential fatty acid supplementation on intradermal test reactivity in atopic dogs: A preliminary study. Vet. Dermatol. 4:191–197.

Boufaïed, H., P. Y. Chouinard, G. F. Tremblay, H. V. Petit, R. Michaud, and G. Bélanger. 2003. Fatty acids in forages. I. Factors affecting concentrations. Can. J. Anim. Sci. 83:501–511.

Briggs, C. J. 1986. Evening primrose. Can. Pharm. J. 119:249–254.

Calder, P. C. 2006. Polyunsaturated fatty acids and inflammation. Prostaglandins Leukot. Essent. Fatty Acids 75:197–202.

Certik, M., and S. Shimizu. 1999. Biosynthesis and regulation of microbial polyunsaturated fatty acid production. J. Biosci. Bioeng. 87:1–14.

Chanussot, B., J. P. Poisson, J. Leclerc, and J. Belleville. 1988. Hepatic microsomal delta 6 and delta 5 desaturations of linoleic acid in lactating rats fed with a low-protein diet supplemented or not with methionine. C. R. Acad. Sci. Ser. III Sci. Vi 307:33–36.

Christie, W. W. 1999. The analysis of evening primrose oil. Ind. Crops Prod. 10:73–83.

Clough, P. 2001. Specialty vegetable oils containing γ-linolenic acid and stearidonic acid. Pp. 75–115 in Structured and Modified Lipids, F. D. Gundstone, ed. New York: Marcel Dekker, Inc.

Court, W. A., J. G. Hendel, and R. Pocs. 1993. Determination of the fatty acids and oil content of evening primrose (*Oenethera biennis* L.). Food Res. Int. 26:181–186.

Craig, M. 1992. Use of an evening primrose oil and fish oil mixture in the management of sweet-itch in horses (abstr.), in Workshop Report 14. Fatty acid supplements and skin disease. P. 458 in Advances in Veterinary Dermatology, Volume 2, P. J. Ihrke, I. S. Mason, and S. D. White, eds. New York: Pergamon Press.

Craig, J. M., D. H. Lloyd, and R. D. Jones. 1997. A double-blind placebo-controlled trial of an evening primrose and fish oil combination vs. hydrogenated coconut oil in the management of recurrent seasonal pruritis in horses. Vet. Dermatol. 8:177–182.

Cunnane, S. C., M. S. Manku, and D. F. Horrobin. 1984. Accumulation of linoleic and γ-linolenic acids in tissue lipids of pyridoxine-deficient rats. J. Nutr. 114:1754–1761.

Cunnane, S. C., J. Vogt, S. S. Likhodii, G. Moine, R. Muggl, K. H. Tovar, G. Kohn, and G. Sawatzki. 1996. Metabolism of [3-^{13}C] γ-linolenic acid in the suckling piglet and rat. Pp. 66–83 in γ-Linolenic Acid Metabolism and Its Roles in Nutrition and Medicine, Y. S. Huang and D. E. Mills, eds. Champaign, IL: AOCS Press.

Das, U. N., V. V. Prasad, and D. R. Reddy. 1995. Local application of gamma-linolenic acid in the treatment of human gliomas. Cancer Lett. 94:147–155.

Davidson, B. C., and J. Haggan. 1990. Dietary polyenoic fatty acids change the response of cat blood platelets to inductions of aggregation by ADP. Prostaglandins Leukot. Essent. Fatty Acids 39:31–37.

De La Cruz, J. P. 1997. Effect of evening primrose oil on platelet aggregation in rabbits fed an atherogenic diet. Thromb. Res. 87:141–149.

Deferne, J. L., and D. W. Pate. 1996. Hemp seed oil: A source of valuable essential fatty acids. J. Int. Hemp Assoc. 3:1,4–7.

Dines, K. C., M. A. Cotter, and N. E. Cameron. 1996. Effectiveness of natural oils as sources of γ-linolenic acid to correct peripheral nerve conduction velocity abnormalities in diabetic rats: Modulation by thromboxane A2 inhibition. Prostaglandins Leukot. Essent. Fatty Acids 55:159–165.

Dobbin, S. 1992. Evening primrose oil and epilepsy. Vet. Rec. 131(25–26):591.

Dove, D., and P. Johnson. 1999. Oral evening primrose oil: Its effect on length of pregnancy and selected intrapartum outcomes in low-risk nulliparous women. J. Nurse Midwifery 44:320–324.

Dunbar, B. L., and J. E. Bauer. 2002. Conversion of essential fatty acids by delta-6 desaturase in dog liver microsomes. J. Nutr. 132:1701S–1703S.

Engler, M. M. 1993. Comparative study of diets enriched with evening primrose, black currant, borage or fungal oils on blood pressure and pressor responses in spontaneously hypertensive rats. Prostaglandins Leukot. Essent. Fatty Acids 49:809–814.

Everett, D. J., R. J. Greenough, C. J. Perry, P. MacDonald, and P. Bayliss. 1988a. Chronic toxicity studies of Efamol evening primrose oil in rats and dogs. Med. Sci. Res. 16:863–864.

Everett, D. J., C. J. Perry, and P. Bayliss. 1988b. Carcinogenicity studies of Efamol evening primrose oil in rats and mice. Med. Sci. Res. 16:865–866.

Fahy, E., S. Subramaniam, H. A. Brown, C. K. Glass, A. H. Merrill, Jr., R. C. Murphy, C. R. H. Raetz, D. W. Russell, Y. Seyama, W. Shaw, T. Shimizu, F. Spener, G. van Meer, M. S. VanNieuwenhze, S. H. White, J. L. Witztum, and E. A. Dennis. 2005. A comprehensive classification system for lipids. J. Lipid Res. 46:839–861.

Fan, Y. Y., and R. S. Chapkin. 1998. Importance of dietary γ-linolenic acid in human health and nutrition. J. Nutr. 128:1411–1414.

Fan, Y. Y., R. S. Chapkin, and K. S. Ramos. 1996. Dietary lipid source alters murine macrophage/vascular smooth muscle cell interactions in vitro. J. Nutr. 126:2083–2088.

Fieldsend, A. F. 1996. Evening primrose–from garden flower to oilseed crop. Horticulturalist 5:2–5.

Fischbach, W., W. Becker, J. Mossner, H. Ohlemuller, W. Koch, and W. Borner. 1987. Leucocytic elastase in chronic inflammatory bowel diseases: A marker of inflammatory activity. Digestion 37:88–95.

Frankel, T. L., and J. P. W. Rivers. 1978. The nutritional and metabolic impact of γ-linolenic acid (18:3n6) on cats deprived of animal lipid. Br. J. Nutr. 39:227–231.

Frankel, T. L., and J. P. W. Rivers. 1988. Fatty acid composition of tissues from ω3-deficient and normal kittens. Proc. Nutr. Soc. Aust. 13:141.

Gawdzik, J., Z. Suprynowicz, M. Mardarowicz, J. Poszytek, R. Lodkowski, and K. Pilorz. 1998. Supercritical fluid extraction of oil from evening primrose (*Oenothera paradoxa* H.) seeds. Chem. Anal. (Warsaw) 43:695–702.

German, J. B., and C. J. Dillard. 2006. Composition, structure and absorption of milk lipids: A source of energy, fat-soluble nutrients and bioactive molecules. Crit. Rev. Food Sci. Nutr. 46:57–92.

Ghasemnezhad, A., and B. Honermeier. 2007. Seed yield, oil content and fatty acid composition of Oenothera biennis L. affected by harvest date and harvest method. Ind. Crops Prod. 25:274–281.

Gibson, R. A., D. R. Lines, and M. A. Neumann. 1992. Gamma linolenic acid (GLA) content of encapsulated evening primrose oil products. Lipids 27:82–84.

Gurr, M. I., J. L. Harwood, and K. N. Frayn. 2002. Lipid Biochemistry: An Introduction, 5th Edition. Oxford, UK: Blackwell Science, Ltd.

Hall, I. V., E. Steiner, P. Threadgill, and R. W. Jones. 1988. The biology of Canadian weeds. 84. *Oenothera biennis* L. Can. J. Plant Sci. 68:163–173.

Hamburger, M., U. Riese, H. Graf, M. F. Melzig, S. Ciesielski, D. Baumann, K. Dittmann, and C. Wegner. 2002. Constituents in evening primrose oil with radical scavenging, cyclooxygenase, and neutrophil elastase inhibitory activities. J. Agric. Food Chem. 50:5533–5538.

Hanczakowski, P., B. Szymczyk, and T. Wolski. 1993. The nutritive value of the residues remaining after oil extraction from seeds of evening primrose (*Oenothera biennis* L). J. Sci. Food Agric. 63:375–376.

Harvey, R. G. 1991. Management of feline miliary dermatitis by supplementing the diet with essential fatty acids. Vet. Rec. 128:326–329.

Harvey, R. G. 1993a. Effect of varying proportions of evening primrose oil and fish oil on cats with crusting dermatosis ('miliary dermatitis'). Vet. Rec. 133:208–211.

Harvey, R. G. 1993b. A comparison of evening primrose oil and sunflower oil for the management of papulocrustous dermatitis in cats. Vet. Rec. 133:571–573.

Harvey, R. G. 1999. A blinded, placebo-controlled study of the efficacy of borage seed oil and fish oil in the management of canine atopy. Vet. Rec. 144:405–407.

Hassam, A. G., J. P. W. Rivers, and M. A. Crawford. 1977. The failure of the cat to desaturate linoleic acid: Its nutritional implications. Nutr. Metab. 21:321–328.

Heinemann, K. M., M. K. Waldron, K. E. Bigley, G. E. Lees, and J. E. Bauer. 2005. Long-chain (n-3) polyunsaturated fatty acids are more efficient than alpha-linolenic acid in improving electroretinogram responses of puppies exposed during gestation, lactation, and weaning. J. Nutr. 135:1960–1966.

Hoffmann, P., C. Taube, T. Bartels, S. Heinemann, and W. Förster. 1984. Cardiovascular effects of antihypertensive drugs as affected by dietary polyunsaturates. Biomed. Biochim. Acta 43:S195–S198.

Holman, C. P. 1983. A trial of evening primrose oil in the treatment of chronic schizophrenia. J. Orthomol. Psychiatry 12:302–304.

Horrobin, D. F. 1992. Nutritional and medical importance of gamma-linolenic acid. Prog. Lipid Res. 31:163–194.

Horrobin, D. F. 1993. Fatty acid metabolism in health and disease: The role of Δ6-desaturase. Am. J. Clin. Nutr. 57:732S–737S.

Horrobin, D. F., K. M. Ells, N. Morse-Fisher, and M. S. Manku. 1991. The effects of evening primrose oil, safflower oil and paraffin on plasma fatty acid levels in humans: Choice of an appropriate placebo for clinical studies on primrose oil. Prostaglandins Leukot. Essent. Fatty Acids 42:245–249.

Høy, C. E., and M. S. Christensen. 1996. Absorption of γ-linolenic acid from borage, evening primrose, and black currant seed oils: Fatty acid profiles, triacylglycerol structures, and clearance rates of chylomicrons in the rat. Pp. 54–65 in γ-Linolenic Acid: Metabolism and Its Roles in Nutrition and Medicine, Y.-S. Huang and D. E. Mills, eds. Champaign, IL: AOCS Press.

Høy, C. E., G. Hølmer, N. Kaur, I. Byrjalsen, and D. Kirstein. 1983. Acyl group distributions in tissue lipids of rats fed evening primrose oil (gamma-linolenic acid plus linoleic acid) or soybean oil (alpha-linolenic acid plus linoleic acid). Lipids 18:760–771.

Huang, Y. S., K. R. McAdoo, J. Mitchell, and D. F. Horrobin. 1988. Effects of calcium deprivation on n-6 fatty acid metabolism in growing rats. Biochem. Med. Metab. Biol. 40:61–67.

Huang, Y. S., P. R. Redden, D. F. Horrobin, S. Churchill, B. Parker, R. P. Ward, and D. E. Mills. 1992. Effects of repeated gestation and lactation on milk n-6 fatty acid composition in rats fed on a diet rich in 18:2*n-6* or 18:3*n-6*. Br. J. Nutr. 68:337–347.

Huang, Y. S., X. Lin, P. R. Redden, and D. F. Horrobin. 1995. In vitro hydrolysis of natural and synthetic gamma-linolenic acid-containing tryacylglycerols by pancreatic lipase. J. Amer. Oil Chem. Soc. 72:625–631.

Huang, Y. S., D. E. Mills, R. C. Cantrill, and J. P. Poisson. 1996. In vivo and in vitro metabolism of linoleic and γ-linolenic acids. Pp. 84–105 in γ-Linolenic Acid: Metabolism and Its Roles in Nutrition and Medicine, Y.-S. Huang and D. E. Mills, eds. Champaign, IL: AOCS Press.

Huang, Y. S., P. Mukerji, and D. S. Knutzon. 2001. Transgenic production of long-chain polyunsaturated fatty acids. World Rev. Nutr. Diet. 88:243–248.

Hudson, B. J. F. 1984. Evening primrose (*Oenothera* spp.) oil and seed. J. Amer. Oil Chem. Soc. 61:540–543.

Ide, T., M. Sugano, T. Ishida, M. Niwa, M. Arima, and A. Morita. 1987. Effects of gamma-linolenic acid on fatty acid profiles and eicosanoid production of the hamster. Nutr. Res. 7:1085–1092.

IUPAC-IUB (International Union of Pure & Applied Chemistry-International Union of Biochemistry). 1976. The nomenclature of lipids. IUPAC-IUB Commission on Biochemical Nomenclature. J. Lipid Res. 19:114–128.

Jacobsen, K. L., E. J. DePeters, Q. R. Rogers, and S. J. Taylor. 2004. Influences of stage of lactation, teat position and sequential milk sampling on the composition of domestic cat milk (*Felis catus*). J. Anim. Physiol. Anim. Nutr. 88:46–58.

Jalc, D., A. Potkanski, M. Szumacher-Strabel, A. Cieslak, and M. Certik. 2005. Effect of microbial oil, evening primrose oil and borage oil on rumen fermentation in vitro. Vet. Med. (Czech.) 50:480–486.

Jenkins, D. K., J. C. Mitchell, M. S. Manku, and D. F. Horrobin. 1988. Effects of different sources of gamma-linolenic acid on the formation of essential fatty acid and prostanoid metabolites. Med. Sci. Res. 16:525–526.

Jensen, R. G. 1999. Lipids in human milk. Lipids 34:1243–1271.

Jensen, R. G. 2002. The composition of bovine milk lipids: January 1995 to December 2000. J. Dairy Sci. 85:295–350.

Kapoor, R., and Y. S. Huang. 2006. Gamma linolenic acid: an anti-inflammatory omega-6 fatty acid. Curr. Pharm. Biotechnol. 7:531–534.

Kemper, K. J. 1999. Evening primrose (*Oenethera biennis*). The Longwood Herbal Taskforce and the Center for Holistic Pediatric Education and Outreach. Online at: http://www.mcp.edu/herbal/epo/epo.pdf. Accessed May 5, 2007.

Kienzle, E., C. Thielen, and C. Pessinger. 1998. Investigations on phosphorus requirements of adult cats. J. Nutr. 128:2598S–2600S.

Knorr, R., and M. Hamburger. 2004. Quantitative analysis of anti-inflammatory and radical scavenging triterpenoid esters in evening primrose oil. J. Agric. Food Chem. 52:3319–3324.

Kriese, U., E. Schumann, W. E. Weber, M. Beyer, L. Bruhl, and B. Matthaus. 2004. Oil content, tocopherol composition and fatty acid patterns of the seeds of 51 *Cannabis sativa* L. genotypes. Euphytica 137:339–351.

Kronfeld, D. S., J. L. Holland, G. A. Rich, T. N. Meacham, J. P. Fontenot, D. J. Sklan, and P. A. Harris. 2004. Fat digestibility in *Equus caballus* follows increasing first-order kinetics. J. Anim. Sci. 82:1773–1780.

Lammer-Zarawska, E., B. Hojden, and A. Milan. 1992. Research on heavy metals contamination of evening primrose (paper in Polish). Pp. 48–50 in Proc. Symp.: Evening primrose oil in prophylaxis and therapy. Lodz, Poland.

Lapinskas, P. 1993. Oil crops for the pharmaceutical industry. Pp. 332–342 in Seed Storage Compounds: Biosynthesis, Interactions and Manipulation, P. Shewry and K. Stobart, eds. New York: Oxford University Press.

Lapinskas, P. 2000. Omega-6 fatty acids—What, why, where and how. Presentation given at: A fitter future for fats? Leatherhead Food Research Association, Leatherhead, England. June 6, 2000. Online at: http://www.lapinskas.com/publications/3548.html. Accessed November 18, 2007.

Larson, K. M., M. R. Roby, and F. R. Stermitz. 1984. Unsaturated pyrrolizidines from borage (Borago officinalis), a common garden herb. J. Nat. Prod. 47:747–748.

Lawson, L. D., and B. G. Hughes. 1988. Triacylglycerol structure of plant and fungal oils. Lipids 23:313–317.

Lechowski, R., E. Sawosz, and W. Klucinski. 1998. The effect of the addition of oil preparation with increased n-3 fatty acids on serum lipid profile and clinical condition of cats with miliary dermatitis. J. Vet. Med. 45:417–424.

Leizer, C., D. Ribnicky, A. Poulev, S. Dushenkov, and I. Raskin. 2000. The composition of hemp seed oil and its potential as an important source of nutrition. J. Nutraceut. Funct. Med. Foods 2:35–53.

Levin, J. L., E. W. Spannhake, A. L. Hyman, and P. J. Kadowitz. 1982. Analysis of airway responses to dihomo-γ-linolenic acid in the cat. J. Pharmacol. Exp. Ther. 223:169–176.

Leyton, J., P. J. Drury, and M. A. Crawford. 1987. Differential oxidation of saturated and unsaturated fatty acids in vivo in the rat. Br. J. Nutr. 57:383–393.

Liu, J. W., S. J. DeMichele, J. Palombo, L. T. Chuang, C. Hastilow, E. Bobik, Jr., and Y. S. Huang. 2004. Effect of long-term dietary supplementation of high-gamma-linolenic canola oil versus borage oil on growth, hematology, serum biochemistry, and n-6 fatty acid metabolism in rats. J. Agric. Food Chem. 52:3960–3966.

Logas, D. B., and G. A. Kunkle. 1993. Double-blind study examining the effects of evening primrose oil on feline pruritic dermatitis. Vet. Dermatol. 4:181–184.

López-García, E., M. B. Schulze, J. B. Meigs, J. E. Manson, N. Rifai, M. J. Stampfer, W. C. Willet, and F. B. Hu. 2005. Consumption of *trans* fatty acids is related to plasma biomarkers of inflammation and endothelial dysfunction. J. Nutr. 135:562–566.

Lotti, G., and M. F. Quartacci. 1990. La distribuzione dell'acido γ-linolenico nei fosfolipidi dei semi di *Oenethera biennis* L. Agrochimica 34:243–250.

Manku, M. S., N. Morse-Fisher, and D. F. Horrobin. 1988. Changes in human plasma essential fatty acid levels as a result of administration of linoleic acid and gamma-linolenic acid. Eur. J. Clin. Nutr. 42:55–60.

Martens-Lobenhoffer, J., and F. P. Meyer. 1998. Pharmacokinetic data of gamma-linolenic acid in healthy volunteers after the administration of evening primrose oil (Epogram). Int. J. Clin. Pharmacol. Ther. 36:363–366.

Miller, R. W., F. R. Earle, I. A. Wolf, and A. S. Barclay. 1968. Search for new seed oils. XV. Oils of Boraginaceae. Lipids 3:43–45.

Miller, W. H., D. W. Scott, and J. R. Wellington. 1993. Efficacy of DVM Derm Caps Liquid in the management of allergic and inflammatory dermatoses of the cat. J. Am. Anim. Hosp. Assoc. 29:37–40.

Morris, J. G. 1998. Ineffective vitamin D synthesis in cats is reversed by an inhibitor of 7-dehydrocholesterol-Δ7-reductase. J. Nutr. 129:903–908.

Morse, N. L, and P. M. Clough. 2006. A meta-analysis of randomized, placebo-controlled clinical trials of Efamol evening primrose oil in atopic eczema. Where do we go from here in light of more recent discoveries? Curr. Pharm. Biotechnol. 7:503–524.

NRC (National Research Council). 2006. Nutrient Requirements of Dogs and Cats. Washington, DC: The National Academies Press.

NRC. 2007. Nutrient Requirements of Horses, 6th Revised Ed. Washington, DC: The National Academies Press.

Olson, R. E. 1999. Discovery of the lipoproteins, their role in fat transport and their significance as risk factors. J. Nutr. 128:439S–443S.

Oomah, B. D., M. Busson, D. V. Godfey, and J. C. G. Drover. 2002. Characteristics of hemp (*Cannabis sativa* L.) seed oil. Food Chem. 76:33–43.

Palombo, J. D., S. J. DeMichele, J. W. Liu, B. R. Bistrian, and Y. S. Huang. 2000. Comparison of growth and fatty acid metabolism in rats fed diets containing equal levels of γ-linolenic acid from high- γ-linolenic acid canola oil or borage oil. Lipids 35:975–981.

Pawloski, R., R. Barnes, and N. Salem. 1994. Essential fatty acid metabolism in the feline: Relationship between liver and brain production of long-chain polyunsaturated fatty acids. J. Lipid Res. 35:2032–2040.

Peiretti, P. G., G. B. Palmegiano, and G. Masoero. 2004. Chemical composition, organic matter digestibility and fatty acid content of evening primrose (*Oenothera paradoxa*) during its growth cycle. Anim. Feed Sci. Technol. 116:293–299.

Peluffo, R. O., A. M. Nervi, M. S. Gonzales, and R. R. Brenner. 1984. Lipid effects of different amino acid diets on delta 5, delta 6 and delta 9 desaturases. Lipids 19:154–157.

Peschel, W., W. Dieckmann, M. Sonnenschein, and A. Plescher. 2007. High antioxidant potential of pressing residues from evening primrose in comparison to other oilseed cakes and plant antioxidants. Ind. Crops Prod. 25:44–54.

Phillips, J. C., and Y. S. Huang. 1996. Natural sources and biosynthesis of γ-linolenic acid: an overview. Pp. 1–13 in γ-Linolenic Acid Metabolism and Its Roles in Nutrition and Medicine, Y. S. Huang and D. E. Mills, eds. Champaign, IL: AOCS Press.

Puri, B. K. 2004. The clinical advantages of cold-pressed non-raffinated evening primrose oil over refined preparations. Med. Hypotheses 62:116–118.

Puri, B. K. 2007. The safety of evening primrose oil in epilepsy. Prostaglandins Leukot. Essent. Fatty Acids 77:101–103.

Raederstorff, D., and D. Moser. 1993. Borage or primrose oil added to standardized diets are equivalent sources for γ-linolenic acid in rats. Lipids 27:1018–1023.

Redden, P. R., Y. S. Huang, X. Lin, and D. F. Horrobin. 1995a. Separation and quantification of the triacylglycerols in evening primrose and borage oils by reversed-phase high-performance liquid chromatography. J. Chromatogr. 694:381–389.

Redden, P. R., X. Lin, J. Fahey, and D. F. Horrobin. 1995b. Stereospecific analysis of the major triacylglycerol species containing γ-linolenic acid in evening primrose oil and borage oil. J. Chromatogr. 704:99–111.

Reilly, J. D., L. Hopegood, L. Gould, and L. Devismes. 1998. Effect of a supplementary dietary evening primrose oil mixture on hoof growth, hoof growth rate and hoof lipid fractions in horses: A controlled and blinded trial. Equine Vet. J. Suppl. 26:58–65.

Richard, J. L., C. Martin, M. Maille, F. Mendy, B. Delplanque, and B. Jacotot. 1990. Effects of dietary intake of gamma-linolenic acid on blood lipids and phospholipid fatty acids in healthy human subjects. J. Clin. Biochem. Nutr. 8:75–84.

Rivers, J. P. W., and T. L. Frankel. 1980. Fat in the diet of cats and dogs. Pp. 67–99 in Nutrition of the Dog and Cat, R. S. Anderson, ed. Oxford: Pergamon Press.

Rivers, J. P., A. J. Sinclair, and M. A. Crawford. 1975. Inability of the cat to desaturate essential fatty acids. Nature 258:171–173.

Roeder, E. 1995. Medicinal plants in Europe containing pyrrolizidine alkaloids. Pharmazie 50:83–98.

Saevik, B. K., K. Bergvall, B. R. Holm, L. E. Saijonmaa-Koulumies, A. Hedhammer, S. Larsen, and F. Kristensen. 2004. A randomized, controlled study to evaluate the steroid sparing effect of essential fatty acid supplementation in the treatment of canine atopic dermatitis. Vet. Dermatol. 15:137–145.

Sallmann, H. P., E. Kienzle, H. Fuhrmann, D. Grunwald, I. Eilmans, and H. Meyer. 1991. Metabolic consequences of feeding ponies with marginal amounts of fat. Pp. 81–82 in Proc. 12th Equine Nutr. Physiol. Soc. Symp., Calgary, Alberta.

Scarff, D. H., and D. H. Lloyd. 1992. Double blind, placebo-controlled, crossover study of evening primrose oil in the treatment of canine atopy. Vet. Rec. 131:97–99.

Scott, D. W., W. H. Miller, G. A. Decker, and J. R. Wellington. 1992. Comparison of the clinical efficacy of two commercial fatty acid supplements (EfaVet and DVM Derm Caps), evening primrose oil, and cold water marine fish oil in the management of allergic pruritis in dogs: A double-blinded study. Cornell Vet. 82:319–329.

Schölkens, B. A., D. Gehring, V. Schlotte, and U. Weithmann. 1982. Evening primrose oil, a dietary prostaglandin precursor, diminishes vascular reactivity to renin and angiotensin II in rats. Prostaglandins Leukot. Med. 8:273–285.

Shields, R. G., and J. P. Bennett. 2000. Star-Kist Foods, Inc., assignee. December 5, 2000. Breed Specific Canine Food Formulations. U.S. Patent 6,156,355.

Shimizu, S., and M. Nakano. 2003. Structural characterization of triacylglycerol in several oils containing gamma-linolenic acid. Biosci. Biotechnol. Biochem. 67:60–67.

Shukla, Y. N., A. Srivastava, and S. Kumar. 1999. Aryl, lipid and triterpenoid constituents from *Oenothera biennis*. Indian J. Chem. B. 38:705–708.

Sinclair, A. J., J. G. McLean, and E. A. Monger. 1979. Metabolism of linoleic acid in the cat. Lipids 14:932–936.

Stasiniewicz, T., B. Niwinska, J. A. Strzetelski, J. Kowalczyk, K. Maciaszek, and K. Bilik. 1998. Nutritive value of evening primrose (*Oenothera paradoxa*) cake for ruminants. J. Anim. Feed Sci. 7:187–195.

Stelzleni, E. L. 2006. Effect of dietary n-3 fatty acid source on plasma, red blood cell and milk composition and immune status of mares and foals. Master's thesis. University of Florida, Gainesville, FL.

Stephens, O. A. 1932. The number and weight of seeds produced by weeds. Amer. J. Bot. 19:784–794.

Stone, K. J., A. L. Willis, M. Hart, S. J. Kirtland, P. B. A. Kernoff, and G. P. McNicol. 1979. The metabolism of dihomo-γ-linolenic acid in man. Lipids 14:174–180.

Strzetelski, J. A., J. Kowalczyk, K. Krawczyk, T. Stasiniewicz, and E. Lipiarska. 1998a. Evening primrose (*Oenothera paradoxa*) oil cake or ground rapeseed supplement to diets for dairy cows. J. Anim. Feed Sci. 7:365–375.

Strzetelski, J. A., K. Krawczyk, J. Kowalczyk, T. Stasiniewicz, S. Osieglowski, and E. Lipiarska. 1998b. Performance and body fat composition of fattening bulls fed diets with evening primrose (*Oenothera paradoxa*) oil cake. J. Anim. Feed Sci. 7:261–271.

Strzetelski, J. A., J. Kowalczyk, T. Stasiniewicz, E. Lipiarska, S. Osieglowski, and K. Bilik. 1999. Milk yield and composition in dairy cows fed a diet with evening primrose (*Oenothera paradoxa*) full fat seeds or oil cake. J. Anim. Feed Sci. 8:89–94.

Sture, G. H., and D. H. Lloyd. 1995. Canine atopic disease: Therapeutic use of an evening primrose oil and fish oil combination. Vet. Rec. 137:169–170.

Syed-Rahmatullah, M. S. K., V. K. S. Shukla, and K. D. Mukherjee. 1994. γ-Linolenic acid concentrates from borage and evening primrose oil fatty acids via lipase-catalyzed esterification. J. Amer. Oil Chem. Soc. 71:563–567.

Szabo, J., W. H. Ibrahim, G. D. Sunvold, and G. G. Bruckner. 2003. Effect of dietary protein quality and essential fatty acids on fatty acid composition in the liver and adipose tissue after rapid weight loss in overweight cats. Am. J. Vet. Res. 64:310–315.

Taha, A. Y., B. M. Baghiu, R. Lui, K. Nylen, D. W. Ma, and W. M. Burnham. 2006. Lack of benefit of linoleic and alpha-linolenic polyunsaturated fatty acids on seizure latency, duration, severity or incidence in rats. Epilepsy Res. 71:40–46.

Tauson, A. H., and M. Forsberg. 1991. Effect of evening primrose oil as food supplement on reproduction in the blue fox. Acta Vet. Scand. 32:345–351.

Tauson, A. H., M. Neil, and M. Forsberg. 1991. Effect of evening primrose oil as food supplement on reproduction in the mink. Acta Vet. Scand. 32:337–344.

Traitler, H., H. Winter, U. Richli, and Y. Ingenbleek. 1984. Characterization of -linolenic acid in Ribes seeds. Lipids 19:923–928.

Traitler, H., H. J. Willie, and A. Studer. 1988. Fractionation of blackcurrant seed oil. J. Am. Oil Chem. Soc. 65:755–760.

USDA (United States Department of Agriculture). Undated. PLANTS Database. Plant Guide, Common Evening Primrose (*Oenothera biennis* L.). National Resources Conservation Service. Online at: http://plants.usda.gov/. Accessed March 20, 2007.

Uzzan, A., J. P. Helme, and J. M. Klein. 1992. Fatty acid composition and quality data for oils rich in GLA. Rev. Fr. Corps Gras 39:339–343.

Vaddadi, K. S. 1981. The use of gamma-linolenic acid and linoleic acid to differentiate between temporal lobe epilepsy and schizophrenia. Prostaglandins Med. 6:375–379.

van Doormaal, J. J., I. G. Idema, F. A. Muskiet, I. A. Martini, and H. Doorenbos. 1988. Effects of short-term high-dose intake of evening primrose oil on plasma and cellular fatty acid compositions, alpha-tocopherol levels, and erythropoiesis in normal and type 1 (insulin-dependent) diabetic men. Diabetologia 31:576–584.

Warren, L. K., and J. Kivipelto. 2007a. Fatty acid content of grass and legume hays commonly fed to horses. J. Anim. Sci. 85 (Suppl. 1):140–141.

Warren, L. K., and J. Kivipelto. 2007b. Effect of season, forage maturity and grazing on the fatty acid composition of bahiagrass pasture. J. Anim. Sci. 85 (Suppl. 1):141.

Warren, L. K., and J. Kivipelto. 2008. Seasonal effects of diet on the omega-6 and omega-3 fatty acid composition of plasma and red blood cells in grazing horses. J. Anim. Sci. 86(E-Suppl. 2):376.

Watson, T. D. G. 1998. Diet and skin disease in dogs and cats. J. Nutr. 128:2783S–2789S.

Watson, T. D. G., C. J. Packard, and J. Shepherd. 1993. Plasma lipid transport in the horse (*Equus caballus*). Comp. Biochem. Physiol. Part B. 106:27–34.

Weems, C. W., Y. S. Weems, and R. D. Randel. 2004. Prostaglandins and reproduction in female farm animals. Vet. J. 171:206–228.

Weems, C. W., Y. S. Weems, and R. D. Randel. 2006. Prostaglandins and reproduction in female farm animals. Vet. J. 171:206–228.

Wettasinghe, M., and F. Shahidi. 1999. Evening primrose meal: A source of natural antioxidants and scavenger of hydrogen peroxide and oxygen-derived free radicals. J. Agric. Food Chem. 47:1801–1812.

Wettasinghe, M., F. Shahidi, and R. Amarowicz. 2002. Identification and quantification of low molecular weight phenolic antioxidants in seeds of evening primrose (*Oenothera biennis* L.). J. Agric. Food Chem. 50:1267–1271.

Wolff, R. L., and J. L. Sebedio. 1994. Characterization of γ-linolenic acid geometrical isomers in borage oil subjected to heat treatments (deodorization). J. Amer. Oil Chem. Soc. 71:117–126.

Yu-Cheng, D., H. Hui-Ming, L. Jun, and P. Lapinskas. 2001. Studies on the cultivation and uses of evening primrose (*Oenothera* spp.) in China. Econ. Bot. 55:83–92.

Zuagg, J., O. Potterat, A. Plescher, B. Honermeier, and M. Hamburger. 2006. Quantitative analysis of anti-inflammatory and radical scavenging triterpenoid esters in evening primrose seeds. J. Agric. Food Chem. 54:6623–6628.

8

Garlic

DESCRIPTION

Common Names and Synonyms

Garlic consists of the fresh or dried compound bulbs of *Allium sativum* Linné (Fam. Liliaceae or Alliaceae).

It is most commonly known as "garlic" but there are a large number of vernacular names including: Ail, camphor of the poor, poor man's treacle, and stinking rose (WHO, 1999).

Synonyms include *Porium sativum* Rehb (WHO, 1999).

Source and Botanical Characteristics

Source

Garlic is thought to have originated in western to central Asia from its progenitor *A. longicuspis Regel* and to have been transported from there originally to the Mediterranean and other areas of cultivation (Maaß and Klaas, 1995). It has been used in the diet of humans for centuries, with evidence that it was eaten in ancient Egypt. Ancient medical texts from Egypt, Greece, Rome, China, and India include prescribed medical applications for garlic (Fenwick and Hanley, 1985a; Rivlin, 2001).

Allium sativum comprises two subspecies, *A. sativum ophioscorodon* and *A. sativum sativum*. The former, commonly referred to as "hardneck garlic," is not significant in commercial garlic production. The U.S. Department of Agriculture (USDA) Economic Research Service (USDA, 2006) noted that "according to the Food and Agriculture Organization of the United Nations, China is by far the top source of garlic, with an estimated 23 billion pounds annually—75 percent of world output. The majority comes from the Shandong Province—a prime agricultural area located just southeast of Beijing. India (4 percent) and South Korea (3 percent) round out the top three producers worldwide. The United States is the fourth leading garlic producer, with 2 percent of the world crop." It goes on to state "in the United States, garlic seems to have gained in popularity as a cash crop over the past 10–15 years. According to the 2002 Census of Agriculture (census), 1,855 farms reported garlic acreage—up from 1,327 farms in 1997 and only 619 farms in 1992." California harvests around 90 percent of the U.S. commercial garlic acreage.

Botanical Characteristics

Garlic varies considerably with respect to its morphological and physiological features (Maaß and Klaas, 1995). The following description is taken from the U.S. Pharmacopeia (USP) Monograph for Garlic (USP, 2007) and may not apply to all types of garlic.

> *Subglobular compound bulbs, 3 to 5 cm in width, consisting of 8 to 20 cloves, the whole surrounded by 2 to 5 layers of white scale leaves attached to a flattened, circular base; cloves ovoid and 3- to 4-sided, summit acute, narrowed into a threadlike portion of fiber base, truncate, each clove covered with a white scale leaf and a pinkish white epidermis, easily separated from the solid portion, consisting of two flaky scale leaves and two yellowish green conduplicate foliage leaves.*

Form

Garlic preparations include the following (Amagase et al., 2001; Staba et al., 2001; Amagase, 2006):

- Whole intact garlic or products that are obtained from raw garlic and used almost immediately;
- Freeze-dried fresh garlic cloves, made by flash evaporation at low temperatures in a partial vacuum (it has been suggested that this results in essentially no changes in chemical composition); and
- Garlic-based commercial products that can in turn be divided into at least four main types including garlic

TABLE 8-1 Proximate Analysis for Various Garlic Forms (Percent Wet Weight)

Form	Moisture (%)	Protein (%)	Fat (%)	Ash (%)	Energy (cal/100 g Wet Weight)
Raw[a]	61.3	6.2	0.2	1.5	137
Raw[b]	61.3–86.3	2.2–6.2	0.2–0.3	0.6–1.5	39–140
Powder[a]	6.1	3.0	6.2	3.5	—
Salt[a]	10	8.8	5.6	82.2	—

[a]SOURCE: Fenwick and Hanley (1985b).
[b]SOURCE: Augusti (1996).

essential oil, garlic oil macerate, garlic powder, and hydroalcoholic extractions.

However, new methods of preparation are constantly being developed, such as combined microwave-vacuum drying preparations that are then microencapsulated (Li et al., 2007).

Chemical Composition

Whole intact garlic contains many chemical substances (Fenwick and Hanley, 1985b,c; Augusti, 1996; Amagase et al., 2001; Rahman, 2007) including:

1. The primary sulfur-containing compounds: γ-glutamyl-S-alk(en)yl-L-cysteines and S-alk(en)yl-L-cysteine sulfoxides (in particular alliin). On average, fresh garlic cloves have been reported to contain around 8 g/kg of alliin.
2. The enzyme CS-lyase: alliinase
3. Small amounts of S-allyl cysteine (SAC: formed by the catabolism of the above sulfur containing compounds)
4. Steroidal glycosides and saponins
5. Lectins
6. Prostaglandins
7. Fructan (polymers up to degree of polymerization 50: DP50), and a particular tetrasaccharide containing 4 fructose residues
8. Pectins
9. Essential oils
10. Adenosine
11. Vitamins B_1 (≈ 0.25 mg/100 g wet weight), B_2 (≈ 0.08 mg/100 g wet weight), B_6 (traces), C (≈ 5–15 mg/100 g wet weight), and E; biotin; nicotinic acid (≈ 0.5 mg/100 g wet weight); and retinol (≈ 15 μg/100 g wet weight).
12. Fatty acids (predominantly C18:2 ≈ 65 percent of total fatty acids)
13. Glucolipids, phospholipids, phenolics, flavonoids, isoflavonoids (including nobiletin, quercetin, rutin, and tangeretin), and some amino acids.

A guide to the proximate composition of garlic is shown in Table 8-1. However, these data are > 20 years old and do not necessarily represent the material present today. For example, a typical dried garlic powder available currently for use in animal feeds has 0.7 percent fat. In addition, garlic has been reported to contain the minerals and trace elements listed in Table 8-2 (Augusti, 1996). It is important to note that garlic has the ability to accumulate and incorporate selenium from the soil (as reviewed by Arnault and Auger, 2006).

Garlic is typified by its characteristic odor. It has been shown that the allyl thiosulfinates (mainly alliin: $C_6H_{11}NO_3S$ and allicin: $C_6H_{10}OS_2$ derived compounds) are responsible for breath allyl methyl sulfide (AMS) and increased breath acetone (Lawson and Wang, 2005; Rahman, 2007). Whole intact garlic bulbs do not contain allicin (diallylthiosulfinate) as this is formed when the garlic clove is damaged, as illustrated in Figure 8-1.

Processed garlic contains a variety of sulfur-containing compounds other than those found naturally in intact garlic cloves, so that if a whole garlic clove is crushed and then ingested the following will be consumed: quantities of alliinase and its primary substrate alliin; allicin and its allyl sulfide volatile conversion products; some γ-glutamyl

TABLE 8-2 Guide to Mineral and Trace Element Analysis for Garlic

Element	Amount (mg per 100 g wet weight)
Ca	50–90
P	390–460
K	100–120
Na	10–22
Mg	43–77
Al	0.5–1
Ba	0.2–1
Fe	2.8–3.9
Sr	0.1–0.7
B	0.3–0.6
Cu	0.02–0.03
Zn	1.8–3.1
Mn	0.2–0.6
Cr	0.3–0.5
S	65
Cl	43

NOTE: Garlic was also reported to contain germanium (14 μg/100 g wet weight), molybdenum (42 μg/100 g wet weight), and selenium (15.1–35.4 μg/100 g wet weight).
SOURCE: Based on data in Augusti (1996).

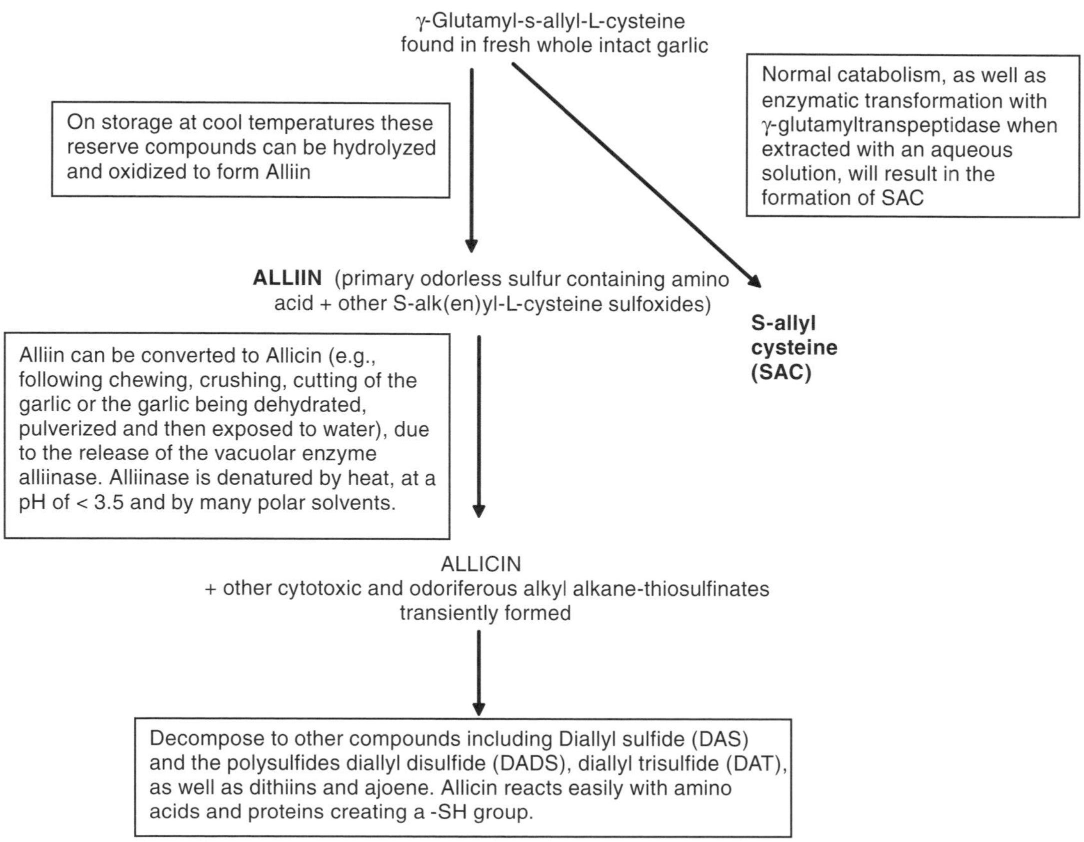

FIGURE 8-1 Guide to some of the effects of storage and other factors on one of the main compounds found in garlic.
SOURCES: Adapted from data in Fenwick and Hanley (1985b,c); Augusti (1996); Amagase et al. (2001); Rahman (2007).

cysteine and S-allyl cysteine; and the largely nonpolar compounds vinyldithiins and ajoene as well as items 4–13 in the above list (steroidal glycosides and saponins through amino acids). Allicin represents approximately 70 percent of the overall thiosulfinates present in garlic cloves upon mechanical crushing (Lawson et al., 1991).

Putative Active Compounds and Proposed Biological Activity

Putative Active Compounds

Putative active ingredients in garlic and garlic-derived preparations include several sulfur compounds. The most important are thought to be allicin, SAC, diallyl sulphide (DAS), and diallyl disulphide (DADS). More recently, the tri- and tetrasulfides have been considered to have a role, as well as a number of nonsulfur compounds, including the steroid saponins, allixin, N-α-fructosyl arginine, and various organoselenium compounds (Fenwick and Hanley, 1985c; Augusti, 1996; Amagase et al., 2001; Kasuga et al., 2001; Kodera et al., 2002; Banerjee et al., 2003; Amagase, 2006; Münchberg et al., 2007; Tsao et al., 2007).

Proposed Biological Activity

The chemistry underlying any potential biological activity of the putative active compounds in garlic is likely to be complex. Recent work, for example, on the polysulfides (biologically active sulfur species, formed by the decomposition of allicin, with more than two sulfide groups) suggests that they might work through a combination of several distinct metabolic transformations. These include oxidation reactions, superoxide radical and peroxide generation, decomposition with release of highly electrophilic S_x species, inhibition of metalloenzymes, disturbance of metal homeostasis and membrane integrity, and interference with different cellular signaling pathways (Münchberg et al., 2007). It has been suggested that the conversion, at least in human red blood cells (RBC), of garlic-derived organic polysulfides into hydrogen sulfide may be related to the vasoactivity of garlic (Benavides et al., 2007). Recent work has concentrated on the influence of garlic-derived organosulfur compounds on the generation of reactive oxygen species, as well as endoplasmic reticulum stress, activation of stress kinases, and cysteine processes promoting apoptosis. Although these activities may protect against certain types of carcinogenesis (Das et al., 2007), the reactive oxygen species generating catalytic cycles may also partially explain the toxicity of garlic polysulfides, but not allicin.

Protection against certain carcinogens may also reflect altered metabolism, specifically increased tissue concentrations of phase 2 detoxification enzymes such as glutathione-S-transferase (GST) and quinone reductase (QR) (Munday et al., 2003). Additionally, at certain concentrations, garlic-derived compounds may inhibit selected cytochrome P450s (CYP450), thus decreasing formation of toxic "metabolites" that may contribute to carcinogenesis. This potential effect on metabolic enzyme activity may also contribute to herb-drug interactions (Zhou et al., 2007).

With regard to the relative beneficial effects of garlic and onions (considered to be the most closely related plant to garlic), Munday et al. (2003) concluded, in a dose-response study, that phase 2 enzymes (QR and GST) were induced by allyl sulfides in rats at a dose equivalent to that expected with human consumption of garlic. In contrast, propyl sulfides (onion equivalents of the allyl sulfides) administration to rats at doses higher than those expected with human onion ingestion had no inductive effect on the same enzymes. The increased presence of granules of oxidatively denatured hemoglobin within RBC (Heinz bodies), following the ingestion of garlic and/or onions above a certain level, suggests that oxidative damage may be involved in the pathophysiology of garlic toxicity. Heinz bodies (HB) are aggregates of denatured, precipitated hemoglobin within the red blood cell. Oxidation of reactive sulfhydryl (S-H) groups creates disulfide bonds that change the conformation of the globin protein chains and result in precipitation of the hemoglobin molecule (Desnoyers, 2000). Munday et al. (2003) suggested that, in vivo, the allyl and propyl di- but especially the tri- and tetrasulfides act as powerful hemolytic agents and therefore contribute to the toxic effects of the allium species. Dogs have been shown to suffer hemolysis and severe anemia after 4–6 days of administration of n-propyl disulfide at 0.067–0.122 ml/kg BW usually after the afternoon feed (active dose not given) (Gruhzit, 1931a). The di-, tri-, and tetrasulfides are readily reduced to thiols by reduced glutathione (GSH). Oxidation in RBC may be initiated by formation of reactive oxygen species during redox cycling, involving hemoglobin, between these polysulfides and their corresponding thiols (Munday et al., 2003).

Importance of Heinz Bodies and Eccentrocytes

When HB are numerous, develop at a fast rate, or are large, the resulting alteration in red blood cell membrane may result in direct intravascular cell lysis. In cats, the hemoglobin molecule contains eight sulfhydryl groups and seems more prone to oxidative damage and HB formation compared to the dog or human, which have four and two sulfhydryl groups, respectively. The ease of dissociation of feline hemoglobin from tetramers to dimers may also play a role. The cat spleen lacks venous sinusoids and does not remove HB-containing RBC efficiently. This may allow damaged RBC to circulate longer, resulting in accumulation of HB to a greater extent than in other species such as the dog. The committee is not aware of data on this in the horse and therefore comparisons between the cat and horse cannot be made. Heinz bodies alter RBC function and shorten half-life. Mechanisms of RBC destruction are thought to include direct cell lysis as RBC membranes with reduced deformability are damaged when traversing the microvasculature, as well as destruction by intracellular proteolysis, glutathione depletion, antibody binding, and alteration of membrane charge distribution (Christopher et al., 1990). In the dog, the reticuloendothelial system of the spleen directly removes damaged RBC or can simply remove HB, by "pitting," without cellular destruction. Like HB, eccentrocytes are believed to be formed as a result of direct oxidative damage to the RBC membrane (Desnoyers, 2000). Eccentrocytes are RBC that have hemoglobin concentrated on one side of the cell, leaving a pale area on the opposite side. Heinz body formation and eccentrocytes both contribute to shortened RBC lifespan or direct destruction of oxidized RBC and represent an adverse effect associated with garlic and/or onion toxicosis in dogs and cats (Desnoyers, 2000).

Method of Analysis

A variety of analytical techniques have been used to detect various garlic-containing or derived compounds (e.g., Iberl et al., 1990; Lawson et al., 1992; Freeman and Kodera, 1995; Fenwick and Henley, 1995a,b,c; Kodera et al., 2002; Lawson and Gardner, 2005). Suggested methods for identifying alliin, allinase activity, and SAC, for example, are given in the USP monographs (USP, 2007).

Standardization

There is a need for the standardization of garlic and garlic-derived products as was pointed out by Staba et al. (2001). However, there has been some debate as to which constituent should form the basis of any such protocols.

It has been stated that U.S. pharmacy-grade garlic contains 0.3 percent (powdered) to 0.5 percent (fresh dried) allicin, while in Europe pharmacy-grade garlic must have at least 0.45 percent allicin (NSRC, 2006). The USP has recently produced a number of garlic monographs (USP, 2000, 2003, 2007), which include their reference standards for the end composition of several but not all garlic preparations based on the levels of alliin, allicin, and SAC as appropriate for the product type as they define them. Examples of these standards include: "Garlic Delayed-Release Tablets are prepared from Powdered Garlic or Powdered Garlic Extract and contain not less than 90.0 percent and not more than 140.0 percent of the labeled amount of alliin ($C_6H_{11}NO_3S$) and not less than 90.0 percent and not more than 140.0 percent of the labeled amount of potential allicin ($C_6H_{10}OS_2$)" and "Powdered Garlic Extract is prepared from fresh Garlic bulbs by extraction with alcohol. The ratio of the starting crude plant material to Powdered Extract is between 9.5:1 and 13.5:1. It contains not less than 4.0 percent of alliin ($C_6H_{11}NO_3S$). It may contain added Powdered Garlic or other suitable substances."

These monographs also provide guidance, where appropriate, as to the maximum level of total ash, acid-insoluble ash, water content, and various contaminants.

There seems to be considerable controversy over the use of allicin in standardization. This is because allicin is a highly unstable and reactive substance that rapidly decomposes to other compounds. Therefore, concentrations of allicin reported in commercial products generally tend to be very low (e.g., < 1 mg/kg; Freeman and Kodera, 1995). One of the reasons given for the enteric coating of certain preparations has been to try and help prevent gastric acid inactivation of the allicin-producing enzyme alliinase. The aim is that such products would then generate more allicin following ingestion resulting in an increased "allicin potential" or "allicin yield" (Freeman and Kodera, 1995). However, one study found that > 80 percent of the enteric-coated products tested released < 15 percent of their stated "potential allicin" content. The low allicin "release" was found to be due both to impaired alliinase activity, in part caused by the tablet excipients, and to slow tablet disintegration (Lawson and Wang, 2001; Lawson et al., 2001). As such it has been proposed that garlic powder supplements should be standardized on dissolution allicin release as defined in the U.S. Pharmacopeia/National Formulary (USP, 2000, 2003) rather than on allicin potential.

Several researchers, particularly those who have evaluated products based on SAC or other compounds rather than allicin, have suggested that even if it survives passage through the stomach following ingestion, only very small quantities of allicin would be available for absorption due to inactivation by alliinase produced by intestinal or other cells (Freeman and Kodera, 1995; Amagase et al., 2001; Rahman, 2007).

An alternative approach to using allicin content has been to evaluate certain metabolic byproducts. For example, allicin and allicin-derived compounds are rapidly metabolized to AMS, a compound that stimulates the production of acetone and that can be used to measure the bioavailability of allicin and allicin-derived compounds, and hence, the ability of garlic supplements to represent fresh garlic (Lawson and Wang, 2005). Other researchers have suggested using the metabolic products of other constituents of garlic, in particular SAC, as biomarkers. For example, urinary N-acetyl SAC has also been suggested as a possible compliance marker for products containing high levels of SAC (Amagase, 2006). However, in another study this marker was not found in human urine after garlic ingestion (Kodera et al., 2002), although this may reflect analytical rather than physiological differences. In addition, marked species differences in the metabolism of SAC (described below) might limit the value of urinary N-Acetyl SAC per se as a marker.

Finally, recently it has been suggested that, at least with respect to possible in vivo vasoactivity, the capacity to produce hydrogen sulfide in vitro might be used to standardize garlic dietary supplements (Benavides et al., 2007). This paper raised the possibility that appropriate standardization may need to vary according to the potential primary purpose of the particular preparation being evaluated.

Related Compounds

Allium (from the Celtic word "all") is the onion genus, with about 1,250 species, making it one of the largest plant genera in the world. They are perennial bulbous plants that produce chemical compounds that give them a characteristic onion or garlic taste and odor, and many are used as food plants. Onions, shallots, leeks, and chives are all members of the genus. Onion (*Allium cepa* L.) is potentially the closest related plant to garlic (Fenwick and Hanley, 1985a).

It is important to note that the nature of the alkyl group in the sulfoxide varies with the Allium species. Garlic contains predominantly allyl cysteine sulfoxide while onions, leeks, and chives contain mainly propyl and prop-1-enyl cysteine sulfoxides. The major sulfide breakdown products from garlic are therefore allyl mono-, di-, tri-, and tetrasulfides, whereas those from the others are the corresponding propyl and prop-1 enyl derivatives. This may affect toxicity as well as efficacy (Munday et al., 2003).

Effect of Manufacturing, Processing, and Storage on Composition

> Effects of processing can be complex and difficult to predict, but it is likely that different preparations will contain different levels of the major compounds.

Stability

Although garlic is not considered in general to be a very perishable product a number of factors can affect its stability, in particular the environmental conditions under which whole garlic or peeled garlic cloves are stored. These affect the dormancy period and the onset of sprout development (Cantwell et al., 2003, Vazquez-Barrios et al., 2006). Prestorage handling as well as the temperature and length of storage influence when sprout development occurs either in the stored garlic or upon removal from storage (Cantwell et al., 2003; Vazquez-Barrios et al., 2006). A number of diseases that affect cultivated garlic may not only reduce the yield and quality but may also affect the bulbs in storage (Fenwick and Hanley, 1985a). A nonparasitic disease referred to as "waxy breakdown" is described for some products in the U.S. Food and Drug Administration (FDA) macroanalytical procedures manual (FDA, 1984). Waxy breakdown is manifested as physical changes in color (yellow to amber) and texture (shrunken and waxy to the touch) in the clove, with the changes increasing in magnitude as the condition progresses. Proposed causes include heat, sunscald, or physiological breakdown.

With respect to the various garlic preparations, stability in storage seems to depend on the preparation being evaluated, as well as the length of storage, but some products are stable for many months (Lawson and Gardner, 2005; Rahman, 2007).

Processing

According to the USDA Economic Research Service (USDA, 2006) garlic sold fresh is hand harvested, whereas seed garlic and garlic designated to be dehydrated are mechanically harvested. The harvesting method may have an impact on quality and stability during storage.

The substances present in any particular garlic product, and therefore any potential activity, will depend on the initial garlic ecotype (Rahman, 2007) and the conditions applied during processing (Fenwick and Hanley, 1985a,b,c; Staba et al., 2001; Banerjee et al., 2003; Lawson and Gardner, 2005; Al-Waili et al., 2007; Cavagnaro et al., 2007) in particular—

- The potential substrate activity of the enzyme allinase that is sequestered within garlic cell vacuoles
- Storage and exposure to heat and ultraviolet light
- Temperature and duration of drying
- The use of polar and/or nonpolar extraction solvents
- Conditions and period of maceration before final extraction.

Certainly, different preparations will tend to have different amounts of the major organosulfur compounds (Banerjee et al., 2003) and as indicated in Table 8-3.

Depending on the nature of the biological test undertaken, studies have shown that processing may (Bordia et al., 1996) or may not (Polasa et al., 2006) affect the biological activity of any particular preparation. Biological activity will also depend on the extent or duration of any processing. For example, Jastrzebski et al. (2007) showed that compared with raw garlic or garlic cooked for 20 minutes at 100°C, garlic cooked for 40 or 60 minutes at 100°C started to lose antioxidant bioactivity. The authors therefore suggested that garlic should be added to cooking dishes within 20 minutes before the end of the cooking to maintain antioxidant potential. However, based on in vitro anti-aggregatory activity of human platelets, Cavagnaro et al. (2007) showed that whether garlic is crushed or not before cooking may also affect final activity. This suggests that the effects of processing can be quite complex and perhaps difficult to predict due to differing effects on particular bioactives.

Potential for Contamination or Adulteration

Although there seems to be general acceptance that external contamination of garlic with yeasts, molds, bacteria, fungal toxins, heavy metals, pesticide residues, and foreign material is possible, there are no globally accepted limits for many potential contaminants. Therefore, for many potential contaminants, national guidelines prevail as stated in the World Health Organization (WHO) monograph for garlic.

Bacterial Contamination

The WHO monograph for garlic (WHO, 1999) states that in garlic products for internal use, salmonella should be negative; aerobic bacteria less than 10^5/g or ml; Enterobacteria and certain gram-negative bacteria not more than 10^3/g or ml and *E. coli* 0/g or ml. The USP monograph (USP, 2000, 2003) for powdered garlic extract states for microbial enumeration "The total bacterial count does not exceed 10,000 cfu (colony forming unit) per gram, and the total combined molds and yeasts count does not exceed 1,000 cfu per gram. It meets the requirements of the tests for absence of *Salmonella* species and *Escherichia coli.*"

In 1989, the FDA warned that botulism food poisoning may occur with certain commercial and homemade chopped garlic-and-oil mixes if left at room temperature. It noted that their studies had shown that garlic in an oil mixture could support bacterial growth and toxin production even when very few *Clostridium botulinum* spores were present (FDA, 1989).

Insect/Fungal/Mycotoxin Contamination

The FDA macroanalytical procedures manual (FDA, 1984), in its section on garlic, noted that "garlic is susceptible to insect and mite infestation, and to several types of decomposition, including bulb rot (caused by *Aspergillus alliaceus*), blue mold rot (*Penicillium* spp.), and white rot (*Sclerotia cepivorum*)." This technical bulletin (FDA, 1984) provides a procedure for the determination of insect-damaged, moldy, and otherwise decomposed garlic bulbs. Fungal disease is a major factor affecting the production, productivity, and quality of garlic. Rust caused by *Puccinia allii*, neck rot caused by various *Botrytis* species, and, in particular, white rot have been described as the most important fungal diseases worldwide (Zewde et al., 2007).

Rot of the basal plate of garlic has been suggested to most commonly occur due to infection by *Fusarium culmorum*, This is often considered to be a minor disease but it can be responsible for up to 40 percent of the losses of garlic cloves in the field and an even higher amount in storage. However, *F. proliferatum* can also be a potentially serious pathogen

TABLE 8-3 Suggested Differences Between Some of the Different Types of Garlic Preparations

Type of Product	How Produced	Main Compounds	Alliin	Standardization
Garlic essential oil	Whole garlic cloves ground in water are heat-distilled or extracted in an organic solvent (e.g., Hexane).	< 1 percent oil-soluble sulfur compounds (e.g., DAS or DADS) plus ≈ 99 percent vegetable oil. Alliicin is volatile and commonly lost or converted to the allyl sulfide degradation products. Over 20 sulfides have been identified in steam-distilled garlic oil and oil-soluble extract of garlic. The actual composition will vary according to the extraction temperature and time.	Little if any alliin or allicin	Little
Garlic oil macerate	Encapsulated mixtures of whole garlic cloves are ground into vegetable oil.	Oil-soluble sulfur compounds DAS, DADS, DATS (but often in low levels) including some allicin-decomposition compounds, such as vinyldithins, allyl sulfides, and ajoene.	Residual amounts	Little
Garlic powder	Garlic cloves are sliced or crushed, dried, and pulverized into powder.	Although supposedly similar to raw garlic, can be highly variable. Fresh crushed raw garlic is high in allicin (≈ 3.7 mg/g) but it has been reported that some preparations contain significantly lower levels e.g., < 1.0 mg/g allicin due to its instability.	Suggested that much of the alliin may be lost during the dehydration process.	Little
Hydroalcoholic extractions Short-term resultant product often called a tincture—and may be made in 10, 20, 30 percent wt/v concentrations in 70 percent ethanol or produced as fluid or dry extracts	Whole or sliced garlic cloves are soaked in an extracting solution (e.g., purified water and diluted alcohol) for short periods of time	Highly variable	—	Stability has been questioned.
Hydroalcoholic extractions Long-term aged garlic extract (AGE)	Whole or sliced garlic cloves are soaked in an extracting solution (e.g., purified water and diluted alcohol) for longer periods of time (≈ 6–20 months). After separation of the solution the extract is generally concentrated and used either in liquid or powdered form. Aged garlic extract is aged for up to 20 months.	Mainly water-soluble compounds (e.g., SAC, SAMC, or saponins) Small amounts of oil-soluble sulfur compounds Allicin is completely converted to allyl sulfides, which are largely all volatized or converted to other compounds.	—	Currently standardized through SAC content

NOTE: DAS: diallyl sulphide; DADS: diallyl disulphide; DAT: diallyl trisulfide; SAC: S-allyl-l-cysteine; SAMC: S-allyl mercaptocysteine.

as the fungal isolates recovered in one study were able to produce a number of potentially serious toxins of concern to human and animal health, including fumonisin B_1 (Stankovic et al., 2007). Other studies have apparently shown fumonisin contamination in cloves of garlic grown in soil artificially inoculated by *F. proliferatum,* suggesting that this fungus can accumulate mycotoxins in the edible part of garlic plants. It highlights the potential for mycotoxin contamination of naturally supplied garlic (Stankovic et al., 2007).

Pesticide Residues

Because of the problems with fungal contamination in particular, pesticides are commonly used during garlic production. In California alone, it has been estimated that at least 24,000 kg of chemicals were used in 2005. Details of the main pesticides used can be found at www.pesticideinfo.org/DS.jsp?sk=14007.

The pesticide residues committee (European Commission, 2005) recently reported residues of two fungicides (carbendazim and iprodione) not permitted for use on organic crops and produce in one sample of whole organic garlic. This is therefore a potential area of concern.

A number of agreed extraneous maximum residue limits are listed under the CODEX Alimentarius (e.g., Pesticide: Maleic Hydrazide - Commodity: Garlic - MRL - 15 mg/kg; Codex Alimentarius, 2008). In the United States, the list of tolerances and exemptions for pesticide residues for foods is compiled in the Code of Federal Regulations (CFR), Chapter 40, Part 180. This is reviewed annually (http://www.access.gpo.gov/nara/cfr/waisidx_02/40cfr180_02.html). Examples of some tolerance limits for insecticides and fungicides are shown in Table 8-4.

The WHO (1999) monograph for garlic stated that pesticide residues should be established in accordance with national requirements but noted that the maximum residue limit of aldrin and dieldrin for garlic was normally not more than 0.05 mg/kg. For other pesticides, *Guidelines on Quality Control Methods for Medicinal Plant Materials* (WHO, 1998) and *Guidelines for Predicting Dietary Intake of Pesticide Residues* (WHO, 1997) should be consulted. It is important to note that such levels have not been set for animal intake as far as the committee is aware.

One of the main issues that has been identified in the analysis of herbicide residues within garlic is interference from sulfur compounds produced through the action of allinase on alliin, which is then rapidly degraded (see Figure 8-1). A number of different methods have been described in an attempt to overcome this problem. For example, a rapid multiresidue method, based on the deactivation of the allinase enzyme using microwave heating, has been developed for the determination of 16 herbicides in garlic (Chen et al., 2007).

Heavy Metals

The potential for garlic to provide a novel method for the removal of cadmium from contaminated waters has been explored (Jiang et al., 2001). This includes sewage and ground water used for irrigation, industrial wastes, and landfill leachates. However, this does mean that there is a potential for garlic preparations to contain varying amounts of heavy metals, with the risk depending on the environment in which the garlic was grown. The actual risk may be small because garlic apparently only transports a small amount of cadmium to its bulbs and shoots (Jiang et al., 2001).

The WHO (1999) monograph for garlic stated the "recommended lead and cadmium levels are no more than 10 and 0.3 mg/kg in the final dosage form of the plant material. Limits for heavy metal contamination vary from country to country and are currently being updated in many countries."

Adulteration

The strong odor of garlic, even when present in relatively low levels, has the potential to mask nongarlic components or adulterants. It is therefore possible, unless labeling is based on the amount of a specific active ingredient (section above on Standardization), that adulteration could occur resulting in more or less of the putative active ingredient being present in any particular preparation or product (Lawson et al., 1992; Ruddock et al., 2005). However, the committee does not know whether there are any specific adulterants that could mimic the effects of any of the compounds used in any current screening or standardization method and whether this would be likely to occur in practice.

BIOLOGY

Absorption, Distribution, Metabolism, and Excretion

Overall, it seems that many of the active compounds in garlic have not been well characterized, and their bioavailability has not been confirmed (Amagase, 2006). For example, various garlic-derived, oil-soluble, organosulfur compounds (allicin, sulfides, vinyldithiins) were apparently not found in the blood or urine of humans even after consumption of a large amount of garlic (25 g) (Lawson et al., 1992). However, definitive bioavailability investigations have not been carried out. The relevance of quantification of allicin in blood has been questioned (Rahman, 2007), especially as it has been reported to be formed by human liver microsomes from DADS (Teyssier et al., 1999) and, therefore, its rapid disappearance from the bloodstream may be associated with intracellular movement of metabolites and resynthesis of the bioactive product (Rahman, 2007). Others have suggested that allicin and allicin-derived compounds are rapidly metabolized to breath AMS (Lawson and Wang, 2005) and cleared by expiration. Finally, in mice and rats it has been suggested that although there is some evidence for absorption of orally administered synthetic alliin, it is

TABLE 8-4 Examples of Tolerances for Residues (ppm)

Item	Captan	Dicloran	Malathion	Parathion	Folpet
Garlic	25[a]	5	8	1	15[a]

[a]Represented by onion dry bulb.
NOTE: These are reviewed annually and may only apply to residues from preharvest application.
SOURCE: Code of Federal Regulations (CFR), Chapter 40, Part 180.

without conversion to allicin or its degradation compounds (Amagase, 2006). It therefore, may not reflect the fate of natural alliin, thereby adding to the confusion.

In contrast to allicin, the pharmokinetics of SAC seem to be more established (Nagae et al., 1994; Rahman, 2007). S-allyl cysteine is rapidly absorbed from the gastrointestinal tract with a peak plasma concentration, occurring at 0.25 hour in dogs, 0.5 hour at doses of 12.5 and 25 mg/kg in rats, and at 1 hour in rats given 50 mg/kg (Nagae et al., 1994). Bioavailability has been described as 103 percent in mice, 98.2 percent in rats, and 87.2 percent in dogs (adult female Beagles ≈ 10 kg BW). S-allyl cysteine is distributed mainly in the liver, kidney, and plasma of rats, mice, and dogs (Nagae et al., 1994). In rats, SAC levels are highest in the kidney, and plasma and tissue levels peak 15–30 minutes after oral SAC administration (Nagae et al., 1994). S-allyl cysteine is thought to be metabolized to N-acetyl SAC in the liver and kidney. In the rat, kidney N-acetyl SAC may partially deacylate back into SAC by acylase in the kidney. In addition, in rats 30–50 percent of the SAC dose is excreted in the urine as N-acetyl SAC and < 1 percent as unchanged SAC. However, in dogs, < 1 percent of the dose was found in the urine as either SAC or N-acetyl SAC, suggesting marked species differences in the elimination of SAC. This is supported by species differences in elimination half-life. The half-life approximates 1 hour (0.77 hour) in mice when given orally and half an hour (0.43 hour) for intravenous (i.v.) administration, whereas in dogs it is approximately 10 hours after either oral or i.v. administration. In humans, the T_{max} of SAC (from ingested aged garlic extract rather than SAC alone) has been shown to be approximately 1 hour, the half-life estimated to be greater than 10 hours, and clearance time more than 30 hours (Kodera et al., 2002).

It is probable that the differing contents and bioavailabilities of the active ingredients within any particular garlic product and species will result in similarly different biological responses as well as potential risk of adverse effects.

Purported Role in Health and Disease

There is a plethora of publications available that have examined the potential health benefits of eating garlic or garlic preparations (Fleischauer et al., 2000; Amagase et al., 2001; Kasuga et al., 2001; Rivlin, 2001; Banerjee et al., 2003; Lee and Park, 2003; Bhattacharyya et al., 2007; Fisher et al., 2007; Howard et al., 2007). These have suggested, with varying levels of scientific proof, that garlic has the potential to—

- Reduce the risk of cardiovascular diseases and cancer (e.g., antithrombotic, antilipolytic, antimetastatic, and improves circulation)
- Stimulate immune function
- Mitigate the effect of oxidants
- Provide antimicrobial and antiviral protection
- Enhance foreign compound detoxification
- Improve radioprotection
- Restore physical strength
- Improve resistance to various stresses
- Have an anti-aging effect.

Despite the large number of studies focusing on the efficacy of garlic, results are inconsistent. Factors contributing to the inconsistencies include differences in preparation used, including active ingredients, vehicles, and doses; differences in storage conditions that may affect the concentration of active components; failure to identify biologically available constituents; inappropriately short study durations; inadequate randomization; and poor blinding procedures, reflecting, in part, the nature of garlic (Fleischauer et al., 2000; Lawson et al., 2001). Das et al. (2007) noted that "many of the effects are observed at concentrations much higher than what is normally ingested by humans and clinical trials will be needed to define the effective dose that has no toxicity in humans."

Drug Interactions

Clinical studies evaluating garlic-drug interactions are limited (Greenblatt et al., 2006). Approaches to investigations regarding pharmacokinetic herb-drug interactions include in vitro studies measuring CYP450 content or biotransformation activity. Biotransformation activity often is based on changes in disappearance of a substrate, which is assumed to be specifically biotransformed by the enzyme of interest. Other types of studies include those that have demonstrated changes in the assumed substrate specificity and in vivo studies based on the area under the plasma concentration time curve (AUC) and maximum plasma concentration of the drug of interest. However, as with many aspects of garlic assessment, data regarding its impact on drug biotransformation are complex and incomplete. Markowitz et al. (2003) noted that comparing studies investigating the metabolic effects of garlic is limited by the use of different garlic formulations, treatment durations, and probe substrates. Hu et al. (2005) supported this concern, particularly as it relates to modulation of CYP enzyme activity and expression, because conclusions are likely to depend on the type and chemical composition of the garlic supplements and dosage regimen used.

The therapeutic effects of garlic compounds have been suggested by some to be, at least in part, due to their interaction with -SH group containing compounds such as enzymes, especially in the liver. As the liver is a major site of metabolic processes, including drug metabolism, altered drug biotransformation could be an expected sequelae of garlic intake. Several in vitro, ex vivo, and in vivo studies have demonstrated herb-drug interactions between garlic or its organosulfur constituents and drugs through modulation of CYP450 (Zhou et al., 2007). Not surprisingly, results varied with the model, dose, preparation, and other variables. For example, ex vivo studies using preparations from livers of rats treated with DAS demonstrated a dose or duration-dependent effect (Dalvi, 1992). A single high dose (500 mg/kg in corn oil) administered intraperitoneal (i.p.) significantly decreased CYP450 microsomal content (in nanomoles/milligram protein), aminopyrine N-demethylase, and aniline hydroxylase activity, whereas repeated low to moderate (50 mg/kg BW for 5 days) doses increased CYP450 content and aminopyrine N-demethylase and benzyphetamine N-demethylase activities. Both induction and decreased degradation of CYP450 was suggested at the low dosage. Other authors using either in vitro or in vivo methods have demonstrated that DAS, diallyl trisulfide (DATS), and DADS, each a major constituent of certain garlic preparations, can induce drug metabolism enzymes, including CYP450, epoxide hydrolyase, glutathione-S-transferase, and NAD(P)H quinone oxidoreductase (Pan et al., 1993; Fisher et al., 2007). Authors have postulated that the effect involves activation of constitutive androstane receptor (CAR) and nuclear factor E2-related factor 2 (Nrf2) transcription factors (Fisher et al., 2007). As such, garlic preparations, including garlic oil, may affect transcriptional regulation of hepatic phase I and phase II drug metabolizing enzymes. This is supported by work in rats receiving short-term high (300 mg/kg) oral doses of garlic oil, but not mice receiving a lower dose (175 mg/kg orally: Fisher et al., 2007). However, the failure to demonstrate a similar effect in mice may reflect the dose-limiting toxicity seen with the garlic oil in mice.

There have been reports that suggest that garlic administration may alter the pharmacokinetics of several therapeutic drugs, including the HIV protease inhibitor saquinavir, the analgesic/antipyretic acetaminophen (paracetamol), and the anticoagulant warfarin (Izzo and Ernst, 2001; James, 2001; Piscitelli et al., 2002). These conclusions are disputed by some due to the size of the studies, the protocols used, and whether the effects just relate to high levels of DAS, DAT, and DAD intake (Wu et al., 2002) rather than garlic per se. Hu et al. (2005) concluded from their review of the literature that garlic decreased the AUC and maximum plasma concentration of saquinavir, but not ritonavir and paracetamol (acetaminophen). Again, the importance of the type of garlic preparation being fed has been raised as it has been questioned whether the same effects would be seen with SAC (and other water-soluble sulfur compounds). This question of relevance to SAC and its analogs is supported by in vitro studies of CYP450 isoenzymes in human hepatic microsomes exposed to aged garlic extract components (Greenblatt et al., 2006). Although SAC reduced CYP3A activity by 60 percent (without evidence of a classical concentration effect), the authors (Greenblatt et al., 2006) concluded that the risk of pharmacokinetic drug interactions, including inhibition of the specific cytochrome isoforms evaluated, was very low as the doses used were higher (100 μmol/L) than would be anticipated in vivo. However, it would seem that further work is required to confirm this, especially as applicability of in vitro studies to in vivo situations is perhaps questionable. In one in vivo study, in healthy volunteers, limited impact of one commercially available garlic product (3 × 600 mg for 14 days: SAC content ≈ 0.03 mg and "allicin potential" ≈ 0.3 mg/600 mg tablet) was found on the disposition of coadministered medications whose clearance is primarily dependent on the CYP2D6 or CYP3A4 activity (Markowitz et al., 2003).

Summarizing, the effects of garlic or its active components on CYP450 or other drug metabolizing enzyme activity is likely to be further complicated by its apparent paradoxical effect, as was suggested by Gallicano et al. (2003). Garlic might act as an enzyme inhibitor or an enzyme inducer on the same enzyme, depending on the circumstances, leading to effects that are complex and, at times, opposite. Although less specific than pharmacokinetic studies in identifying a cause and effect mechanism, an advantage of pharmacodynamic studies is their potential relevance to clinical use. For example, Hu et al. (2005) in their review concluded that *A. sativum* increased the clotting time and international normalized ratio of warfarin and caused hypoglycemia when taken with chlorpropramide. Further, two HIV-infected people receiving garlic or garlic supplements for > 2 weeks developed severe gastrointestinal tract (GIT) toxicity after beginning therapy with ritonavir, whose clearance is dependent primarily on biotransformation by CYP3A4. Symptoms resolved after discontinuing either the drug or the garlic (as reviewed by Gallicano et al., 2003). These authors showed that acute dosing of garlic over 3 days did not significantly alter the single dose pharmacokinetics of ritonovir in healthy volunteers, although there were nonsignificant changes that may or may not have been due to an effect of the garlic on CYP3A4.

Staba et al. (2001) noted it is possible that excess (not defined) intake of garlic products may promote orthostatic hypertension when consumed in patients treated with antihypertensive drugs, or hypoglycemia when consumed in patients treated with insulin or oral hypoglycemic medications. However, although the authors noted that the vast majority (not defined) of individuals are unlikely to experience these difficulties, determining the true incidence of these possible interactions would seem to be prudent. It is clear that further research is needed before the impact of garlic or its active components on drug disposition or response can be reliably predicted.

The textbook *Veterinary Herbal Medicine* (Wynn and Fougère, 2007), states that garlic by virtue of its effect on the CYP450 enzymes, CYP3A, CYP2B1, CYP2C, CYP2D, and CYP2E1 could potentially interact with the following drugs: acetaminophen, antacids, anticoagulants, antihypertensives, doxorubicin, insulin, and oral hypoglycemic agents, isoprenaline, and saquinavir. Garlic is likely to have an additive effect with certain oxidizing drugs, thereby increasing the potential for oxidative damage or lysis of RBC. Drugs associated with Heinz body formation include acetaminophen, phenacetin, urinary acidifiers/antiseptics (DL-methionine, phenazopyridine), propofol, methimezole, zinc, copper, benzocaine, and vitamin K (Gossett et al., 2000).

Finally, it is important to note that herb-drug interactions in general may be significantly underreported and underestimated for a number of reasons, as discussed by Hu et al. (2005).

Diet Interactions

There may be differences in response to garlic administration in the fed or fasted animal. For example, garlic oil fed to rats at a dose of 100 mg/kg after a 24-hour fast could be lethal, most probably due to causing acute pulmonary edema with severe congestion. However, this dose was apparently well tolerated in the fed rat or in those adapted to garlic feeding (Joseph et al., 1989). This observation could have practical implications for dogs, cats, and horses. While cats and horses eat many small meals, dogs tend to consume their food in one or two large meals. Therefore, garlic potentially would be more likely to be consumed by dogs when in a fasting state.

Impact of Disease and Vulnerable Populations

Horses

To the committee's knowledge there is no published information with respect to the impact of disease or vulnerable populations on the ADME of garlic in horses.

Dogs

To the committee's knowledge there is no published information with respect to the impact of disease or vulnerable populations on the ADME of garlic in dogs.

Cats

To the committee's knowledge there is no published information with respect to the impact of disease or vulnerable populations on the ADME of garlic in cats. In theory, limitation of hepatic glucuronidation due to the natural deficiency of glucuronyl transferase in the cat could extend the half-life of toxic components or metabolites from garlic, thereby increasing its toxicity in the cat compared to other species.

SAFETY

Toxicity Studies

Target Species

Horses

To the committee's knowledge no classical LD_{50} toxicity studies have been undertaken in horses. However, there has been one published paper whose primary purpose was to evaluate safety. Pearson et al. (2005) reported on a small study in four animals: two control and two treated animals (2–12 years of age, one Thoroughbred and three Standardbreds, two females and two geldings, BW 475–557 kg). Before the study, the animals had been treated with vitamin E and selenium to correct an apparent selenium deficiency, but they were considered normal at the study start (and continued to receive vitamin E and selenium supplementation throughout the trial). The original dose of garlic (0.1 g/kg) provided as a topdressing was refused. Thus, dosing began, after a 1-week washout, at 0.05 g/kg twice daily mixed with molasses into their concentrate pellet ration and was increased once or twice a week until the maximum dose that would not result in feed refusal was reached. The final dose of 0.25 g/kg initial BW twice daily was achieved at day 41 and continued through day 71 (terminated because the predetermined minimum hematocrit (HCT) of 20 percent had been reached). The garlic fed (230 kg) had been peeled, sliced, and stored at –80°C before being freeze-dried (FDG) and immediately grated to a variable particle size. It was stored in a 95-liter (25-gallon) plastic-covered container until use. The apparent allicin content (the freeze-dried or fresh garlic samples were homogenized in water and then analyzed after centrifugation and filtration) was 3.192 mg/g in the fresh garlic and 9.2 mg/g as fed in the FDG (the water content was 62 and 6.3 percent, respectively, in the two preparations). The authors therefore estimated that horses received 460 μg/kg of "allicin" on day 1 and 2,300 μg/kg on day 21. Blood samples were taken periodically for various analyses, and blood smears were made and stained with cresyl blue for HB. By day 28, approximately 75 percent of all RBC in smears from the garlic-treated (GT) horses had visible projections compared with two or less projections/ocular view (the highest prevalence seen in the control animals over the whole study) on day 21. On day 59, essentially all the RBC from the GT horses had visible projections. The RBC, hemoglobin, and HCT decreased, reaching nadirs on days 49–62, depending on the index. The RBC was below the normal reference range from days 49–71. Other RBC abnormalities included decreased mean corpuscular hemoglobin concentration (MCHC) with an increased mean corpuscular hemoglobin (MCH) and mean corpuscular volume (MCV). There was no change in white blood cell (WBC) or serum liver enzyme activities. Unconjugated serum bilirubin and haptoglobin were increased, whereas serum creatinine was decreased. Sweating was evident in both GT animals only (from day 42 and 49, respectively). Following cessation of the garlic administration, platelet numbers (which had increased in the GT animals) and MCHC recovered within 1 week, most biochemistry by 2 weeks, hemoglobin by 3 weeks, and RBC within 4 weeks. Despite the small number of horses studied, the authors concluded that biochemical and hematologic findings that were indicative of garlic toxicosis were evident 4 days after consuming 0.2 g of freeze dried garlic/kg BW twice daily. They stated that "as a result of the increasing amount consumed over time in our study, a safe dose for dietary consumption of garlic cannot be determined, although it is certainly < 0.4 g FDG/kg daily. It is unlikely that horses would normally ingest toxic quantities of garlic on a daily basis. However, the potential for garlic toxicosis is present when FDG is fed to horses" (Pearson et al., 2005).

This is a useful study as it confirms that garlic can cause hemolytic anemia in horses. However, there are a number of methodological issues with the study including the fact that one of the GT horses was a 2-year-old, which according to the authors was in a growth phase of development and therefore the diets in the control and GT horses were not isocaloric. It is important to note that initially the horses refused the garlic at 0.1 g/kg BW, but after a period of time on lower amounts they tolerated up to 0.25 g/kg original BW. This suggests that with acclimation horses may tolerate high intake levels of garlic.

Dogs

To the committee's knowledge, no classical LD_{50} toxicity studies have been undertaken in dogs.

Early studies (Nordio, 1952, 1953a,b, as quoted by Kamel, 1966) described anemia, hemoglobinuria, and icterus in dogs eating wild cultivated allium species. Later, the hematologic effects of large doses of garlic were characterized by Lee et al. (1994) and Lee et al. (2000). While evaluating the effect of garlic on cadmium accumulation in tissues. Lee and coworkers observed that ingesting large quantities of raw garlic (7 percent of the diet) induced hemolytic anemia and HB. Assuming a 15-kg dog consumes 1,000 kcal per day (NRC, 2006), this equates to 1,167–1,556 mg garlic/kg BW.

Researchers (Lee et al., 2000) administered 1.2 ml of garlic extract/kg BW to adult mixed-breed dogs via nasogastric tube daily for 7 days. The authors stated that this dose was equivalent to 5 g whole garlic/kg BW. Control dogs received water via nasogastric tube. Blood measurements were obtained throughout the supplementation period and continued until 30 days after the initial dose. RBC counts and HCT decreased significantly in dogs consuming garlic with a maximum effect at 9 days. None of the dogs developed clinical hemolytic anemia (criterion not described), intravascular hemolysis, or hemoglobinuria. White blood cells and neutrophils were higher in the garlic group on days 6 and 9. The concentration of GSH in RBC increased (increased GSH can be an indicator of oxidative stress within a cell) almost immediately after garlic consumption was initiated, being significantly higher than the control the day after supplementation started and significantly higher than initial values by day 5. Heinz bodies were present in the RBC of the garlic-fed dogs, but not the control dogs, reaching a maximum on day 8. Eccentrocytes (morphologically abnormal RBC with dense contracted hemoglobin on one side of the cell) were not present in the control dogs and reached a maximum on day 7 in the garlic-fed dogs. All blood values slowly returned to initial values after termination of garlic consumption. These data indicate that consumption of large doses of whole garlic (5 g/kg BW) cause oxidative damage in RBC of dogs.

Jin et al. (2001) investigated the effects of hereditary differences in erythrocyte potassium and sodium concentrations and Na,K-ATPase activity on susceptibility to oxidative damage in Japanese Jindo dogs consuming garlic. Dogs were fed 5g/kg BW as a garlic solution by stomach tube once a day for 7 days. Dogs with high potassium and low sodium concentration and high Na,K-ATPase activity (HK erythrocyte phenotype) had significant decreases in HCT, hemoglobin, RBC, MCV, MCHC, white blood cells, GSH, and methemoglobin in response to the garlic administration. In contrast, LK phenotype dogs had no significant changes in response to garlic administration.

Garlic preparations have been shown to cause direct damage to the dog's gastric and ileal mucosa (Hoshino et al., 2001). In this study, three different garlic preparations (raw garlic powder, boiled garlic powder, and aged garlic extract and two commercial enteric-coated tablets (whole and pulverized) were tested for evidence of gastrointestinal irritation in anesthetized Beagle dogs (n = 6; body weight ≈ 10 kg) receiving 40 mg of either garlic preparation applied endoscopically directly to the gastric mucosa. Twenty-four hours after application, gastric mucosal changes were evaluated endoscopically. Using one of the commercial enteric-coated tablets, three tablets were administered at 2-hour intervals to a single dog. That dog was euthanized and necropsied 3 hours after the last tablet administration. Neither the cellulose control nor the aged garlic extract (AGE) caused a significant change in the stomach mucosa (see Table 8-5). However, redness and erosion were noted in four of six dogs given raw and dehydrated garlic powder. Erosions were confirmed by histopathology. Direct administration of pulverized enteric-coated products in two dogs caused reddening of the mucosa. In the one dog given oral tablets, the mucosa of the ileum was congested and irregular, with loss of epithelial cells. This suggests that enteric coating may protect the upper GI tract following oral administration but exposure to garlic as the enteric coating is lost could result in lower intestinal damage. It was not stated whether the

TABLE 8-5 Effect of Various Garlic Preparations on the Gastric Mucosa when Applied Directly via an Endoscope

Preparation	Alliin (mg/g)	"Allicin Potential" (mg/g)	SAC (μg/g)	No change/3 sites per dog = 18 sites	Redness 18 sites	Erosion 18 sites
Control	0	0	0	18	0	0
Raw garlic powder	23.3	11.3	162	0	3	15
Dehydrated boiled garlic powder	6.6	< 0.2	67	6	12	0
Aged garlic extract	1.6	< 0.2	671	18	0	0

SOURCE: Based on data in Hoshino et al. (2001).

dogs were in the fasting state when the garlic preparations were applied; however, the dogs were anesthetized during the procedure and the garlic was applied directly to the gastric mucosa. Animals are typically fasted prior to anesthesia and application of the garlic directly onto the mucosa would have been difficult if food had been present in the stomach. It is likely, therefore, that the garlic was administered in the absence of food. Consequently, these results may have limited relevance to consumption of garlic in a dog food, as part of a dog treat, or as a supplement administered along with the dog's food. They do, however, indicate that consumption of garlic during the fasting state could cause gastrointestinal damage.

Cats

To the committee's knowledge no classical LD_{50} toxicity studies have been undertaken in cats.

No known studies have been undertaken in cats where the primary purpose was to evaluate safety.

Nontarget Species

A few studies have determined an LD_{50} in rodents for garlic or garlic-derived compounds. Kamel (1966) established a minimum lethal dose of 100 mg/kg BW and an LD_{50} of 128 mg/kg BW, respectively, for an alkaloidal extract (details not provided) of 1 percent Egyptian garlic injected subcutaneously in white rats of similar age and weight under variable temperature and humidity. Clinical signs also included colic, diarrhea, vomiting, incoordination, icterus, leucocytosis, hemoglobinuria, and anemia. Death was associated with inflammation in all internal organs (which the author suggested could be due to the irritant properties of the garlic). In contrast, no rats (n = 20) died after 10 days of oral dosing at 10 mg/kg BW. Both environmental temperature and relative humidity influenced mortality rates: the LD_{50} dose resulted in deaths in 70 percent of animals following 24 hours exposure to high temperature, and 85 percent following exposure to both high humidity and high temperature with no preacclimatization (60 and 70 percent respectively with 24 hours acclimatization to the environment). The mortality of control non-garlic-administered animals was not determined. A second independent study found a similar LD_{50} of 100 mg/kg BW using garlic oil (given intragastrically), although the clinical sign was acute pulmonary edema, which may not be related to the garlic per se (as reviewed by Kodera et al., 2002).

The LD_{50} of allicin has been reported to be 60 mg/kg BW i.v. and 120 mg/kg BW subcutaneous (s.c.) in mice (as reviewed by Kodera et al., 2002). Acute toxicity studies of SAC in mice and rats enabled LD_{50} to be determined as shown in Table 8-6 (Kodera et al., 2002). Interestingly, this study did show a sex effect with i.p. administration in mice, with the LD_{50} being about 1.7 times higher in males than in females. (There were also some sex effects during subacute toxicity tests.)

Several other reports on garlic toxicity in rodents have been published (e.g., Nakagawa et al., 1984a,b; Yoshida et al., 1984), although the protocols used have been questioned (Alnaqeeb et al., 1996). In general, the studies did not always report the toxic effects in sufficient detail. For example, one study investigating the antithrombotic effect of garlic and onions (Bordia et al., 1996) noted that high doses (i.e., 500 mg/kg presumed BW but not stated) but not low doses (50 mg/kg presumed BW but not stated) of garlic

TABLE 8-6 The LD_{50} Values of Synthetic S-Allyl cysteine (SAC) in Rats and Mice (mg/kg BW)

Route	Sex	Mice		Rat	
Oral	Male	8,890	(7,600–10,220)	10,940	(9,500–12,660)
	Female	9,390	(8,600–10,130)	9,500	(8,080–11,150)
Intraperitoneal	Male	6,910	(6,020–8,000)	3,340	(2,890–4,090)
	Female	3,650	(2,640–4,410)	3,340	(2,930–3,850)

NOTE: 95% confidence limits expressed in parentheses. Most deaths occurred within 24 hours of the oral or intraperitoneal administration.
SOURCE: Based on data in Kodera et al. (2002).

had a toxic effect on the organs of the animals (unpublished observation). There are also apparent species differences in that rats were apparently able to tolerate four consecutive days of garlic oil at 300 mg/kg (presumed BW but not stated) orally but mice could not tolerate this dose (Fisher et al., 2007).

Hemolytic Anemia

Laboratory animals seem to be relatively refractory to the hemolytic action of allium vegetables although anemia has been induced in rabbits, rats, and guinea pigs through the feeding of large amounts of onions (as reviewed by Munday et al., 2003). Garlic or chemicals found within garlic preparations can also induce hemolytic anemia in rats (Umar et al., 1996, 1998), although, interestingly, this finding often is not reported, even in studies that establish LD_{50}. In one subacute toxicity study, up to 2,000 mg/kg of SAC given orally to 10 male and 10 female rats for 1 month had little effect on the RBC, although the HCT, MCV, and hemoglobin tended to be significantly decreased at the 500 mg/kg dose and above (some differences were described in the responses between the males and females). In contrast, no effects occurred when either the males or females were fed 250 mg/kg SAC (Kodera et al., 2002).

Prolonged feeding of high levels of raw garlic to rats can result in lysis of the RBC, anemia, weight loss, and failure to grow (Augusti, 1996). Wistar strain albino rats showed a significant decrease in packed cell volume (PCV), hemoglobin, RBC, and WBC plus an increase in MCV (Oboh, 2004) when fed a basal diet containing 4 percent of a garlic compound (compared to the basal diet or a garlic plus leafy vegetable diet). In a study by Munday et al. (2003), female rats (Sprague Dawley; 12 weeks of age) given ad libitum access to feed in groups of six were orally given various sulfides that could be derived from garlic or onion (equivalent to 500 µmol/kg BW/day: 57 and 59 mg/kg/day for the diallyl and dipropyl monosulfides; 73 and 75 mg/kg/day for the equivalent disulfides; 89 or 91 mg/kg/day for the equivalent trisulfides; and 105 or 107 mg/kg/day for the equivalent tetrasulfides), all provided as freshly prepared solutions in soybean oil for 5 days. The control group was fed the soybean oil only. The HB were determined turbidometrically by the decrease in optical density of RBC lysates at 700 nm following centrifugation. All of the rats remained healthy with no signs of toxicity. However, rats dosed with the diallyl di-sulfide and both the tri- and tetrasulfides developed anemia (with significantly reduced PCV and hemoglobin associated with pronounced HB formation). Splenic enlargement in the absence of apparent intravascular hemolysis suggested the hemolysis was extravascular. There were some changes in the liver (both gross and on histology), but again the extent and nature depended on the sulfide. This study confirmed that many of the sulfides produced by garlic can induce moderate hemolytic anemia as indicated by decreased blood cell volumes and hemoglobin levels. The tri- and tetrasulfides were more powerful hemolytic agents than was diallyl disulfide in rats, as would be expected from the greater oxidative activity of these compounds in vitro. The results of the study confirm that diallyl tri- and tetrasulfides are highly toxic to RBC, suggesting that these compounds are an important cause of garlic-induced hemolytic anemia. Similarly, dipropyl tri- and tetrasulfides together with dipropenyl disulfide may be largely responsible for the toxicity of onions.

Carcinogenesis

Several studies have shown inhibitory effects of garlic components on tumor development in rodents when given prior to the administration of several carcinogens (Takada et al., 1994). However, Lee and Park (2003) noted that several studies have suggested that the organosulfur compounds and selenium from garlic may under certain circumstances have enhancing effects on, for example, the tumor promotion stage. For example, DAS may promote hepatocarcinogenesis by enhancing the development of diethynitosamine-induced GST placental form-positive foci, and high doses of various organosulfur compounds within garlic may promote preneoplastic lesion development in the rat liver (Takahashi et al., 1992; Takada et al., 1994). Yet individual organosulfur compounds may, in fact, be inhibitors of tumor growth or development.

The committee noted that garlic is not listed as a carcinogen under the IARC carcinogen, US NTP carcinogen, California Proposition 65 known carcinogens, US EPA carcinogens, or the TRI carcinogen databases (as reviewed by Kegley et al., 2007 in the Pesticides Action Network [PAN] Pesticides database).

Other Effects

Dipropyl disulfide can affect thyroid function in rats (as reviewed by Fenwick and Hanley, 1985c). However, the majority of the side effects of garlic administration in rats reported have targeted the gastrointestinal tract and the liver (Banerjee et al., 2003; Oboh, 2006). Unfortunately, many reports do not provide sufficient information to determine the actual amount of garlic or active component/kg BW fed or do not fully evaluate potential adverse effects. For example, Jastrzebski et al. (2007) showed no effect on bodyweight gain in growing rats but did not evaluate liver function. A few studies have provided more detailed information. For example, significant liver and lung damage occurred in rats given garlic at 500 mg/kg BW either by gavage or intraperitoneally, but little effect was seen when they were given 50 mg/kg BW by gavage. This level given intraperitoneally, however, still caused abscess formation (Alnaqeeb et al., 1996). In another study, rats fed fresh garlic homogenate for 28 days at doses from 100 to 5,000 mg/kg

BW had deterioration in liver function at all doses, although the authors concluded that a safe dose could be up to 250 mg/kg BW (Rana et al., 2006). A different study, also in rats, suggested that doses of either 300 or 600 mg/kg BW of a garlic bulb aqueous extract for 21 days would result in reduced weight and growth with tissue damage (Fehri et al., 1991). Together, these two studies suggest that approximately 250–300 mg/kg BW might be the level above which significant tissue damage may occur in rats. This is supported by another study in rats that showed suppression of spermatogenesis linked with reduced concentration of sialic acid in the testes, epididymis, and seminal vesicle with ≈ 300 mg/kg garlic powder given by gavage (Dixit and Joshi, 1982). Lower levels, however, were not evaluated, which would have helped confirm the LOAEL for such changes. Finally, in a recent study (Jastrzebski et al., 2007), growing rats were given 25 mg of lyophilized nonprocessed garlic at 25 mg/kg BW, which according to the authors was equivalent to 500 mg of raw garlic/kg BW, for 30 days with no apparent detrimental effects on feed intake, body weight gain, or feed efficiencies. Although no other adverse effects were noted, liver enzymes and any effects on spermatogenesis, for example, were not monitored, again making it difficult to confirm that this level would not have adverse effects on any system. This study also highlights the importance of confirming the type of garlic preparation being used when suggesting "safe" limits.

Another factor that may be important in the development of adverse events is timing of garlic administration in relation to the ingestion of other food and with what type of meal it is fed. For example, one study showed that garlic oil fed at a dose of 100 mg/kg after a 24-hour fast could be lethal, most probably due to causing acute pulmonary edema with severe congestion. However, this dose was apparently well tolerated in the fed rat or in those adapted to garlic feeding (Joseph et al., 1989). Another study looking at the effect of garlic oil (GO) fed at 200 mg/kg with a low- or high-fat diet), DADS (200 mg/kg BW with a high-fat diet only), and DAS (100 mg/kg with a high-fat diet only), showed that there was a significantly reduced body weight gain when GO or DADS were fed at 200 mg/kg BW three times a week for 7 weeks with the high-fat diet or when the same dose of GO was fed with a low-fat diet. However, there was no effect of DAS at 100 mg/kg (Sheen et al., 1999). The authors concluded that the action of GO seemed to be independent of dietary lipid content. Kodera et al. (2002) undertook both acute and subacute toxicity tests using SAC. These tests showed a number of effects depending on the dosage, the type of rodent, and in some cases the sex. For example, high doses increased glucose and caused atrophy of the pancreas in female, but not male, rats. These studies suggested that the nontoxic dose for SAC in rats under experimental conditions is at least 250 mg/kg.

The above work suggests that an upper limit would need to be determined for a particular garlic preparation under typical conditions and that a "general" upper limit of safety that encompasses all garlic preparations may not be possible to determine. However, the studies do suggest that rodents can be fed garlic or garlic preparations safely if fed at an appropriate dose but "high" levels will be harmful to one or more body systems.

In conclusion, it seems that studies undertaken in rodents may be of value in the screening process for a particular garlic preparation, but it is not possible to extrapolate fully to other species and/or other preparations or doses.

In Vitro

The potential for in vitro tests to be used as a screening tool was investigated by Charles et al. (2002) on a number of common food ingredients, including garlic. They used a standard juicer to juice garlic (whole, peeled), which was then diluted 1:6 with culture medium before being filtered and filter-sterilized. It was then further diluted with the treatment medium (maximum dose tested was 10 percent volume/volume: v/v). The following were evaluated:

- Cytotoxicity: Proliferation of CHO-K_1-BH_4 cells was inhibited by 50 percent in the presence of < 1 percent juice. Garlic extract was actually one of the most cytotoxic materials evaluated, exhibiting significant inhibition of cellular growth at concentrations as low as 0.05 percent (v/v);
- Chromosomal aberration test: Garlic at 0.05 percent induced significant levels of chromosomal damage, relative to control treatments in CHO-K_1-BH_4 cells, leading to a clastogenic classification by the authors;
- Limb bud micromass assay: Garlic was considered to be a nonspecific inhibitor (producing cytotoxicity), suggesting that cytotoxicity and inhibition of differentiation seemed to parallel each other;
- Estrogen receptor transactivation assay: Garlic was not considered to be estrogenic.

These studies confirmed that garlic can be toxic under certain circumstances; however, these authors concluded that these tests are not directly useful to predict human or animal risk from eating such materials.

In vitro studies have also been conducted in canine models. Sundaram and Milner (1993) administered various organosulfur compounds, isolated from garlic, to canine mammary tumor cells (CMT-13) in culture. They discovered that oil-soluble organosulfur compounds (diallyl sulphide, diallyl disulfide, and diallyl trisulfide) had antineoplastic activity and that their efficacy was attenuated by glutathione.

A series of in vitro studies was conducted to determine the effect of organosulfur compounds from garlic on oxidation of canine RBC (Hu et al., 2002; Yamato et al., 2003; Yang et al., 2003). Isolated canine RBC were incubated with various garlic components. Oxidation was assessed through methemoglobin measurement. These researchers determined that a variety of compounds are responsible for the hemoglobin and RBC membrane oxidizing effect of garlic, including bis-2-propenyl trisulfide, bis-2-propenyl tetrasulfide, bis-2-propenyl pentasulfide, bis-2-propenyl thiosulfonate, 2-propene-1-sulfinothioic acid *S-(E)*-1-propenyl ester, and *trans*-sulfurous acid allyl ester 3-allylsulfanyl-allyl ester.

While in vitro tests are useful in establishing mechanisms of action, they are of limited use in establishing a safe intake level.

Nonsafety Studies

When evaluating the use of nonsafety studies, it is important to understand the likelihood of any particular adverse event being identified if it is not specifically included as part of the study design. As discussed above, a common effect of garlic (allium) toxicity is oxidative damage to red blood cell membranes resulting in Heinz body or eccentrocyte formation. Heinz bodies are not easily visible during microscopic evaluation of blood slides stained by Romanowsky stains or Wright's-Giemsa stains unless large and abundant. The use of vital stains such as new methylene blue will stain HB deep blue, enhancing their detection (Desnoyers, 2000). When determining the proportion of RBC with HB, the latter staining technique is best used. Importantly, automated hematology analyzers do not detect these abnormalities in erythrocyte cellular morphology, and therefore microscopic examinations of peripheral blood smears are required. Only when RBC damage is sufficient to result in lysis or increased destruction will anemia, hemolysis, or RBC regeneration (reticulocytosis) become obvious when using an automated hematology analyzer.

Target Species

Horses

Garlic is anecdotally added to horse feed for its aroma, as a flavorant, and/or palatant; for its assistance in respiratory health; and for its antiparasitic or fly-repellent properties. However, there is little if any research to support any of these potential benefits, although there are a few reports on palatability. A trial by Horton et al. (1991), suggested that garlic increased the palatability of the feed offered when added at 1,500 or 3,000 mg/kg feed (estimated by the committee to be < 60 mg/kg BW). However, Goodwin et al. (2005) showed that garlic was ranked 11 out of the 12 flavors tested (based on consumption times) when added at 1 percent garlic flavor to a standard 100 g cereal byproduct. Furthermore, Cairns et al. (2002), investigating responses to orosensory characteristics of foods through preference choice tests between mint and garlic, reported that mint was preferred in isocaloric diets. No adverse effects were reported in these relatively short-term trials with low intake levels.

A number of studies have been published looking at the effect of feeding a particular antioxidant supplement, which contains garlic, on lung antioxidant status in Thoroughbred horses. No adverse events were reported in studies in which the particular supplement was fed for up to 4 weeks in thoroughbred horses in hard exercise. For example, in one study (Deaton et al., 2002), six Thoroughbreds, (four geldings and two mares, 7.5 ± 2.7 years, 466 ± 16 kg BW) were fed a mean daily amount of garlic of ≈ 3 mg/kg BW. Hematology was not reported. However, the lack of adverse effects might be inferred by the lack of adverse effects on the RBC, as this was a key factor in determining hemolysate glutathione analysis and therefore any significant decrease would have been noted.

Dogs and Cats

In vivo studies in dogs and cats are generally divided into two categories of evidence: those designed to demonstrate potential beneficial effects of ingesting garlic or its chemical components and those demonstrating toxic effects. While not specifically designed to evaluate safety, studies designed to evaluate physiological effects can sometimes be useful in determining a presumed safe intake level for a compound, particularly if relevant safety parameters were measured and adverse events, or lack thereof, were reported. Many scientific articles have been published concerning the physiological effects of garlic in dogs and cats. Some examples of these are presented in Tables 8-7 and 8-8. The committee found these studies to be of limited use in establishing a safe intake level for garlic in dogs and cats for the following reasons:

- Typically, a single dose of garlic or a purified garlic extract was administered. As a result, long-term, cumulative effects of daily ingestion of garlic could not be evaluated in these studies.
- Often the compound was administered intravenously or directly onto the tissue of interest. Toxic effects of compounds can be exacerbated under these conditions. When consumed as part of a food matrix, very little of the garlic will come into direct contact with the gastrointestinal mucosa, and when it does contact the mucosa, the amount contacting any particular mucosal site will be much less than if the entire dose was applied directly to that site. In addition, absorption of most compounds is less than 100 percent, lowering the dose that will enter the bloodstream and contact the target tissue. Likewise, direct application to an internal organ bypasses any potential metabolism that might increase or decrease toxicity that may otherwise occur.
- Application of a single compound isolated from a complex ingredient such as garlic ignores the presence and

TABLE 8-7 Examples of Studies Evaluating the Effect of Garlic Compounds on Physiological Response in Dogs and Cats

Sources	Garlic Form	Dose	Route	Effect	Duration	Model	Comment
Bastidas (1969)	Raw garlic mixed with food	7–10 g/days (0.7–1 g/kg BW/d)	Oral	Decreased *Ancylostoma caninum* larvae in feces, dead eggs in feces, no effect on egg production	5 days	1 dog infected with *Ancylostoma caninum*	Indicators of safety (e.g., Heinz bodies, HB) were not reported
Chang et al. (2004)	Synthetic 2-propenyl thiosulfate	0.01–10 μM	Ex vivo	Increased superoxide generation and respiratory burst in PMNs, ↓ platelet aggregation	—	Ex vivo canine PMNs	Difficult to extrapolate dose to in vivo
Chang et al. (2005)	Synthetic 2-propenyl thiosulfate	0.01–10 μM	Ex vivo	↓ COX 1 at 0.1 mM ↓ GSH at 0.1 mM	—	Ex vivo – canine platelets	Difficult to extrapolate dose to in vivo
Dixit et al. (1980)	Garlic powder	25 mg/kg BW	—	Decreased serum cholesterol, phospholipids and triglycerides	Single dose-effects measured for 48 hours	Dogs	Very short-term trial. No indicators of safety
Kaye et al. (1995)	Allicin	0.1–1.0 mg 0.1 mg 0.3 mg 0.6 mg 1.0 mg	Intrathoracic artery	Dose related ↓ in pulmonary arterial pressure and systemic pressure; pulmonary vasodilation	Single dose	Intact cat chest	Difficult to extrapolate doses to in vivo
Nagae (1994)	SAC	—	Oral	Orally absorbed, bioavailable (87.2%), excreted in urine, half life longer in dogs	—	Dogs Rats Human	—
Pantoja et al. (1991)	Garlic powder capsules	2.5–15 mg/kg BW 15–20 mg/kg BW	Directgastric administration	Naturesis, diuresis ↓ arterial pressure, transient bradycardia and T wave inversion at 15 and 20 mg/kg BW which returned to normal after the first 15 minutes of the trial	Single administration, effects monitored for > 250 minutes	Anesthetized dogs	—
Pantoja et al. (2000)	Purified, dialyzed biologically active fraction of garlic	6 μg/kg BW	Intravenous	Naturesis, diuresis	Single injection	Anesthetized dogs	—
Turek et al. (2000)	Garlic powder	0.5% DM of diet; approximately 80–110 mg/kg BW	Oral	Increased lymphocyte blastogenesis; no effect on cytokine production	77 days	Dog	No indicators of safety reported

thus possible additive, exacerbatory, or inhibitory effects of other compounds within that garlic preparation.

- While specific physiological responses were evaluated, HB and other potential indicators of safety were not reported. For example, a study was conducted to evaluate the immunomodulatory effect of garlic-supplemented dog food (garlic powder as 0.5 percent of the dry formula; approximately 80–110 mg/kg BW) for over 77 days (Turek et al., 2000). Blood samples were collected for evaluation of immune response, however, the authors did not state whether other blood measurements (e.g., hemoglobin and HCT) were evaluated. Therefore, published information

TABLE 8-8 Examples of Studies Reporting Potential Adverse Effects of Garlic in Dogs

Sources	Garlic Form	Dose	Route	Effect	Duration	Dog
Hoshino et al. (2001)	Raw, boiled, or aged garlic	4 mg/kg BW	Direct application onto stomach mucosa	Reddening, ulceration, swelling, loss of epithelial layer of ileum in all but aged garlic	Single application with observation 24 hours later	6 adult males
Lee et al. (1994)	Raw garlic	7% of diet; equivalent to approximately 1167–1556 mg/kg BW	Oral via diet	Hemolytic anemia, HB	50 days	—
Lee et al. (2000)	Water soluble extract of boiled garlic	1.2 ml garlic extract/kg BW; equivalent to 5 g whole garlic/kg BW	Via nasogastric tube	Decreased RBC counts and HCT, increased % of RBC with HB, neutrophils, erythrocyte GSH and eccentrocytes in RBC	7 days; measurements taken for 30 days after initial dose	Mixed breed
Pantoja et al. (1991)	Garlic powder	15 and 20 mg/kg BW	Intragastric	Transient bradycardia and T-wave inversion immediately after dosing	Single dose; effects monitored for > 250 minutes	Anesthetized
Pantoja et al. (2000)	Garlic dialysate	6 µg/kg BW	Intravenous right femoral vein	Diuretic, no change in arterial blood pressure or electrocardiogram	Single injection	Anaesthetized

from this study is not sufficient to draw conclusions as to long-term safety at the levels administered.

The committee therefore was not able to find published nonsafety studies that provided sufficient evidence to help establish a presumed safe intake level for garlic in dogs or cats.

Table 8-8 outlines example publications describing adverse or potentially adverse effects of garlic administration in dogs.

As data regarding garlic intake in cats are extremely limited in all categories, the available studies are described in more detail. They represent acute interventional trials designed to evaluate the vasodilatory properties of allicin using the anesthetized cat as an in situ vascular model. The first study by Mayeux et al. (1988) utilized a feline mesenteric vascular bed model to demonstrate that allicin induced a dose-related decrease in vascular resistance (vasodilation) by mechanisms independent of B-adrenoceptor activation or prostaglandin production. An undefined number of adult cats were anesthetized, and an extracorporeal circuit was established to perfuse the mesentery via the superior mesenteric artery at a constant rate. Chemically synthesized allicin was injected at 100, 300, and 1,000 µg intra-arterially and vascular resistance measured. The vasodilatory response was dose dependent and nearly immediate with a peak reduction in mesenteric pressure within 10 seconds. This study suggested that the cat mesenteric vascular bed is sensitive to the vasodilatory properties of allicin. A similar study was conducted by Kaye et al. (1995) to test the effect of allicin on pulmonary vascular response. The study models included the intact chests of anesthetized cats and isolated rat lung (Kaye et al., 1995). Twenty-two adult cats, weighing between 3.0–4.6 kg, were anesthetized and intubated following ketamine sedation. Systemic blood pressure was measured from a femoral artery catheter. A perfusion catheter was placed from the external jugular vein into the artery of the left lower lung lobe. Left atrial pressure was measured via a catheter placed in the vein draining the left lower lobe. Pulmonary vascular responses of allicin (chemically synthesized), sodium nitroprusside, and isoproterenol were compared when lobar tone was increased. Allicin was perfused into the lobar artery at 0.1–1.0 mg, causing a significant dose-related decrease in lobar arterial pressure. System arterial pressure was decreased in a dose-related manner as well. The relative vasodilator action of allicin compared to other vasodilators was significantly less. Sodium nitroprusside was 100-fold, and isoproterenol 10,000-fold more potent than allicin in dilating the lobar vascular bed. The authors noted that allicin is immediately converted to allyl mercaptan in whole blood and that this analog possesses significant pulmonary vasodilatory activity in the cat and rat similar to allicin. While these studies demonstrate that garlic compounds possess significant vasodilator activity in mesenteric and pulmonary vasculature of the cat, the relevance to safety and natural exposure are uncertain.

Nontarget Species

Humans

Intakes of approximately 300 mg/day of garlic powder do not seem to be associated with significant adverse effects at least in healthy individuals. For example, 300 mg of garlic powder in tablet form (n = 20) or placebo (n = 22) was fed three times a day to 42 patients with high serum total cholesterol levels for 12 weeks. The authors noted that in general the garlic tablets were quite well tolerated without any significant odor problems. The authors, however, pointed out that this may have been related to the "expectation" of a garlic smell or taste from the garlic pills (although the study was blind) and therefore it was not recognized/reported as an adverse effect. Reported adverse effects included one of the 20 patients who received garlic treatment complaining of increased belching with garlic taste. Most of the issues, however, seemed to be with the placebo and consisted of mild abdominal discomfort (n = 2), a mild rash (n =1), and prolonged oozing from a razor cut during shaving (n = 1) (Jain et al., 1993).

No significant adverse effects were noted in a study looking at the efficacy of garlic as a cholesterol-lowering agent. Raw garlic, a powdered garlic supplement, aged garlic extract supplement (at an approximate dose equivalent to a 4-g clove per day), or placebo were given 6 days/week for 6 months to a group of adults (Gardner et al., 2007). Previous work by this group had suggested that the products used would be consistent over the time period studied (Lawson and Gardner, 2005). There were rare reports of individual symptoms possibly linked to the garlic administration—including rash, heartburn, and mouth ulcers in one participant each; flatulence was reported in up to four participants in each group. Bad breath and body odor were reported often or almost always in 57 percent of the raw garlic group and one with the aged garlic.

Bad odor is a commonly reported undesirable side effect of garlic ingestion. In a multicentric placebo-controlled double-blind study in Germany, for example, 21 percent of patients ingesting 800 mg garlic powder (providing 1.3 percent alliin—i.e., ≈ 10.4 mg alliin) for 16 weeks exuded a mild garlic smell, compared to 9 percent of placebo participants (Mader, 1990).

It should be noted that in the PAN pesticide database (Kegley et al., 2007) garlic was not listed under any of the carcinogen, endocrine disruption, reproduction, and developmental toxicity, or chemicals of special concern lists. It was given a slightly toxic rating from the US EPA product label (suggesting the LD_{50} for oral ingestion in rats is 500–5,000 mg/kg), but it was not clear how this rating had been determined.

Ex Vivo

The alkyl thiosulfate 2-propenyl thiosulfate (2PTS) has been identified as a causative agent in the production of hemolytic anemia in dogs consuming garlic. Recent work (Chang et al., 2004) suggests that the alkyl thiosulfates (sodium n-propyl thiosulfate and 2-propenyl thiosulfate) have a bimodal dose-dependent effect on oxygen radical generation in canine polymorphonuclear cells up to 1 mM, with a return to normal activity at a very high concentration (10 mM). The increased superoxide generation indicated an increase in respiratory burst, a marker of a very active innate immune system. Therefore, while implicated in the toxic side effects of garlic in dogs, 2PTS may also help stimulate immune function in dogs. In addition, the attenuation of this effect at high levels of 2PTS indicated protection against excessive superoxide production, and resultant damage, in polymorphonuclear neutrophils (PMN). Neither compound impacted oxygen generation in human PMN at any concentration used in the study, suggesting species differences in susceptibility to alkyl thiosulfates by PMN. In contrast, 2PTS inhibited platelet aggregation in both species, a potentially beneficial effect in the prevention of cardiovascular disease, The mechanism of decreased platelet aggregation was identified in further research (Chang et al, 2005). The 2PTS inhibited cyclooxygenase (COX) activity as well as modulating GSH concentration in platelets.

Use, Risk, and Exposure as a Supplement

Target Species

Horses

Garlic has apparently been fed to horses since Roman times (Hyland, 1990). Harris et al. (1999) reported that before 1733 the diet [of racehorses] consisted of barley, beans, wheat-sheaves, butter, white wine and up to 25 cloves of garlic per feed. However, there is very little published information available to support its use, although there are a few published reports that describe potential adverse effects. One case report suggests that the feeding of garlic can cause urticaria in horses (Miyazawa et al., 1991). A 7-year-old Thoroughbred stallion had been imported from Ireland to a quarantine station in Japan where it was fed more than 50 g of a feed additive containing sesame, ginseng, wild yeast, beer yeast, honey, and garlic. Ten days after arrival, it developed apparently nonpainful and nonitchy wheals initially around the neck and then over the whole body. Its RBC, hemoglobin, and other measures were all within the normal range. Glucocorticioid administration only resulted in short-term resolution. The serum from this horse gave a precipitin line against an extract from the garlic (but not the other ingredients in the ration). In addition, when this extract was inoculated into the dermis of the neck of the affected horse (but not a control horse), it resulted in a small induration unlike the injection of extracts from other ingredients. Removing garlic from the feed resulted in a disappearance of the wheals within 13 days. Five other stallions fed the same ration showed no signs of any urticaria. Although neither the exact amount nor type of garlic fed to the horse is known, assuming less than 50 g was fed and that the stallion was at least 500 kg, this report suggests that an allergic reaction may be associated with the feeding of ≈ 100 mg/kg

BW of some types of garlic to some individual horses. However, it is not known whether the initial sensitization was a response to the garlic alone or to the combination of ingredients within the feed additive.

Valle et al. (2006) reported that a 10-year-old Standardbred mare showed apathy, water and food rejection, staggering, and alteration of her biochemical and hematological profile following supplementation with 100 g of dehydrated flaked garlic (considered to be equivalent to 500 g of whole fresh garlic/day) for 10 days. The mare was in poor condition (and had apparently been so prior to the garlic supplementation) and weighed around 500 kg, but was not apparently anemic although she was dehydrated at the time of sampling (E.Valle, personal communication, 2007). The blood smear was evaluated as part of an investigation into possible parasitic involvement and showed HB (E.Valle, personal communication, 2007). The mare responded to veterinary treatment plus cessation of the garlic administration. The diagnosis was garlic intoxication. As a guide, the estimated daily dose was 200 mg/kg BW of dehydrated flaked garlic.

The committee was not able to find any specific published data regarding the safe feeding of garlic per se to horses, despite many garlic-rich products being on the market with apparently poor guidance as to the feeding levels for animals of different bodyweights (see Table 8-9).

A database maintained by the National Animal Supplement Council (NASC) suggests that typical recommended dosages for their members' equine garlic products range from 0.01 to 14.68 mg/kg BW. Further, the NASC has received no reports of adverse effects despite over 9 million doses being sold since 1998 (NASC, personal communication, 2007). The types of garlic products (i.e., garlic form, top-dress supplement vs. feed inclusion) included in the NASC database were not available to the committee. Nonetheless, the daily intake described by NASC is far lower than would be expected from the recommended doses given by the manufacturers of the products listed in Table 8-9 (often > 100 mg/kg BW), which are designed to be added to the horse's core ration. However, the NASC intake values fall within the range of that provided when garlic is included as part of certain commercial horse feeds (and thus makes up

TABLE 8-9 Examples of Dietary Garlic Supplements Marketed to be Fed to Horses in the United States by Addition to the Basal Ration

Product	Description of Garlic Form	Manufacturer Recommended Dosage	Other Notes
1	Low-temp, air-dried garlic powder (granular form)	21 g/day per 1,000 lb BW "In areas of heavy infestation, dosage may be doubled or tripled"	Reported alliin content = 1.31 percent; 100 percent pure garlic
2	Mixture of air-and freeze-dried garlic	Up to 250 kg BW: 26 g/day 250–400 kg BW: 35 g/day 400–600 kg BW: 52 g/day Over 600 kg BW: 70 g/day	100 percent pure garlic
3	Described only as "garlic granules"	35 g/day for "average horse"	100 percent pure garlic
4	Garlic powder	28 g/day; amount may be doubled if needed No BW qualification given	100 percent pure garlic
5	Dehydrated garlic powder	20 g/day No BW qualification given	Garlic combined with rice bran (bran 10 percent of product)
6	Garlic powder	28.4–56.8 g/day for mature horses weighing 1,100 lb 14.2–28.4 for ponies or smaller breeds	Also contains grain byproducts, yeast culture, apple cider vinegar, brewers yeast, dried distillers' grains (DDG), diatomaceous earth, various vitamins, and minerals. Garlic listed as third ingredient.
7	Garlic powder and "garlic liquid"	4–8 g/day No BW qualification given	Also contains dried *Lactobacillus acidophilus* fermentation product, diatomaceous earth, yeast culture, bifidobacterium, *Lactobacillus plantarum, Enterococcus faecium, Lactobacillus acidophilus*, and brewers yeast. Garlic powder listed as second ingredient; garlic liquid listed as ninth ingredient.
8	Garlic powder	Give 14–28 g/day or more daily per 1,000 lb BW For difficult situations, up to 112 g/day.	Also contains ground dried grape and seed pomace, distillers grains, diatomaceous earth, brewers yeast, soybean oil. Garlic powder is listed as fourth ingredient.

a part of the horse's core ration). For example, dehydrated garlic powder has been included in certain specific commercial feeds at 2.5 g/kg of feed, resulting in daily intakes of approximately 15 mg/kg BW in horses and ponies. These feeds have been successfully available in the marketplace for a prolonged period of time (> 5 years) with no reports of any adverse effects (C. Barfoot, personal communication, 2007). Higher daily intake levels of garlic in one trial also resulted in no apparent adverse effects when sedentary ponies with varying body condition scores were allowed ad libitum access to a feed containing 2.5 g/kg feed of dried powdered garlic (average daily intake of 88 mg/kg BW) for 12 weeks (A. Dugdale, personal communication, 2007). In a subsequent study in another 5 ponies, no change in the number of HB was seen after 12 weeks with ad libitum access to the same feed and an average garlic intake of 74 mg/kg BW (A. Dugdale, personal communication, 2008).

Dogs and Cats

Garlic for dogs and cats can be supplied as a raw ingredient, as a supplement, or as a component of table foods, prepared meals, or commercial pet foods or treats. Garlic has also been used for centuries to treat or prevent a variety of ailments in humans and is commonly used as a flavor enhancer (see Wynn and Fougère, 2007 for a review of historical use of garlic in humans and livestock). Therefore, it is possible that garlic has been fed to domesticated dogs and cats intentionally or accidentally for hundreds of years, if not longer. Despite this, reports of accidental garlic poisoning are rare, particularly in cats (Aldrich, 2007). The committee was only able to find three published reports of suspected garlic toxicity in dogs (Edwards and Belford, 1996; Caldin et al., 2005; Yamato et al., 2005) and possibly one published case report for cats (Edwards and Belford, 1996).

In one report, 60 cases of canine eccentrocytes were reviewed by Caldin et al. (2005). One of the cases was associated with garlic ingestion. Details of the garlic source, amount consumed, or severity of symptoms were not given.

A second report detailed the case of a 4-year-old Miniature Schnauzer that developed dark urine one day after ingesting Chinese steamed dumplings containing Chinese chive and garlic (Yamato et al, 2005). The amount of garlic or Chinese chive (a source of allium) consumed by the dog was unknown. The next day the dog began vomiting and had diarrhea. The dog was admitted to a veterinary clinic 2 days after consuming the dumplings. At time of admission, the dog had a slightly low HCT, hemolysis, moderate leukocytosis, and neutrophilia. Over 37 percent of the dog's RBC were eccentrocytes and many of the cells had projections that resembled HB. By the fourth day postdumpling ingestion, HCT had decreased to 19 percent, 21.6 percent of the RBC were eccentrocytes, and 44.3 percent of the RBC had HB. Methemoglobin concentration in the blood was abnormally high and the dog was anorectic. The dog was given erythropoietin, fluids, a high-calorie liquid diet, and vitamin and mineral supplements. The dog began to show signs of remission on day 5 and had nearly returned to normal by day 22. Osmotic fragility and antioxidative status (reduced glutathione, superoxide dismutase, catalases, glutathione peroxidise, glutathione reductase, reduced NAD methemoglobin reductase, glucose-6-dehydrogenase, and 6-phosphogluconate dehydrogenase) tests indicated no predisposition of the dog to oxidative stress. The authors stated that to their knowledge, this was the first report of naturally occurring hemolytic anemia in a dog caused by Chinese chive and/or garlic (Yamato et al., 2005).

Edwards and Belford (1996) described cases of hemolytic anemia in five dogs and one cat with a history of eating onions and/or garlic. The cat had a history of consuming both garlic and onions, one of the dogs consumed only garlic, and the other four dogs consumed garlic and onions from a variety of human foods (pizza, Chinese food, mincemeat). Unfortunately, the amount of garlic and/or onion consumed was unknown. The animals showed signs of abdominal pain, vomiting, pale membranes, hemoglobinuria, diarrhea, and an enlarged spleen (in the cat). Three of the dogs and the cat had HB, although the percentage of HB was not noted in the cat. All of the animals had decreased RBC, hemoglobin, and HCT.

Garlic has been used as a palatant in pet foods for more than 30 years (Pet Food Institute, personal communication). Garlic powder and garlic oil seem to be the most common sources in pet foods plus treats. A recent search of the Mintel Global New Products Database (GNPD, www.gnpd.com) identified garlic as an ingredient in 363 of 2,604 dog and cat foods and treats in the United States. Of these, 127 products contained garlic powder and 61 contained garlic oil. Additional sources included whole garlic (3), garlic salt (3), and garlic extract (6). Many products listed garlic without identifying the source. Unfortunately, published data on the concentration of garlic in commercial pet foods are not readily available despite the common usage. Typical use levels have been reported to be 0.05 to 0.25 percent on a dry matter basis as a palatant in pet foods for dogs (G. Aldrich, personal communication, 2007). This equates to approximately 8–56 mg garlic/kg BW for dogs. One pet food company reported that it has tested dog foods containing up to 0.1 percent garlic (either as garlic powder or garlic oil) in AAFCO protocol tests (Pet Food Institute, personal communication, 2007). These products passed AAFCO protocol tests, including reproduction and growth tests. The researchers observed no adverse effects that could be associated with excess garlic consumption. Assuming a 15-kg dog requires 1,000 kcal/day (NRC, 2006) and a dietary energy density range of 3–4 kcal/g, these foods would have provided approximately 17–22 mg garlic/kg BW/day.

Numerous natural care and holistic-themed pet care texts recommend garlic inclusion to home-prepared diets or daily supplements. Dosage recommendations vary widely from one-half to three garlic cloves (≈ 1.5–9 g) per day depending on the size of the pet (Pitcairn and Pitcairn, 1982; Frazier and Eckroate, 1990; Orey, 1998).

Wynn and Fougère (2007) suggested the following dosages and noted that anemia in dogs and cats has not been reported with this level of use:

Small Animal (dogs and cats) Dosage:

- Fresh garlic: 1 clove (≈ 3–4 g) per 20–25 kg BW (equating to approximately 120–200 mg/kg BW/day);
- Dried/powdered garlic: 15–20 mg/kg, divided daily;
- Tinctures/extractions (25–40 percent alcohol): 1:2–1:3 at 0.5 mL per 10 kg, divided daily.

When corrected for the moisture difference between fresh garlic and garlic powder (see Table 8-1), Wynn and Fougère's recommendations for fresh and dried garlic are comparable.

The National Animal Supplement Council (NASC, personal communication, 2007) indicated that garlic-containing supplements have been on the market for 18 years. The dosage range for their members' products were:

- Dogs: 1.5–33.1 mg/kg (mean: 22.8 mg/kg)
- Cats: 2.1–30.1 mg/kg (mean 17.4 mg/kg)

Mean values are again similar to those recommended by Wynn and Fougère (2007) and to levels provided by commercial pet foods containing garlic as a flavor enhancer. NASC reported that while over 161 million administrations of garlic were sold for use in dogs since 1997, only 77 adverse events have been reported, resulting in an adverse event rate, as reported by NASC, of 0.48 per million administrations. This adverse event rate is similar to that for evening primrose oil (0.61 per million administrations) in dogs (see Chapter 7). No serious adverse events were reported during this time frame. Despite the sale of over 4.5 million administrations for cats, only one adverse event was reported between 1999 and 2007, resulting in an adverse event rate, as reported by NASC, of 0.22 per million administrations sold. No serious adverse events were reported for cats during this time frame. The actual amount of garlic consumed by the animals experiencing the adverse events, whether the animal was also consuming a garlic-containing pet food, and the actual nature of the adverse events were not reported. In addition, the source of garlic (e.g., powder or oil) was not reported for any of the NASC-monitored supplements.

Nontarget Species

Humans

The USDA Economic Research Service (USDA, 2006) stated that garlic was introduced into America sometime in the 1700s, but that its use was only slowly accepted. The first estimates of use were made in 1919 when per capita use annually was < 0.02 kg, compared to a peak use of 1.5 kg in 1999 and 1.3 kg averaged during the three-year period 2003–2005.

The WHO monograph on *Bulbus Allii Sativi* (WHO, 1999) gave the following recommendations with respect to daily intake in humans "unless otherwise prescribed average daily dose is as follows: fresh garlic 2–5 g, dried powder 0.4–1.2 g, oil 2–5 mg, extract 300–1,000 mg (as solid material). Other preparations should correspond to 4–12 mg of alliin or about 2–5 mg of allicin. Bulbus Allii Sativi should be taken with food to prevent gastrointestinal upset."

The committee was not able to find either a NOAEL or a LOAEL for garlic or its active constituents for humans. Estimates are often made as to intake in long-term trials, which limits accurate interpretation, for example, in a study that inversely correlated consumption of raw or cooked garlic (but not the garlic supplements used) with the incidence of stomach or colorectal cancers in humans. Fleischauer et al. (2000) assumed that one serving size was equal to one clove of garlic or ≈ 3 g. As such, the highest mean (± SD) intake of garlic across all published reports in this review was 18.3 ± 14.2 g/week or ≈ 6 cloves of garlic/week. Adverse events were not reported or commented upon, another major limitation. Storage may affect the composition of garlic (see above), further complicating interpretation of doses used in more long-term studies unless specifically allowed for, as was the case in the long-term study by Gardner et al. (2007). Raw garlic, a powdered garlic supplement, aged garlic extract supplement, or a placebo were studied as potential cholesterol-reducing supplements (4 g (one average clove) raw garlic, for example, per day) taken 6 days/week for 6 months by a group of adults. Previous work by this group had suggested that the particular products used would be consistent in their content of key active components over the time period studied (Lawson and Gardner, 2005). However, this dose was associated with adverse events (although these were not considered by the authors to be serious), including rare reports of rash, heartburn, and mouth ulcers (1 participant each out of at least 144) and flatulence (3/48 with raw garlic; 4/47 with the powdered garlic; 4/48 with the aged garlic; and 1/48 in the placebo group). Bad breath and body odor were, however, reported as being "often" or "almost always" present in a high proportion of those receiving raw garlic (57 percent: n = 28/49) but only 1 (out of 48) with the aged garlic.

Irritant/Allergen

Garlic allergy seems to be manifested as occupational asthma, contact dermatitis, urticaria, angioedema, rhinitis, and/or diarrhea (Allman and Cupp, 2000). Garlic can also cause "burns" when topically applied (as reviewed by Allman and Cupp, 2000). Allergic contact dermatitis in response to garlic has been recognized since the early 1950s and garlic-sensitive patients show positive tests to DAS, allylpropyldisulfide, allymercaptan, and allicin (Papageorgiou et al., 1983), although Papageorgiou et al. (1983) could not rule out garlic acting both as an irritant and a sensitizer.

Raw garlic can result in painful burning and/or prickling sensations when cut and placed on the tongue or lips (Rahman, 2007). The reaction may reflect allicin and DADS exciting an allyl isothiocyanate-sensitive subpopulation of sensory neurons and inducing vasodilation by activating capsaicin-sensitive perivascular sensory nerve endings (Bautista et al., 2005).

Raw garlic, due most likely to its high allicin content, but not oven-roasted garlic, activates two transient receptor potential (TRP) receptors, TRPA1 and TRPV1. These thermo TRP are present in the pain-sensing neurons that innervate the mouth and allicin has therefore been suggested to be one of the major irritants in raw garlic, especially to the mouth (Macpherson et al., 2005; Rahman, 2007).

Asthma

Several cases of occupational allergy and asthma have been reported in the literature (Allman and Cupp, 2000). Many are linked to people closely involved with the production of garlic preparations. Included is a case report in one individual who worked at a spice (including garlic) processing plant for 9 years. Asthma developed during the seventh and eighth summers and then when eating foods containing garlic. The patient's serum contained a high level (14.8 percent) of apparently garlic-specific immunoglobulin E (IgE). Ingestion of 1,600 mg garlic produced overt clinical signs (Lybarger et al., 1982).

Gastrointestinal Tract Issues

Reported signs of gastrointestinal tract (GIT) disturbances vary from burning sensations and diarrhea when large amounts are ingested to vomiting. For example, more than 25 ml of garlic extract caused vomiting and severe burning sensations in the esophagus and the stomach in one study (Caporaso et al., 1983).

Bleeding

Again, the potential for garlic to have positive or potential adverse effects on blood clotting may depend on the dose and preparation. For example, microwaved garlic had no effect on platelet aggregation, and the addition of raw garlic juice was needed to restore full complement of antiplatelet activity (Cavagnaro et al., 2007).

Various constituents of garlic have been shown, under certain circumstances, to possess antioxidant properties and to inhibit the production and/or release of mediators such as platelet activating factor (PAF), adenosine, prostaglandins, and thromboxanes (as summarized by Abebe, 2002). It has been suggested that the inhibitory effect of garlic on the production and/or release of one or more of these mediators may decrease platelet function: sodium 2-propenyl thiosulfate (2PTS), as an example, has an anti-aggregatory effect in vitro on both canine and human platelets at relatively low concentrations, but the extent of aggregation tends to return to the control level at high concentrations (Chang et al., 2005). Spontaneous bleeding/excessive bleeding associated with surgery has been reported on occasions (Rose et al., 1990; Burnham, 1995; Abebe, 2002).

Bruising was noted in a survey of complementary and alternative medicine use by patients attending an emergency department in Australia, but the dose and nature of garlic used was not provided (Taylor et al., 2004).

Hemolytic Anemia

There is apparently no evidence that consumption of garlic, at the doses studied or commonly ingested, causes hemolytic anemia in humans, although it is known to result in hemolytic anemia in dogs and horses as described above. The committee, however, was not able to find specific studies in humans that used high doses of garlic and monitored for HB. Sodium n-propyl thiosulfate and sodium 2-propenyl thiosulfate have been suggested to be two of the hemolytic agents responsible for both onion- and garlic-induced anemia in dogs. This difference in susceptibility between species may be due to differences in sensitivity to oxidative damage between humans and dogs (Chang et al., 2004) or an effect of dosage.

It has however, been suggested that even though hemolytic effects have not been reported in humans, the potent hemolytic activity of the tri- and tetrasulfides suggest that they should be treated with caution (Munday et al., 2003).

Rodents

In addition to the studies referred to above, there have been many publications with respect to the possible antibacterial effects of various garlic preparations as reviewed by Fenwick and Hanley (1985a,c) and Sivam (2001), although many of the studies are in vitro evaluations. A number of papers have reported that garlic administration can influence the gut microflora of rats, in particular resulting in decreased gut flora (as reviewed by Shashikanth et al., 1986), although the effects seem to depend on the nature of the garlic fed. For example, Shashikanth et al. (1986) showed that after feeding raw garlic extract for 4 weeks to rats, there was a significant decrease in total Streptococci, coliforms, lactobacilli, aerobes, and anaerobes, but there was no effect of feeding boiled garlic. Another study also potentially indicates that SAC may have some effect on intestinal flora at high dosages (Kodera et al., 2002).

Impact of Disease and Vulnerable Populations on Safety

Horses

To the committee's knowledge there is no published information with respect to the impact of disease or vulnerable populations in horses. However, it should be pointed out that the adverse events described by Valle et al. (2006) were seen in an animal that was in poor condition prior to supplementation, and the stallion with urticaria (Miyazawa et al., 1991) had relatively recently arrived in Japan from Europe. Whether these factors influenced the development of the apparent adverse events is not known.

Dogs

Animals with medical conditions associated with oxidative stress are likely to be more sensitive to excess garlic ingestion. Caldin et al. (2005) evaluated 60 cases of canine eccentrocytosis; eccentrocytes are indicators of oxidative damage to RBC. Eccentrocytes were significantly associated with drug administration, diabetes mellitus, ketoacidotic diabetes, T-cell lymphomas, untreated vitamin K antagonist intoxication as well as presumptive onion and garlic ingestion (11/60: 18.3 percent). There were no differences in eccentrocytes between healthy dogs and dogs with genitourinary, gastrointestinal, or respiratory infections; chronic renal failure; or bone marrow aplasia. While not specifically noted, it is logical to consider animals with disorders causing hemolytic anemia (e.g., immune mediated, metabolic defects) being at greater risk of hemolysis during garlic ingestion.

Cope (2005) suggested that treatment with propofol, sulfonamides, sulfapyridine, benzocaine, and acetaminophen can increase susceptibility to garlic toxicity because they can induce erythrocyte oxidative damage or diminish erythrocyte oxidative defenses. Likewise, glucose-6-phosphate dehydrogenase deficiency, zinc deficiency, and other inborn errors in metabolism or nutritional deficiencies that result in decreased erythrocyte antioxidant defense are also expected to exacerbate the oxidative effects of garlic compounds (Cope, 2005).

In canine RBC, high concentrations of potassium and reduced glutathione increase susceptibility to oxidative damage (Yamato et al., 1999). Thus, dogs with this hereditary HK phenotype (high potassium, low sodium, high Na, K-ATPase activity, high GSH) have been shown to be more susceptible to erythrocyte oxidative damage caused by garlic or onion ingestion (Maede et al., 1991; Yamato and Maede, 1992; Jin et al., 2001). This hereditary condition has been described in several Japanese dog breeds (Maede et al., 1991; Jin et al., 2001), as well as indigenous mongrel dogs in Japan (Maede et al., 1991). Whippets, Maremmano-Abruzzese Shepherds, Boxers, and English Setters seemed to have a high incidence of eccentrocytosis (Caldin et al., 2005) and could potentially be more sensitive to oxidative stress.

Little information is available in reproducing animals; however, both young animals and pregnant or lactating animals consume greater amounts of food compared to adult animals of the same body size. As such, increased garlic intake may be expected in growing and reproducing dogs and cats.

Caldin et al. (2005) noted no differences in incidence of oxidative stress (as indicated by presence of eccentrocytes) between males and females or between intact and neutered dogs. Young dogs were slightly more likely to have eccentrocytes than adult or old dogs (3.4 percent of young dogs vs. 0.8–1.5 percent of senior or adult dogs).

Cats

Medical disorders known to promote high oxidative stress (e.g., diabetes mellitus, hyperthyroidism, and lymphoma) or the use of certain medications (e.g., propofol, sulfonamides, and benzocaine) can potentially increase the susceptibility to garlic toxicity (Christopher, 1989; Cope, 2005). For example, diabetic ketoacidotic cats seem be at oxidative risk, having increased HB (Christopher et al., 1995).

The feline erythrocyte is more susceptible to oxidation and damage than the erythrocyte of other species. This is thought to be due to the increased number of sulfhydryl groups in feline hemoglobin that are more readily oxidized (Harvey and Kaneko, 1976) in combination with ease of hemoglobin dissociation (Desnoyers, 2000). Therefore, cats in general, seem to be at risk of being highly sensitive to RBC damage from allium species.

Nontarget Species

Humans

There have been many studies that have tried to evaluate the efficacy of garlic ingestion on various diseases or conditions, as mentioned above, although adverse effects tend to be rarely reported. This lack could reflect the protocols/reporting structure within the various trials or a real absence of significant adverse effects. It is also important to note that although efficacy studies (e.g., Markowitz et al., 2003; Gallicano et al., 2003) may not show any significant adverse effects, they do not necessarily reflect long-term use, use at different doses, or the effects in vulnerable populations rather than healthy volunteers.

Few studies have examined the long-term effects in vulnerable populations. One study looking at the potential protective effects of chronic garlic intake on the elastic properties of the aorta in the elderly examined the impact of garlic ingested for 2 years at a dose of 300 mg or more/day of standardized (details not given) garlic powder on the elastic properties of the aorta. Subjects were middle-aged to elderly, healthy, nonsmoking adults (n = 101: aged 50–80 years) with controls age and sex matched. No adverse effects were noted, although the study did not specifically look for or discuss this aspect (Breithaupt-Grogler et al., 1997).

The risk of increased bleeding in patients who simultaneously received anticoagulants and a particular garlic preparation has been studied. A double-blinded, randomized, placebo-controlled study in patients (n = 48 patents; 30 men and 18 women) receiving warfarin therapy for various reasons and either a placebo (n = 26) or AGE (n = 22) at a dose of 5 ml or 7.35 mg/dose of SAC (BW ≈ 90 kg) for 12 weeks found that the need for warfarin dose adjustment did not differ between the two treatment groups. Under this very closely monitored study (biweekly telephone follow-up and monthly study visits with maintenance of appropriate international normalized ratio levels), no increased incidence of bleeding was noted. The investigators concluded that with close, careful monitoring, AGE may be carefully administered in combination with anticoagulant therapy (Macan et al., 2006). However, this conclusion may only relate to AGE given under such circumstances. This view is supported by Vaes and Chyka (2000), who reviewed interactions between warfarin and garlic and concluded that the true risks of these interactions and effects are difficult to characterize due to the limited number and nature of existing reports. The WHO monograph on garlic (WHO, 1999) provided the warning that consumption of large amounts of garlic may increase the risk of postoperative bleed and notes the following precaution that patients on warfarin therapy should be warned that garlic supplements may increase bleeding times.

The WHO monograph on garlic (WHO, 1999) however, commented the level of safety for *Bulbus Allii Sativi* is reflected by its world-wide use as a seasoning agent, although it pointed out its administration is contraindicated in human patients with a known allergy to garlic. It did not note any objections to the use of garlic during pregnancy and lactation, and garlic was not considered to be mutagenic in vitro. In the section on adverse reactions it states

> Bulbus Allii Sativi *has been reported to evoke occasional allergic reactions such as contact dermatitis and asthmatic attacks after inhalation of the powdered drug. Ingestion of fresh garlic bulb extracts on an empty stomach may occasionally cause heartburn, nausea, vomiting, and diarrhea. Garlic odor from breath and skin may be perceptible. One case of spontaneous spinal epidural hematoma, which was associated with excessive ingestion of fresh garlic cloves, has been reported.*

Other Species

Several reports have involved rodents with particular diseases receiving garlic. Unfortunately, control nondiseased populations generally are not included and numbers tend to be small. For example, Ruffin and Hunter (1983) administered a concentrated garlic extract (no indication of level of actives) to spontaneously hypertensive rats (211–384 g; n = 8) at either 0.25 ml/kg or 0.5 ml/kg by oral injection once, twice, or three times a day for up to 28 days. Several rats exhibited lethargy and weakness; four of them died (all receiving more than one dose per day), potentially due to continuously lowered blood pressures, although toxic effects of garlic per se could not be ruled out. All rats had soft feces and showed signs of dehydration and weight loss, especially those that were given the extract more than once a day. No control group (without spontaneous hypertension) was given garlic for comparison. The authors concluded that garlic when used as an antihypertensive agent can cause side effects in rats and that further research was needed to determine whether such side effects would occur if such a concentrated garlic extract was administered to humans (Ruffin and Hunter, 1983).

Consumption as Part of a Normal Diet

Target Species

Horses

Potentially horses have the opportunity to ingest garlic or onions in the wild, although it is perhaps unlikely in large amounts. There is evidence of at least one incidence involving toxicity associated with the ingestion of wild onions (Pierce et al., 1972) in paddock-kept horses, suggesting that under certain circumstances, horses will eat wild onions.

Dogs

Foraging for wild or commercially grown garlic has not been described for dogs, and it is reasonable to expect that on an evolutionary basis, dogs would not have ingested garlic or onion bulbs.

Mason et al. (1994) reported that diallyl disulfide (garlic) and propane thiosulfoneate (onions) are attractants and palatants to carnivores such as dogs and cats. He observed that successful coyote lure contains sulfurous compounds and thus are attractive to wild canids, as well. Thus, the potential for limited natural exposure would seem plausible.

Cats

Foraging for wild or commercially grown garlic has not been described for cats. It is reasonable to expect that on an evolutionary basis, cats would not have ingested garlic or onion bulbs.

Safety of Similar Compounds

Target Species

Horses

Acute hemolytic anemia has been reported in horses following the ingestion of onions (Thorp and Harshfield, 1939; see Pierce et al., 1972). A small outbreak of wild onion poisoning (Pierce et al., 1972) occurred in a group of nine horses kept in a small, overgrazed pasture covered with wild onions (*Allium canadense*). All horses became sick, weak, and icteric; some had passed coffee-colored urine; and one had already died when two others were referred to the diagnostic laboratory. One of the referred horses was euthanized on arrival but apparently showed signs considered to be indicative of an acute hemolytic disease. The other referred case was hospitalized and found to have very marked HB anemia. She was managed conservatively; after 1 week, she started to improve and 2 weeks later gave birth to a foal. Based on these animals, onion tops collected from the field were fed to a normal Quarterhorse by stomach tube at a rate of 0.45 kg per day for 3 days, then 0.9 kg to day 9. On the ninth and tenth days, it was fed 1.8 kg of the tops with grain and hay. The PCV gradually decreased from the fourth to the eighth day from 30 to 23 percent and by the day 11 was 13 percent, by which time the horse was anorexic, icteric, and weak.

Dogs

Numerous cases of onion toxicity have been reported in dogs, and accidental onion poisoning seems more common than garlic poisoning. Aldrich (2007) and Tang et al. (2008) recently summarized these reports. Typically the dogs consumed human foods such as onion soup or raw or boiled onions. While it is difficult to estimate actual intake in a case of accidental toxicity, Cope (2005) reported that consumption of 0.5 percent of an animal's body weight as onions will consistently cause onion toxicity and that 15–30 g/kg BW results in hematological changes that are clinically important. Signs of onion toxicity in dogs include HB, hemolytic anemia, hematuria, anorexia, and tachycardia.

Tang and et al. (2008) recently investigated the progression of hemolysis in dogs consuming onion. They fed adult, clinically normal, Pekingese dogs 30 g cooked onions/kg BW, apparently with no other food, for 2 days and then took samples 1, 3, 5, 8, 12, 18, and 24 days post (P) this feeding. Dogs developed HB (≈ 73 percent in the 1 P samples) and a rapid decrease in RBC counts (significant in all the post samples), hemoglobin, and HCT (both significantly lower in all but the 1 P sample). In addition, erythrocyte glucose-6-phosphate dehydrogenase and the reduced form of NADP were significantly decreased in the 1–12 P samples. Catalase was significantly increased on days 5 and 8 P, whereas malondialdehyde was significantly increased in the 1–8 P samples. While reduced glutathione initially decreased (1 and 3 P) and then increased (8 P), hydrogen peroxide was increased in the 1P but then was significantly decreased until the 18 P. Fluorescence polarization and microviscosity of erythrocyte membranes increased (from 1–12 P) whilst the decreased erythrocyte deformity was associated with decreased erythrocyte lifespan. The study confirmed that the anemia was caused by hemolysis.

Interestingly, in one early study dogs apparently developed a tolerance to fresh or autoclaved onions or their juice (Gruhzit, 1931b). Four adult dogs of mixed breeds were fed either ground onions or autoclaved ground onions initially for 6 days at 15 g/kg BW or the equivalent in onion juice derived from the same amount of autoclaved onions, for 8 days (10 ml/kg BW). The RBC decreased significantly reaching their lowest 1–2 days after cessation of the onion administration. The maximum number of reticulocytes was seen 4–6 days post this cessation. Onion administration at the same dose was started again for a further 5 days on the 15th day of the study. During this period, there were no adverse effect on the blood parameters measured.

Cats

In response to reports of onion toxicity in cats consuming baby food, Robertson et al. (1998) investigated HB formation in cats fed baby food with or without onion powder. Cats fed the commercial baby food containing onion powder developed up to 55 percent HB, but there was no change in HCT or glutathione concentration. However, the authors reported at least two cats with apparent and one cat with definitive, hemolytic anemia caused by ingestion of baby food with an estimated concentration of onion powder of 1.8 percent. They then conducted a dose-response study, feeding cats canned cat food containing 0, 0.3, 0.75, 1.5, or 2.5 percent (dry basis) onion powder. A dose-dependent increase in HB was observed. Consumption of 2.5 percent onion powder decreased HCT and increased punctuate reticulocyte percentage. The HCT of cats fed lower doses of onion powder were not significantly different from the control. Based on reported average food intake of 46.1 g/kg BW (as is basis) and a dietary moisture content of 78 percent, it is estimated that cats had mean onion powder intake of approximately 30, 76, 152, and 254 mg/kg BW/day. The authors concluded that "baby food or other foods containing similar amounts of onion powder should be avoided for use in cats because of HB formation and the potential for development of anemia, particularly with high food intake" (Robertson et al., 1998). Other reports have described hemolytic anemia and enlarged livers and spleens of cats that have ingested onion soup or ether extracts of raw onions at levels equivalent to 28 and 56 g raw onions/kg BW (Kobayashi, 1981). Cope (2005) reported that consumption of 0.5 percent of a cat's body weight as onions will consistently cause onion toxicity in the animals. This is equivalent to 5,000 mg onions/kg BW. In one experimental study five 4-month-old cats were fed a single dose of dried onion (10,000 mg/kg BW). All cats showed clinical signs that included apathy, tachycardia, tachypnea, and cyanosis. One cat diet within 24 hours of ingestion of the onion. Laboratory findings included hemolytic anemia (with HB) and methemoglobinaemia. Histopathological findings included splenic and hepatic hemosiderosis and extramedullary hematopoiesis (Fighera et al., 2002). Such doses, however, cannot be directly related to garlic administration and safety. The relative toxicity between garlic and onion has not been studied in the dog or cat. The studies do, however, confirm that the genus *Allium* can cause toxicity in cats and dogs and demonstrate a comparable mechanism of toxicity.

CURRENT REGULATORY STATUS

Garlic is codified in FDA regulations as GRAS (generally recognized as safe) for use in animal feeds under 21 CFR 582.10 (Spices and other natural seasonings and flavorings). Further, essential oils, oleoresins (solvent-free), and natural extractives of garlic (for intended use as a "natural flavor" as defined in 21 CFR 501.22) are codified as GRAS under 21 CFR 582.20. For the pertinent regulation to apply, however, the substance must be used in accordance with good manufacturing and feeding practice, e.g., of appropriate grade, prepared and handled as a food ingredient, and not added in excess of the amount reasonably required to accomplish its intended effect. Therefore, garlic or its derivatives added for purposes other than flavoring or in amounts exceeding that needed for flavoring are not GRAS under FDA regulations. A minimum or maximum quantity of garlic inclusion in animal food has not been established but instead is given as "the quantity of a substance added to animal food does not exceed the amount reasonably required to accomplish its intended physical, nutritional, or other technical effect in food" (21 CFR 582.1).

These listings in FDA regulations may not be based on documented histories of safe use or submission of data to support use specifically in animal feed, but rather seem to be the result of circumstance. Garlic and its derivatives, along with a host of other herbs, spices, and natural flavors, were first codified as GRAS for use in food as a result of passage of the Food Additives Amendment of 1958. Substances added to food that were in substantive use prior to passage of the Act were reviewed by experts for evidence of toxicity, and only those deemed to have a safe history of use were codified as GRAS. However, at that time, a single set of regulations applied to both human food and animal feed. The regulations pertaining to human food or animal feed were subsequently codified into separate sections of the CFR approximately a decade later. During this process, further review by or on behalf of FDA resulted in some substances listed in the earlier joint regulations to be excluded from the GRAS regulations for animal feed. However, for the substances remaining on the GRAS list for use in animal feed, it is unclear to what extent histories of safe use in animal feeds were documented.

LIMITATIONS TO THE ASSESSMENT OF SAFETY

Many garlic preparations are available on the market, and they differ in their constituents plus pharmacological properties. This means that they also differ in their potential health benefits and possible adverse effects. In addition, it seems that adverse effects in general appear to be frequently underreported or inadequately reported in many human clinical studies involving garlic. Most of the work on garlic has been carried out in humans and rodents, but it seems that the major toxicity or safety issues that affect other species such as the dog, cat, and horse may not be as apparent in these studies due to differing sensitivities of cells to processes such as oxidative damage, the dosages used, or the target organs or systems evaluated. This means that while potential side effects detected in other species may be useful to consider for companion animals, safety limits cannot necessarily be set based on the available data in rodents or humans. Metabolism of the main sulfur components of garlic also differ considerably between species. For example, SAC has a half-life of $\approx$ 10 hours after oral administration in dogs but 0.77 hour in mice. The pharmacokinetics do not seem to be known in horses or cats. Unfortunately there is a lack of safety data in target species and nonclinically apparent adverse events may not be noticed during certain trials due to the design or other factors.

This review has, therefore, not tried to establish a NOAEL or LOAEL for humans, rodents, or other species in order to help establish such levels in horses, dogs, and cats.

RISK ASSESSMENT

Due to the variability in the nature of garlic and garlic preparations, the lack of standardization of commercial garlic preparations, plus a general lack of standardization regarding the level of potential actives, it is difficult to determine a realistic LOAEL for either short- or long-term administration for any species based on the literature currently available for garlic as a generic material. It might be possible, with more in-depth reviews of the literature, to determine levels for various specific preparations or active components for rodents and potentially humans, but there is insufficient information available for horses, dogs, and cats. Problems and concerns arise due to intrinsic toxicity, contamination, potential unfavorable garlic-drug interactions, lack of standardization, and other factors.

> Above certain intake levels, which will vary according to the garlic preparation (including processing) being fed as well as the individual animal being fed, the committee believes that garlic administration will result in an adverse event in horses, dogs, and cats. However, at low levels of administration garlic can be fed safely to such animals.

Microscopic evaluations of blood smears are not currently required as a component of AAFCO testing protocols to establish nutritional adequacy, and most modern laboratories use automated hematology analyzers. Therefore, the committee could not automatically assume that an AAFCO trial for nutritional adequacy is suitable to assess the safety of garlic-flavored pet foods. Additional supportive data, such as measurements of HB, are required.

Horses

Two studies have confirmed that garlic administration over a certain amount will cause HB hemolytic anemia in horses and another report suggested that in certain individuals skin reactions may occur. The committee is also concerned about the potential for the putative antibacterial action of garlic to have an adverse consequence on the horse due to effects on the microfloral balance of the gastrointestinal tract. It is appreciated that in the Valle et al. (2006) study, the horse did not show any signs of GIT disturbance as the feces were apparently within acceptable limits and diarrhea was not reported (E. Valle, personal communication, 2007) and diarrhea was not reported in the report by Pearson et al. (2005). However, these reports do not provide sufficient evidence to prove that GIT disturbances may not occur with garlic administration above a certain threshold. Similarly, the committee is concerned that the background level of oxidative stress and other factors may influence the level of risk for garlic administration for any individual. In addition, it should be emphasized that total garlic intake needs to be taken into consideration (i.e., that present within the core ration as well as any that is provided as a top dressing).

Although more data are needed, the committee believes that intake levels of dried garlic powder of 15 mg/kg BW/day on a long-term basis are unlikely to result in a risk of an adverse event in horses under normal circumstances and that levels up to 90 mg/kg BW/day may not be associated with any adverse events in healthy, nonexercising, nonoxidatively stressed adult horses. The threshold level above which the risk of an adverse event will increase significantly is likely to be between 15 and 200 mg/kg BW of dried garlic and most probably between 90 and 200 mg/kg BW, potentially depending on the health and oxidative status of the individual horse involved (see Table 8-10).

TABLE 8-10 Historical Safe Intake (HSI) and Presumed Safe Intake (PSI) of Garlic in Horses, Dogs, and Cats (mg/kg BW per day)

Species	HSI	PSI
Horses[a]	15	90[b]
Dogs[c]	22	56
Cats[c]	17	ND[d]

[a]For garlic powder.
[b]Nonoxidatively stressed healthy animals.
[c]For garlic powder or garlic oil.
[d]Not determined (insufficient data).

Dogs

Allium species are associated with toxicoses and adverse events in dogs, but have also been used for a long time as flavorings and health supplements. While most reports of toxicity concern ingestion of onions (*Allium cepa*), a number of reports of adverse effects of garlic in dogs are also available. Toxic effects included gastrointestinal disturbances when applied directly to the gastric mucosa and hemolytic anemia (HB, methemoglobenimia, and hemoglobinuria) (Cope, 2005).

Garlic has a long history of safe use as a supplement, with mean levels of ≈ 22 mg/kg BW being reported with apparently no serious adverse events. This level is similar to the 0.1 percent level used without any overt adverse events in long-term AAFCO trials and has therefore been given as the historical use level. Levels of up to 56 mg/kg BW of garlic powder or garlic oil seem to have been included in foods for dogs with no apparent adverse events reported.

Cats

The cat lacks sufficient data to support a generic recommendation that covers all the types of garlic preparations. Mean intake levels of 17 mg/kg BW have been reported with apparently no serious adverse events, which is similar to the levels recommended for long-term use by some nutritionists with no apparent problems.

Currently, however, there seems to be less supportive data for the long-term feeding of cats with garlic-supplemented feeds above this level. This gap, coupled with the potential for an increased susceptibility in cats, means that more data are needed to support the safety of inclusion of garlic at levels above those historically used as a flavor.

It was not possible for the committee to provide values for whole garlic or aged garlic for horses, dogs, or cats due to the lack of sufficient published or historical data.

OTHER RECOMMENDATIONS

> The committee recommends that due to the complexity and variability within garlic preparations, safety evaluations should ideally be undertaken for each type of product especially if it is to be fed above the levels recommended herein.

Because of the high potential for biological activity of garlic and garlic-derived compounds that can be either beneficial or detrimental (Zhou et al., 2007; Münchberg et al., 2007), further work is required to define more accurately the safe dose of specific garlic preparations that have known levels of core active ingredients. Standardization of preparations based on agreed active compound(s) is essential. However, clarification as to what should be considered an adverse event and over what period of time a trial should be undertaken (e.g., half-life of the RBC), is required for the most benefit to be gained from this work.

Due to the wide use and easy availability of garlic, further research should be conducted to determine the safety and quality of garlic preparations. In the future, in reports of garlic administration in any species, including humans, more complete information is required with respect to the nature and type of garlic provided, time of administration, and a more complete evaluation of potential adverse effects. These should include the more commonly recognized adverse events as well as potential consequences including—

- Exacerbation of any gastric ulceration in horses and, in particular, in racehorses where > 90 percent may suffer from some level of gastric ulceration;
- Adverse effects of garlic on microflora within the equine gastrointestinal tract, given that the horse is a nonruminant herbivore that utilizes microflora as part of the normal digestive process.

It is also noted that it may be important in future safety or efficacy studies to clearly define what would constitute an adverse event or overt toxicity for any particular substance. With respect to garlic, this poses a number of questions including—

- Is "anemia" the adverse event or is it the finding of an increased percentage of HB? Does the animal have to become clinically anemic before a study would be reported as showing an adverse event?
- What RBC/HB level would be considered an adverse event? And is this or does it have to be of any clinical significance?
- What would be reported if, for example, the RBC decreased but did not reach the predefined level?
- If animals are not obviously anemic, but no specific check of the level of HB had been made, can the paper report no adverse events?
- Should an increase in the percentage of HB be considered an adverse event, whereas clinical anemia represents toxicity?

> It is important to note that the committee believes that human- or rodent-based garlic safety data may not guarantee safety in horses, dogs, or cats.

REFERENCES

Abebe, W. 2002. Herbal medication: Potential for adverse interactions with analgesic drugs. J. Clin. Pharm. Ther. 27:391–401.

Aldrich, G. 2007. Ingredient issues: Onions and garlic offer flavor in the right amounts. Pet Food Ind. 48(11):40–41.

Ali-Waili, N. S., K. Y. Saoom, M. Akmal, T. N. Al-Waili, A. N. Al-Waili, H. Al-Waili, A. Ali, and K. Ali-Sahlani. 2007. Effects of heating storage and ultraviolet exposure on antimicrobial activity of garlic juice. J. Med. Food. 10:208–212.

Allman, J., and M. Cupp. 2000. Garlic. Pp. 107–122 in Toxicology and Clinical Pharmacology of Herbal Products, M. J. Cupp, ed. Totowa, NJ: Humana Press.

Alnaqeeb, M. A., M. Thomson, T. Bordia, and M. Ali. 1996. Histopathological effects of garlic on liver and lung of rats. Toxicol. Lett. 85:157–164.

Amagase, H. 2006. Clarifying the real bioactive constituents of garlic. J. Nutr. 136:716S–725S.

Amagase, H., B. L. Petesch, H. Matsuura, S. Kasuga, and Y. Itakur. 2001. Intake of garlic and its bioactive components. J. Nutr. 131:955S–963S.

Arnault I., and J. Auger. 2006. Seleno-compounds in garlic and onion. J. Chromatography A. 1112:23–30.

Augusti, K. T. 1996. Therapeutic values of onion (*Allium cepa* L.) and garlic (*Allium sativum* L.). Indian J. Exp. Biol. 34:634–640.

Banerjee, S. K., P. K. Mukherjee, and S. K. Maulik. 2003. Garlic as an antioxidant: The good, the bad and the ugly. Phytother. Res. 17:97–106.

Bastidas, G. J. 1969. Effect of ingested garlic on *Necator Americanus* and *Ancylostoma Caninum*. Am. J. Trop. Med. Hyg. 18:920–923.

Bautista, D. M., P. Movahed, P. A. Hinman, H. E. Axelsson, O. Sterner, E. D. Högestätt, D. Julius, S. E. Jordt, and P. M. Zygmunt. 2005. Pungent products from garlic activate the sensory ion channel TRPA1. Proc. Nat. Acad. Sci. (USA) 102:12248–12252.

Benavides, G. A., G. L. Squadrito, R. W. Mills, H. D. Patel, T. S. Isbell, R. P. Patel, V. M. Darley-Usmar, J. E. Doeller, and D. W. Kraus. 2007. Hydrogen sulfide mediates the vasoactivity of garlic. Proc. Nat. Acad. Sci. U. S. A. 104:17977–17982. Online at: http://www.pnas.org/cgi/content/short/104/46/17977.

Bhattacharyya, M., G. V. Girish, S. K. Karmohapatra, S. A. Samad, and A. K. Sinha. 2007. Systemic production of IFN-a by garlic (Allium sativum) in humans. J. Interferon Cytokine Res. 27:377–381.

Bordia, T., N. Mohammed, M. Thomson, and M. Ali. 1996. An evaluation of garlic and onion as antithrombotic agents. Prostaglandins Leukot. Essent. Fatty Acids 54:183–186.

Breithaupt-Grogler, K., M. Ling, H. Boudoulas, and G. G. Belz. 1997. Protective effect of chronic garlic intake on elastic properties of aorta in the elderly. Circulation 96:2649–2655.

Burnham, B. E. 1995. Garlic as a possible risk for postoperative bleeding. Plast. Reconstruct. Surg. 95:213–219.

Cairns, M. C., J. J. Cooper, H. P. B. Davidson, and D. S. Mills. 2002. Association in horses of orosensory characteristics of foods with their-post-ingestive consequences. Anim. Sci. 75:257–265.

Caldin, M., E. Carli, T. Furlanello, L. Solano-Gallego, S. Tasca, C. Patron, and G. Lubas. 2005. A retrospective study of 60 cases of eccentrocytosis in the dog. Vet. Clin. Pathol. 34:224–231.

Cantwell, M. I., J. Kang, and G. Hong. 2003. Heat treatments control sprouting and rooting of garlic cloves. Postharv. Biol. Technol. 30:57–65.

Caporaso, N., S. M. Smith, and R. H. K. Eng. 1983. Antifungal activity in human urine and serum after ingestion of garlic (Allium sativum). Antimicrob. Agents Chemother. 23:700–702.

Cavagnaro, P. F., A. Camargo, C. R. Galmarni, and P. W. Simon. 2007. Effect of cooking on garlic (*Allium sativum* L.) antiplatelet activity and thiosulfinates content. J. Agric. Food Chem. 55:1280–1288.

Chang, H. S., O. Yamato, Y. Sakai, M. Yamasaki, and Y. Maede. 2004. Acceleration of superoxide generation in polymorphonuclear leukocytes and inhibition of platelet aggregation by alk(en)yl thiosulfates derived from onion and garlic in dogs and humans. Prostaglandins Leukot. Essent. Fatty Acids 70:77–83.

Chang, H. S., O. Yamato, M. Yamasaki, and Y. Maede. 2005. Modulatory influence of sodium 2-propenyl thiosulfate from garlic on cylcooxygenase activity in canine platelets: Possible mechanism of the anti-aggregatory effect. Prostaglandins Leukot. Essent. Fatty Acids 72:351–355.

Charles, G. D., V. A. Linscombe, B. Tornes, J. L. Mattson, and B. B. Gollapudi. 2002. An in vitro screening paradigm for extracts of whole foods for detection of potential toxicants. Food Chem. Toxicol. 40:1391–1402.

Chen, Z., H. Zhang, B. Liu, G. Yang, H. Y. Aboul-Enein, W. Wang, R. Ding, H. Du, and H. Li. 2007. Determination of herbicide residues in garlic by GC-MS. Chromatographia 66:887–891.

Christopher, M. M. 1989. Relation of endogenous Heinz bodies to disease and anemia in cats: 120 cases (1978–1987). J. Am. Vet. Med. Assoc. 194:1089–1095.

Christopher, M. M., J. G. White, and J. W. Eaton. 1990. Erythrocyte pathology and mechanisms of Heinz body-mediated hemolysis in cats. Vet. Pathol. 27:299–310.

Christopher, M. M., J. D. Broussard, and M. E. Peterson. 1995. Heinz body formation associated with ketoacidosis in diabetic cats. J. Vet. Intern. Med. 9:24–31.

Codex Alimentarius. 2008. Rome, Italy: Food and Agriculture Organization and World Health Organization. Online at: http://www.codexalimentarius.net/web/index_en.jsp#. Accessed March 6, 2008.

Cope, R. B. 2005. *Allium* species poisoning in dogs and cats. Vet. Med. 100:562–566.

Dalvi, R. R. 1992. Alterations in hepatic phase 1 and phase 11 biotransformation enzymes by garlic oil in rats. Toxicol. Lett. 60:299–305.

Das, A., N. L. Banik, and S. K. Ray. 2007. Garlic compounds generate reactive oxygen species leading to activation of stress kinases and cysteine proteases for apoptosis in human glioblastoma T98G and U87MG cells. Cancer 110:1083–1095.

Deaton, C. M., D. J. Marlin, C. A. Roberts, N. Smith, P. A. Harris, F. J. Kelly, and R. C. Schroter. 2002. Antioxidant supplementation and pulmonary function at rest and exercise. Equine Vet. J. Supp. (34):58–65.

Desnoyers, M. 2000. Anemias associated with Heinz bodies. Pp. 178–184 in Schalm's Veterinary Hematology, 5th edition, B. F. Feldman, J. G. Zinkle, and N. C. Jain, eds. Philadelphia, PA: Lippencott Williams and Wilkins.

Dixit, V. P., and S. Joshi. 1982. Effects of chronic administration of garlic (allium sativum linn) on testicular function. Indian J. Exp. Biol. 20:534–536.

Dixit, V. P., S. Joshi, R. Sinha, S. K. Bharvava, and M. Varma. 1980. Hypolipidemic activity of guggal resin (Commiphora mukul) and garlic (Alium sativum linn.) in dogs (Canis familiaris) and monkeys (Presbytis entellus entellus Dufresne). Biochem. Exp. Biol. 6:421–424.

Edwards, C. M., and C. J. Belford. 1996. Six cases of Heinz body haemolytic anaemia induced by onion and/or garlic ingestion. Aust. Vet. Pract. 26:18–22.

European Commission. 2005. Monitoring of Pesticide Residues in Products of Plant Origin in the European Union, Norway, Iceland and Liechtenstein. Brussels, Belgium: European Commission. Online at: http://ec.europa.eu/food/fvo/specialreports/pesticide_residues/summary_2005_en.pdf. Accessed March 6, 2008.

FDA (U.S. Food and Drug Administration). 1984. FDA Technical Bulletin Number 5: Macroanalytical procedures manual, vegetable and vegetable products. Online at: http://www.cfsan.fda.gov/~dms/mpm-toc.html. Accessed November 20, 2007.

FDA. 1989. Chopped Garlic in Oil Mixes. Online at: http://www.fda.gov/bbs/topics/NEWS/NEW00130.html. Accessed September 19, 2007.

Fehri, B., J. M. Aiaches, S. Korbi, M. Monkni, M. Ben Said, A. Memmi, B. Hizaoui, and K. Boukef. 1991. Toxic effects induced by the repeat administration of Allium sativum L. J. Pharm. Belg. 46:363–374.

Fenwick, G. R., and A. B. Hanley. 1985a. The genus Allium—Part 1. Crit. Rev. Food Sci. Nutr. 22:199–271.

Fenwick, G. R., and A. B. Hanley. 1985b. The genus Allium—Part 2. Crit. Rev. Food Sci. Nutr. 22:273–377.

Fenwick, G. R., and A. B. Hanley. 1985c. The genus Allium—Part 3. Crit. Rev. Food Sci. Nutr. 23:1–74.

Fighera, R. A., T. M. Souza, L. Ingeborg, and C. S. L. Barros. 2002. Intoxicação experimental por cebola, *Allium cepa* (liliaceae), em gatos. Pesq. Vet. Bras. 22(2):79–84.

Fisher, C. D., L. M. Augustine, J. M. Maher, D. M. Nelson, A. L. Slitt, C. D. Klaassen, L. D. Lehman-McKeeman, A. T. Fleischauer, C. Poole, and L. Arab. 2007. Garlic consumption and cancer prevention: Meta-analyses of colorectal and stomach cancers. Am. J. Clin. Nutr. 72:1047–1052.

Fleischauer, A. T., C. Poole, and L. Arab. 2000. Garlic consumption and cancer prevention: Metaanalysis of colorectal and stomach cancers. Am. J. Clin. Nutr. 72:1047–1052.

Frazier, A., and N. Eckroate. 1990. The New Natural Cat: A Complete Guide for Finicky Owners. New York: Plume.

Freeman, F., and Y. Kodera. 1995. Garlic chemistry: Stability of S-(2-Popenyl) 2 –propene-1-sulfinothioate (Allicin) in blood solvents and simulated physiological fluids. J. Agric. Food Chem. 43:2332–2338.

Gallicano, K., B. Foster, and S. Choudhri. 2003. Effect of short-term administration of garlic supplements on single dose ritonavir pharmacokinetics in healthy volunteers. Br. J. Clin. Pharmacol. 55:199–202.

Gardner, C. D., L. D. Lawson, E. Block, L. M. Chatterjee, A. Kiazand, R. R. Balise, and H. C. Kraemer. 2007. Effect of raw garlic vs. commercial garlic supplements on plasma lipid concentrations in adults with moderate hypercholesterolemia: A randomized clinical trial. Arch. Intern. Med. 167:346–353.

Goodwin, D., H. P. B. Davidson, and P. A. Harris. 2005. Sensory varieties in concentrate diets for stabled horses: Effects on behaviour and selection. Appl. Anim. Behav. Sci. 90:337–349.

Gossett, K. A. 2000. Anemias associated with drugs and chemicals. Pp. 185–189 in Schalm's Veterinary Hematology, 5th edition, B. F. Feldman, J. G. Zinkle, and N. C. Jain, eds. Philadelphia, PA: Lippencott Williams and Wilkins.

Greenblatt, D. J., R. A. Leigh-Pemberton, and L. L. Von Moltke. 2006. In vitro interactions of water soluble garlic components with human cytochromes P450. J. Nutr. 136:806S–809S.

Gruhzit, O. M. 1931a. Anemia in dogs produced by feeding disulphide compounds. Am. J. Med. Sci. 181:815–820.

Gruhzit, O. M. 1931b. Anemia of dogs produced by feeding of the whole onions and of onion fractions. Am. J. Med. Sci. 181:812–815.

Harris, P. A. 1999. Changes in equine feeding practices. Pp. 149–152 in Guardians of the Horse: Past, Present, and Future: A Millennium Celebration, P. D. Rossdale, T. R. C. Greet, P. A. Harris, R. E. Green, and S. Hall, eds. Newmarket and London, UK: Romney Publications and British Equine Veterinary Association.

Harvey, J. W., and J. J. Kaneko. 1976. Oxidation of human and animal haemoglobins with ascorbate, acetylphenylhydrazine, nitrite, and hydrogen peroxide. Br. J. Haematol. 32:193–203.

Horton, G. M., D. B. Blethen, and B. M. Prasad. 1991. The effect of garlic (*Allium sativum*) on feed palatability of horses and feed consumption, selected performance and blood parameters in sheep and swine. Can. J. Anim. Sci. 71:607–610.

Hoshino, T., N. Kashimoto, and S. Kasuga. 2001. Effects of garlic preparations on the gastrointestinal mucosa. J. Nutr. 131:1109S–1113S.

Howard, E. W., M. T. Ling, C. W. Chua, H. W. Cheung, X. Wang, and Y. C. Wong. 2007. Garlic derived S-allymercaptocysteine is a novel antimetastatic agent for androgen-independent prostate cancer. Clin. Cancer Res. 13:1847–1856.

Hu, Q., Q. Yang, O. Yamato, M. Yamasaki, Y. Maede, and T. Yoshihara. 2002. Isolation and identification of organosulfur compounds oxidizing canine erythrocytes from garlic (*Allium Sativum*). J. Agric. Food Chem. 50:1059–1062.

Hu, Z., X. Yang, P. C. L. Ho, S. Y. Chan, P. W. S. Heng, E. Chan, W. Duan, H. L. Koh, and S. Zhou. 2005. Herb-drug interactions. Drugs 65:1239–1282.

Hyland, A. 1990. Equus: The Horse in the Roman World. New Haven, CT: Yale University Press.

Iberl, B., G. Winkler, B. Muller, and K. Knobloch. 1990. Quantitative determination of allicin and alliin from garlic by HPLC. Planta Med. 56:320–326.

Izzo, A. A., and E. Ernst. 2001. Interactions between herbal medicines and prescribed drugs: A systematic review. Drugs 61:2163–2175.

Jain, A. K., R. Vargas, S. Gotzkowsky, and F. G. McMahon. 1993. Can garlic reduce levels of serum lipids? A controlled clinical study. Am. J. Med. 94:632–635.

James, J. S. 2001. Garlic reduces saquinavir blood levels 50%; may affect other drugs. AIDS treatment news (375):2–3.

Jastrzebski, Z., H. Leontowicz, M. Leontowicz, J. Namiesnik, Z. Zachwieja, H. Barton, E. Pawelzik, P. Arancibia-Avila, F. Toledo, and S. Gorinstein. 2007. The bioactivity of processed garlic (*Allium sativum* L.) as shown *in vitro* and *in vivo* studies in rats. Food Chem. Toxicol. 45:1626–1633.

Jiang, W., D. Liu, and W. Hou. 2001. Hyperaccumulation of cadmium by roots, bulbs and shoots of garlic (*Allium sativum* L.). Bioresour. Technol. 76:9–13.

Jin, T. W., H. T. Kim, W. S. Chang, T. H. Oh, J. C. Song, K. S. Jeong, S. C. Park, and K. W. Lee. 2001. The effect of short-term administration of excessive amount of garlic on haematology in HK phenotype Jindo-dog. J. Vet. Clin. 18:232–236.

Joseph, P. K., K. R. Rao, and C. S. Sundaresh. 1989. Toxic effects of garlic extract and garlic oil in rats. Indian J. Exp. Biol. 27:977–979.

Kamel, S. H. 1966. Toxicity of the Egyptian garlic alkaloid injected into rats kept under various conditions of temperature and relative humidity. Zentbl. Veterinarmedizin Rehke A 13:662–668.

Kasuga S., N. Uda, E. Kyo, M. Ushijima, N. Morihara, and Y. Itakura. 2001. Pharmacologic activities of aged garlic extract in comparison with other garlic preparations. J. Nutr. 131:1080S–1084S.

Kaye, A. D., B. D. Nossaman, I. N. Ibrahim, C. J. Feng, D. B. McNamara, K. C. Agrawal, and P. J. Kadowitz. 1995. Analysis of responses of allicin, a compound from garlic, in the pulmonary vascular bed of the cat and in the rat. Eur. J. Pharmacol. 276(1-2):21–26.

Kegley, S., B. Hill, and S. Orme. 2007. PAN Pesticide Database, Pesticide Action Network, North America. Online at: http:www.pesticideinfo.org.

Kobayashi, K. 1981. Onion poisoning in the cat. Feline Pract. 11(1):22–27.

Kodera, Y., A. Suzuki, O. Imada, S. Kasuga, I. Sumioka, A. Kanezawa, N. Taru, M. Fujikawa, S. Nagae, K. Masamoto, K. Maeshige, and K. Ono. 2002. Physical, chemical and biological properties of S-allycysteine, an amino acid derived from garlic. J. Agric. Food Chem. 50:622–632.

Lawson, L. D., and C. D. Gardner. 2005. Composition, stability and bioavailability of garlic products used in a clinical trial. J. Agric. Food Chem. 53:6254–6261.

Lawson, L. D., and Z. J. Wang. 2001. Low allicin release from garlic supplements: a major problem due to the sensitivities of alliinase activity. J. Agric. Food Chem. 49:2592–2599.

Lawson, L. D., and Z. J. Wang. 2005. Allicin and allicin-derived garlic compounds increase breath acetone through allyl methyl sulfide: Use in measuring allicin bioavailability. J. Agric. Food Chem. 53:1974–1983.

Lawson L. D., S. G. Wood, and B. G. Hughes. 1991. HPLC analysis of allicin and other thiosulfinates in garlic clove homogenates Planta Medica 57:263–270.

Lawson, L. D., D. K. Ransom, and B. G. Hughes. 1992. Inhibition of whole blood platelet-aggregation by compounds in garlic clove extracts and commercial garlic products. Thromb. Res. 65:141–156.

Lawson, L. D., Z. J. Wang, and D. Papadimitriou. 2001. Allicin release under simulated gastrointestinal conditions from garlic powder tablets employed in clinical trials on serum cholesterol. Plant Med. 67:13–18.

Lee, B. J., E. J. Sung, M. S. Lee, I. H. Jang, and H. B. Lee. 1994. Effects of garlic on cadmium accumulation in the tissue of dogs. Korean J. Vet. Res.34:635–645

Lee, B. M., and K. K. Park. 2003. Beneficial and adverse effects of chemopreventive agents. Mutat. Res. 523–524:265–278.

Lee, K. W., O. Yamato, M. Tajima, M. Kuraoka, S. Omae, and Y. Maede. 2000. Hematologic changes associated with the appearance of eccentrocytes after intragastric administration of garlic extract to dogs. Am. J. Vet. Res. 61:1446–1450.

Li, Y., S. Y. Xu, and D. W. Sun. 2007. Preparation of garlic powder with high allicin content by using combined microwave-vacuum and vacuum drying as well as microencapsulation. J. Food Eng. 83:76–83.

Lybarger, J. A., J. S. Gallagher, D. W. Pulver, A. Litwin, S. Brooks, and I. L. Bernstein. 1982. Occupational asthma induced by inhalation and ingestion of garlic. J. Allergy Clin. Immunol. 69:448–454

Maaß, H. I., and M. Klaas. 1995. Infraspecific differentiation of garlic (*Allium Sativum* L.) by isozyme and RAPD markers. Theor. Appl. Gen. 91:89–97.

Macan, H., R. Uykimpang, M. Alconcel, J. Takasu, R. Razon, H. Amagase, and Y. Niihara. 2006. Aged garlic extract may be safe for patients on warfarin therapy. J Nutr. 136:793S–795S.

Macpherson L. J., B. H. Geierstanger, V. Viswanath, M. Brandell, S. R. Eid, S. Hwang, and A. Patapoutian. 2005. The pungency of garlic: Activation of TRPA1 and TRPV1 in response to Allicin. Current Biol. 15:929–934.

Mader, F. H. 1990. Treatment of hyperlipidaemia with garlic powder tablets. Evidence from the German association of General Practitioners multicentric placebo-controlled double blind study. Arzneim-Forsch. 40:1111–1116.

Maede, Y., Y. Amano, A. Nishida, T. Murase, A. Sasaki, and M. Inaba. 1991. Hereditary high-potassium erythrocytes with high Na, K-ATPase activity in Japanese Shiba dogs. Res. Vet. Sci. 50:123–125.

Markowitz, J. S., L. DeVane, K. D. Chavin, R. M. Taylor, Y. Ruan, and J. L. Donovan. 2003. Effects of garlic (*Allium sativum* L.) supplementation on cytochrome P450 2D6 and 3A4 activity in healthy volunteers. J. Clin. Pharm. Ther. 74:170–177.

Mason, J. R., G. Epple, and D. L. Nolte. 1994. Semiochemical and improvements in pest Control. P. 335 in Behavioral Aspects of Feeding, B. G. Galef, M. Mainardi, and M. Valsecchi, eds. Newark, NJ: Harwood Academic Publishers.

Mayeux, P. R., K. C. Agrawal, J. S. H. Tou, B. T. King, H. L. Lippton, A. L. Hyman, P. J. Kadowitz, and D. B. McNamara. 1988. The pharmacological effects of allicin, a constituent of garlic oil. Agents Actions 25(1-2):182–190.

Miyazawa, K., M. Ito, and K. Ohsaki. 1991. An equine case of urticaria associated with dry garlic feeding. J. Vet. Med. Sci. 53:747–748.

Munday, R., J. S. Munday, and C. M. Munday. 2003. Comparative effects of mono-di-tri-and tetra sulfides derived from plants of the allium family: Redox cycling in vitro and hemolytic activity and phase 2 enzyme induction in vivo. Free Radic. Biol. Med. 34:1200–1211.

Münchberg, U., A. Anwar, S. Mecklenburg, and C. Jacob. 2007. Polysulfides as biologically active ingredients of garlic. Org. Biomol. Chem. 5:1505–1518.

Nagae, S., M. Ushijima, S. Hatono, J. Imai, S. Kasuga, H. Matsuura, Y. Itakura, and Y. Higashi. 1994. Pharmocokinetics of the garlic compound S-allyl cysteine. Planta Med. 60:214–217.

Nakagawa, S., H. Sumiyoshi, and K. Masamoto. 1984a. Acute and subacute toxicity tests of a ginseng and garlic preparation containing vitamin B1 (LEOPIN-FIVE®). Pharmacometrics 27:1133–1150.

Nakagawa, S., K. Masamoto, H. Sumiyoshi, and H. Harada. 1984b. Acute toxicity test of garlic extract. J. Toxicol. Sci. 9:57–60.

Nordio, C. B. 1952. Studies on hematological responses in fowl treated with Allium cepa. Boll. Soc. Ital. Biol. Sper. 28:1008–1009.

Nordio, C. B. 1953a. Boll. Soc. Ital. Biol. Sper. 29:12.

Nordio, C. B. 1953b. Anemia caused by feeding rats on onions. (Original Title: Nuove richerche su l'anemia da cipolle.) Arch. Vet. Ital. 4:201–206.

NRC (National Research Council). 2006. Nutrient Requirements of Dogs and Cats. Washington, DC: The National Academies Press.

NSRC (National Standard Research Collaboration). 2006. National Standard Research collaboration: Garlic (*Allium sativum* L). Online at: http://www.mayoclinic.com/health/garlic/NS_patient-garlic. Accessed on January 7, 2008.

Oboh, G. 2004. Prevention of garlic induced haemolytic anaemia by some commonly consumed green leafy vegetables in Nigeria. Biomed. Res. 1:134–137.

Oboh, G. 2006. Tropical green leafy vegetables prevent garlic induced hepatotoxicity in the rat. J. Med. Food 9:545–551.

Orey, C. 1998. Cancer: Essential Guide to Natural Pet Care for Cats & Dogs. Irvine, CA: BowTie Press.

Pan, J., J. Y. Hong, B. L. Ma, S. M. Ning, S. R. Paranawithara, and C. S. Yang. 1993. Transcriptional activation of cytochrome P450 2B1/2 genes in rat liver by diallyl sulfide, a compound derived from garlic. Arch. Biochem. Biophys. 302:337–342.

Pantoja, C. V., L. C. Chiang, B. C. Norris, and J. B. Concha. 1991. Diuretic, natriuretic and hypotensive effects produced by *Allium sativum* (garlic) in anesthetized dogs. J. Ethnopharmacol. 31:325–331.

Pantoja, C. V., N. T. Martin, B. C. Norris, and C. M. Contreras. 2000. Purification and bioassays of a diuretic and natriuretic fraction from garlic (*Allium sativum*). J. Ethnopharmacol. 70:35–40.

Papageorgiou, C., J. P. Coret, F. Menezes-Brandao, M. Pecegueiro, and C. Benezra. 1983. Allergic contact dermatitis to garlic (*Allium sativum* L.) identification of the allergens: The role of mono –di and trisulfides present in garlic. Arch. Dermatol. Res. 275:229–234.

Pearson, W., H. J. Boermans, W. J. Bettger, B. W. McBride, and M. Lindinger. 2005. Association of maximum voluntary dietary intake of freeze-dried garlic with Heinz body anemia in horses. Am. J. Vet. Res. 66:457–465.

Pierce, K. R., J. R. Joyce, R. B. England, and L. P. Jones. 1972. Acute hemolytic anemia caused by wild onion poisoning in horses. J. Am. Vet. Med. Assoc. 160:323–327.

Piscitelli, S. C., A. H. Burstein, N. Welden, K. D. Gallicano, and J. Falloon. 2002. The effect of garlic supplements on the pharmacokinetics of saquinavir. Clin. Infect. Dis. 34:234–238.

Pitcairn, R. H., and S. H. Pitcairn. 1982. Dr. Pitcairn's Complete Guide to Natural Health for Dogs & Cats. Emmaus, PA: Rodale Press.

Polasa, K., V. V. Annapurna, T. Prasanna Krishna, and K. Krosjmaswamy. 2006. Inhibitory effect of unprocessed/processed alliums under in vitro/in vivo conditions on carcinogen induced mutagenesis using different assays. Int. J. Cancer Res. 2:199–211.

Rahman, M. S. 2007. Allicin and other functional active components in garlic: Health benefits and bioavailability. Int. J. Food Prop. 10:245–268.

Rana, S. V., R. Pal, K. Vaiphei, and K. Singh. 2006. Garlic hepatotoxicity: Safe dose of garlic. Trop. Gastroenterol. 27:26–30.

Rivlin, R. S. 2001. Historical perspective on the use of garlic. J. Nutr. 131:951S–954S.

Robertson, J. E., M. M. Christopher, and Q. R. Rogers. 1998. Heinz body formation in cats fed baby food containing onion powder. J. Am. Vet. Med. Assoc. 212:1260–1266.

Rose, K. D., P. D. Croissant, C. F. Parliament, and M. B. Levin. 1990. Spontaneous spinal epidural hematoma with associated platelet dysfunction from excessive garlic ingestion: A case report. Neurosurgery 26:880–882.

Ruddock, P. S., M. Liao, B. C. Foster, L. Lawson, J. T. Arnason, and J. A. Dillon. 2005. Garlic natural health products exhibit variable constituent levels and antimicrobial activity against Neisseria gonorrhoeae, Staphylococcus aureus and Enterococcus faecalis. Phytother. Res. 19:327–334.

Ruffin, H., and S. A. Hunter. 1983. An evaluation of the side effects of garlic as an antihypertensive agent. Cytobios. 37:85–89.

Shashikanth, D. N., S. C. Basappa, and V. S. Murthy. 1986. Effect of feeding raw and boiled garlic (*A sativum* L.) extracts on the growth caecal microflora and serum proteins of albino rats. Nutr. Rep. Int. 33:313–319.

Sheen, L.Y., H. W. Chen, Y. L. Kung, C. T. Liu, and C. K. Lii. 1999. Effect of garlic active principle, diallyl disulfide, on cell viability, lipid peroxidation, glutathione concentration and its related enzyme activities in primary rat hepatocytes. Nutr. Cancer 35:160–166.

Sivam, G. P. 2001. Protection against Helicobacter pylori and other bacterial infections by garlic. J. Nutr. 131:1106S–1108S.

Staba, E. J., L. Lash, and J. E. Staba. 2001. A commentary on the effects of garlic extraction and formulation on product composition. J. Nutr. 131:1118S–1119S.

Stankovic, S., J. Levic, T. Petrovic, A. Logrieco, and A. Moretti. 2007. Pathogenicity and mycotoxin production by *Fusarium proliferatum* isolated from onion and garlic in Serbia. Eur. J. Plant Pathol. 118:165–172.

Sundaram, S. G., and J. A. Milner. 1993. Impact of organosulfur compounds in garlic on canine mammary tumor cells in culture. Cancer Lett. 74(1-2):85–90.

Takada, N., T. Matsuda, T. Otoshi, Y. Yano, S. Otani, T. Hasegawa, D. Nakae, Y. Konishi, and S. Fukushima. 1994. Enhancement by organosulfur compounds from Garlic and onions of diethynitrosamine-induced glutathione S-Transferase positive foci in the rat liver. Cancer Res. 54:2895–2899.

Takahashi, S., K. Hakoi, H. Yada, M. Hirose, N. Ito, and S. Fukushima. 1992. Enhancing effects of diallyl sulfide on hepatocarcinogenesis and inhibitory actions of the related diallyl disulfide on colon and renal carcinogenesis in rats. Carcinogenesis 13:1513–1518.

Tang, X., Z. Xia, and J. Yu. 2008. An experimental study of hemolysis induced by onion (*Allium cepa*) poisoning in dogs. J. Vet. Pharmacol. Ther. 31:143–149.

Taylor, D. M., N. Walsham, S. Taylor, and L. Wong. 2004. Use and toxicity of complementary and alternative medicines among emergency department patients. Emerg. Med. Australasia 16:400–406.

Teyssier, C., L. Guenot, M. Suschetet, and M.-H., Siess. 1999. Metabolism of diallyl disulfide by human liver microsomal cytochrome P-450 and flavin-containing monooxygenases. Drug Metab. Disposition 27:835–841.

Thorp, Jr., F., and G. S. Harshfield. 1939. Onion poisoning in horses. J. Am. Vet. Med. Assoc. 94:52–53.

Tsao, S. M., W. H. Liu, and M. C. Yin. 2007. Two diallyl sulphides derived from garlic inhibit meticillin-resistant staphlyococcus aureus infection in diabetic mice. J. Med. Microbiol. 56:803–808.

Turek, J. J., S. P. Massimino, K. P. Boebel, and M. G. Hayek. 2000. Investigation of garlic as an immunomodulator in canines. Pp. 573–582 in Recent Advances in Canine and Feline Nutrition. Volume III. 2000 Iams Nutrition Symposium Proceedings, G. A. Reinhart and D. P. Carey, eds. Wilmington, OH: Orange Frazer Press.

Umar, I. A., E. E. Otukenyong, I. O. Igbokwe, J. J. Omage, and I. B. Buralai. 1996. Garlic induced hemolytic anaemia in garlic fed rats may be associated with decreased levels of erythrocyte. West Afr. J. Biol. Sci. 4:73–81.

Umar, I. A., Z. G. Arjinoma, A. Gidado, and H. H. Hamza. 1998. Prevention of garlic (*Allium sativum* linn.)-induced anaemia in rats by supplementation with ascorbic acid and vitamin E. Nigerian J. Biochem. Mol. Biol. 13:31–40.

United Kingdom Stationary Office. 2007. The Pesticides (Maximum Residue Levels in Crops, Food and Feeding Stuffs) (England and Wales) (Amendment) (No. 4) Regulations 2007. London: United Kingdom Stationary Office. Online at: http://www.pesticides.gov.uk/uploadedfiles/Web_Assets/PSD/uksi_20073297_en.pdf. Accessed March 6, 2008.

USDA (United States Department of Agriculture). 2006. Vegetables and Melons Outlook/VGS-317/October 19, 2006. Economic Research Service. Online at: http://www.ers.usda.gov/publications/vgs/2006/10oct/vgs317.pdf. Accessed February 29, 2008.

USP (United States Pharmacopeia). 2000. Drug release; delayed-release (enteric coated) articles-general drug release standard. P. 1947 in U.S. Pharmacopeial Convention 724. Rockville, MD: U.S. Pharmacopeia.

USP. 2003. Garlic delayed-release tablets. Pp. 2752–2754 in U.S. Pharmacopeial Convention. Rockville, MD: U.S. Pharmacopeia.

USP. 2007. Garlic. P. 927 in USP30–NF25. Rockville, MD: U.S. Pharmacopeia.

Vaes, L. P. J., and R. A. Chyka. 2000. Interactions of warfarin with garlic, ginger, ginkgo or ginseng: Nature of the evidence. Ann. Pharmacother. 34:478–482.

Valle, E., E. Del Moro, and B. Padalino. 2006. Garlic effects in the horse: A clinical report (Original title: Un caso di intossicazione da aglio). Ippologia 17(4):35–39.

Vazquez-Barrios, M. E., G. Lopez-Echevarria, E. Mercado-Silva, E. Castano-Tostado, and F. Leon-Gonzalez. 2006. Study and prediction of quality changes in garlic cv Perla (*allium staivum* L.) stored at different temperatures. Sci. Hortic. (Amst.) 108:127–132.

WHO (World Health Organization). 1997. Guidelines for predicting dietary intake of pesticide residues, 2nd rev. ed. Unpublished document WHO/FSF/FOS/97.7; available from Food Safety, WHO, 1211 Geneva 27, Switzerland.

WHO. 1998. Quality control methods for medicinal plant materials. Geneva, Switzerland: World Health Organization.

WHO. 1999. Pp. 16–32 in WHO Monographs on Selected Medicinal Plants. Geneva, Switzerland: World Health Organization.

Wu, C. C., L. Y. Sheen, H. W. Chen, W. W. Kuo, S. J. Tsai, and C. K. Lii. 2002. Differential effects of garlic oil and its three major organosulfur components on the hepatic detoxification system in rats. J. Agric. Food Chem. 50:378–383.

Wynn, S. G., and B. A. Fougère. 2007. Veterinary Herbal Medicine. St Louis, MO: Mosby Inc.

Yamato, O., and Y. Maede. 1992. Susceptibility to onion-induced haemolysis in dogs with hereditary high erythrocyte reduced glutathione and potassium concentrations. Am. J. Vet. Res. 53:134–137.

Yamato, O., M. Hayashi, E. Kasai, M. Tajima, M. Yamasaki, and Y. Maede. 1999. Reduced glutathione accelerates the oxidative damage produced by sodium n-propylthiosulfate, one of the causative agents of onion-induced hemolytic anemia in dogs. Biochim. Biophys. Acta 1427:175–182.

Yamato, O., Y. Sugiyama, H. Matsuura, K. W. Lee, K. Goto, M. A. Hossain, Y. Maede, and T. Yoshihara. 2003. Isolation and identification of sodium 2-propenyl thiosulfate from boiled garlic (*Allium sativum*) that oxidizes canine erythrocytes. Biosci. Biotechnol. Biochem. 67:1594–1596.

Yamato, O., E. Kasai, T. Katsura, S. Takahashi, T. Shiota, M. Tajima, M. Yamasaki, and Y. Maede. 2005. Heinz body haemolytic anemia with eccentrocytosis from ingestion of Chinese chive (*Allium tuberosum*) and garlic (*Allium sativum*) in a dog. J. Am. Anim. Hosp. Assoc. 41:68–73.

Yang, Q., O. Hu, O. Yamato, K. W. Lee, Y. Maede, and T. Yoshihara. 2003. Organosulfur compounds from garlic (*Allium sativum*) oxidizing canine erythrocytes. Z. Naturforsch. Sect. C J. Biosci. 58:408–412.

Yoshida, S., Y. Hirao, and S. Nakagawa. 1984. Mutagenicity and cytotoxicity tests of garlic. J. Toxicol. Sci. 9:77–86.

Zewde, T., C. Fininsa, P. K. Sakhuja, and S. Ahmed. 2007. Association of white rot (*Sclerotium cepivorum*) of garlic with environmental factors and cultural practices in the North Shewa highlands of Ethiopia. Crop Protect. 26:1566–1573.

Zhou, S. F., C. C. Xue, X. Q. Yu, and G. Wang. 2007. Metabolic activation of herbal and dietary constituents and its clinical and toxicological implications: An update. Curr. Drug Metab. 8:526–553.

9

General Considerations in Determining Safety of Animal Dietary Supplements

This report has taken a two-pronged approach to the consideration of factors important in assessing the safety of animal dietary supplements. Chapters 1 through 5 covered the history of and science behind the determination of safety for animal dietary supplements, as well as the basis for their regulation. This analysis provided important general principles that could be applied to the assessment of the safety of animal dietary supplements. Chapters 6, 7, and 8 attempted to apply these principles to three diverse animal dietary supplements: lutein, evening primrose oil (EPO), and garlic. A formal review of the scientific literature of these three supplements was conducted to assess whether feeding them to horses, dogs, or cats presents a significant adverse health effect that changes normal function in the animals. The knowledge gained from conducting these assessments afforded an opportunity to review and to begin to define factors that should be considered when evaluating safety of animal dietary supplements in general. The goals of these analyses were an attempt to define some measure of safe intake that would avoid the risk of adverse health events (see Chapter 4).

This committee operationally defines animal dietary supplements as "a substance for oral consumption by horses, dogs, or cats, whether in/on feed or offered separately, intended for specific benefit to the animal by means other than provision of nutrients recognized as essential or for provision of essential nutrients for intended effect on the animal beyond normal nutritional needs, but not including legally defined drugs." The committee has deliberately not evaluated evidence of efficacy or utility and offers no recommendations for the use of animal dietary supplements. Efficacy is referenced only in cases where it demonstrates potential biological activity. If an intake level is quoted from a specific study, it was not to evaluate the actual efficacy of these claims or suggested levels of intake. In many cases, feed intakes had to be estimated. The studies were only cited to assess whether adverse effects were noted at the specific exposure level characterizing the study. These studies were also used to determine "common levels of intake." It is important to note that there was no evidence of any well-characterized studies sufficient to conduct meta-analyses of safety in target species. The data are inadequate for reasons fully discussed in previous chapters. Risk-benefit was not dealt with because only safety was evaluated and efficacy was not examined, which is required for a risk-benefit analysis. The committee did not examine probiotics or genetically modified organisms, and it did not assess the potential for transfer of infectious disease agents associated with contaminants in supplement use. It did not consider implications of the use of animal dietary supplements in food-producing animals or the effects on environmental or human health, nor did it examine specific formulation strategies (e.g., nanoformulations) on supplement safety. The committee did not assess the potential impact that labeling deficiencies might have in the development of adverse events (e.g., failure to cite the plant source or part, all potential active ingredients, dose, or content). Finally, the focus was on U.S. regulations, although the scientific principles discussed obviously have implications to other regulatory jurisdictions.

FINDINGS AND RECOMMENDATIONS

1. Although animal exposure to animal dietary supplements is potentially greater than exposure to either drug or food additives, minimal safety data were available. Ideally, the committee would have liked to have the data to define a no observed adverse effect level (NOAEL) for each of the three supplements. Lacking such information, a safe upper limit (SUL) would have been a less desirable, but acceptable, outcome. With the limited data currently available, the committee could only report historical safe intakes (HSI) and estimate presumed safe intakes (PSI) for garlic (except for the cat), EPO, and lutein. The committee has identified a number of data elements that should be considered that may be different from those routinely considered for drugs.

The following 12 factors should be taken into consideration when constructing any framework for assessing animal dietary supplement safety.

a. It is crucial to assess the quality and relevance of data used in studies not specifically defined to detect safety. Bias must be assessed relative to the purpose of the original study. At a minimum, studies require peer review or some level of documented quality assurance. The committee found it very difficult to evaluate the statistical power of the available studies to detect a significant adverse event. This included poor definition of signals, lack of sufficient animal numbers, or failure to evaluate a well-known adverse signal or a potential adverse signal. We could not perform meta-analyses of data that were present in some nontarget animal exposures due to species differences detailed below. We strongly recommend that efficacy studies monitor animal dietary supplements' specific adverse event signals. Efficacy studies should be accompanied by reasonable attempts to identify and evaluate the risk of potential adverse events. Further, data that have been collected that support potential safety should be clearly described and reported. Simply stating "no adverse effects/events" is not acceptable.

b. Validated and publically available analytical methods and standards are often lacking. There is often lack of consensus for what the active compound actually is because "activity" is not clearly defined, making standardization by active compound, de rigueur for drug studies, impossible. This may include failure to identify which compound is active, the existence of multiple active compounds with different biologic effects with respect both to efficacy and safety, the effect of matrix and presentation, and the potential for biotransformation. Even if the active compound is known, an acceptable quality standard and validated matrix-appropriate assay for quantification may not be available or used. Differences in mode of preparation (e.g., solvent vs. mechanical extraction of EPO; proprietary methods of lutein; crushing vs. cooking times in garlic) may further confound this issue. Accuracy of any label data provided must also be assured.

c. There are a number of challenges associated with defining dosage of animal dietary supplements. Supplements are often dosed on the basis of intended use and employ units not directly correlated to putative active ingredients (e.g., cloves of garlic, normal garlic vs. elephant garlic, fresh vs. dried). Units across supplement types and dosage forms are not uniform and the committee did not have sufficient data to make reliable conversions to a consistent metric. The committee also faced the dilemma that doses were neither consistent nor directly related to a common safety endpoint and often varied considerably across studies (e.g., flavor vs. health benefit for garlic). This precluded evaluation of escalating doses to assess safety as, is done with drugs.

d. Dosage of some supplements is intrinsically different than that associated with drugs, which are dosed on a milligram per kilogram of body weight (BW) basis. However, many supplements are incorporated as quantity per unit food. The intake of these supplements incorporated in a complete food/feed is a function of energy intake, which may differ from a stand-alone supplement (e.g., capsule, treat, or top-dressing) whose dosage tends to be more defined. Dosage of animal dietary supplements may be considered an imprecise science. Lack of knowledge of the actual dose of biologically active ingredients given in some studies evaluated by this committee is a major factor that has prevented us from defining exposure levels associated with lack of adverse events. Information needed to accurately calculate doses was often insufficient (e.g., body weight, food intake, quantity of active component per capsule, number of capsules successfully administered, or compliance).

e. Dietary supplements may be given in combination with other supplements or dietary constituents (e.g., multiple vitamin and supplement preparations), making the attribution of a specific adverse effect to one specific supplement difficult. Such combination therapy also often confounds the definition of a precise dosage.

f. Dosages are complicated by the potential for interactions among combined products or other dietary constituents that may impact absorption (e.g., lutein with or without oil) and subsequent metabolism or elimination (e.g., garlic and drug interactions).

g. Contaminants and adulterants are a potential issue for all supplements. Occurrence of contaminants, both natural and artificial (e.g., pesticides), are a function of the source of the supplement as well as the method of harvest and manufacture.

h. Processing techniques are crucial determinants of final composition and properties. These techniques may change over time and thus conclusions made today may not be applicable to the same supplement processed using different techniques in the future. There are also issues for some supplements as to the degree of quality control required in their manufacture (e.g., good manufacturing practice).

i. Failure to provide detailed information on proprietary preparations limits the interpretation of certain studies.

j. In some studies, explanatory information is lacking for adverse events. Signals may be buried in some trials. These datasets lack specificity but may be useful.

k. Sometimes a single case report is all the evidence available for adverse events associated with an animal dietary supplement (e.g., EPO and a potential risk of seizure). Is this a true signal? The answer to this question is dependent on whether there is a biological rationale for the observed effect in the species studied. Such decisions must be based on a supplement- and species-specific basis.

l. Assessment of xenobiotics, which are by definition foreign to the body, needs to be more stringent than assessment of nutrients or endogenous metabolites (e.g., garlic vs. EPO). This is particularly true with respect to the pathways of metabolism and excretion (see Chapter 4).

2. Since the amount of target animal data will probably always be insufficient for safety assessment, it is necessary to look at other species for safety signals. However, based on the specific animal dietary supplements studied, it is clear that safety of the same supplements in humans does not guarantee safety in animals. The clearest example is with garlic, where the potential exists for hemolytic anemia in horses, dogs, and cats, an adverse effect not described in humans. The committee has identified five factors to consider when selecting appropriate surrogates for horses, dogs, and cats:

a. Nutritional, metabolic, pharmacokinetic, and natural dietary patterns must be considered when selecting appropriate animal model species. All three species considered in this report have unique metabolic properties that alter the way supplements are processed in the body, making cross-species extrapolations difficult.

b. Supplements that are naturally occurring in a diet should be considered differently than those not natural for a given species (e.g., lutein for horses vs. cats). However, even if an ingredient is naturally occurring in the diet, the effect of higher "supra-dietary" levels of supplementation and degree of processing must be evaluated.

c. Information gleaned from a study of the evolutionary diets of wild and feral species vs. diets of domestic animals might provide some indications of normal intake. Such studies may also provide guidance on whether adverse signals obtained in a laboratory animal are relevant for horses, dogs, or cats.

d. There are significant digestive, physiologic, and metabolic differences among the species studied, as discussed in previous chapters. The relevance of these factors must be considered on an individual supplement basis.

e. As stated earlier, safety in humans may not translate to safety in animal species. In fact, some signs of adverse events reported for humans (e.g., nausea and headache) may not translate to the target species in this report.

3. As a result of conducting these reviews, the committee could rank the suitability of assessing acceptable and relevant data based on the following broad seven-point scale. Within each of these point scales, more credence would be given to data addressing several populations at risk We believe that compilation of data from a combination of the classes below will be the most practical and reasonable solution.

Class 1. Safety studies conducted in the target species similar to that acceptable for animal drug safety determination (see Chapter 3).

Class 2. Studies in the target species that specifically assess some marker of potential adverse effect. These studies could include clinical, epidemiological, or defined experimental models.

Class 3. Safety studies in a nontarget species closely related biologically to a target species (e.g., wolf for dog, mink for cat, and donkey for horse; see Chapter 5).

Class 4. Nonsafety (e.g., efficacy or long-term feeding) studies in a target species, ideally with a study design that allows for evaluation of potential adverse events.

Class 5. Documented historical or common usage in target species; case reports; adverse event database.

Class 6. Safety studies in a more distantly related species including humans.

Class 7. Ex vivo/in vitro studies.

For all three animal dietary supplements studied in this report, the highest rank of data assessed was class two, with the majority of studies in classes four, five, and six.

4. There is a clear need for a comprehensive adverse event reporting system. Existing systems are deficient often for the factors discussed above related to difficulty of defining dosages, active ingredients, or consistent adverse signals. Some systems require payment to access (e.g., the Poison Control Center of the American Society for the Prevention of Cruelty to Animals) or are limited by membership (e.g., the National Animal Supplement Council). Any system should be easily accessible for reporting and retrieving purposes, generate accurate data with a high level of confidence, and build upon the experience embedded in existing systems. The committee's analysis of these supplements has not uncovered a system for adverse reporting that is similar to those in place for drugs. The committee believes that lack of adverse events being reported to a manufacturer is weak evidence for a lack of adverse effects having actually occurred. Similarly, extensive exposure without specifically monitoring biomarkers of adverse effects does not automatically demonstrate safety.

5. The absence of laws and regulations that specifically address animal dietary supplements causes considerable confusion to the industry and the public.[1] Clarification is required to clearly differentiate the regulation of human and animal dietary supplements as well as factors that differentiate an animal dietary supplement from a food additive or animal drug. A generally recognized as safe (GRAS) designation of an ingredient does not imply general safety, but signifies only safety under intended conditions of use. Additionally, grandfathered GRAS supplements did not differentiate between those intended for humans and animals. Any future animal dietary supplement regulations should take into account existing American Association of Feed Control Officials (AAFCO), Codex, and U.S. Pharmacopeia (USP) standards.

[1]The report contains minor changes from the prepublication version to clarify that in the United States there are currently no laws and regulations that address animal dietary supplements as a specific group or entity.

6. The committee is concerned that use of an ineffective animal dietary supplement, in lieu of using an approved animal drug that could reasonably be expected to lead to a cure or amelioration of disease, is in itself an adverse event. This concept is similar to the requirement that human dietary supplement labels declare "this product is not intended to diagnose, treat, cure, or prevent any disease."

COMMENTS ON SPECIFIC ANIMAL DIETARY SUPPLEMENTS REVIEWED

The previous chapters review the committee's analyses of three supplements in great detail. The summary below presents only the major findings on whether we believe these supplements are safe for use in horses, dogs, or cats and what is unique about each supplement as it applies to animal dietary supplements in general. Suggested areas of research are also stressed. Where a PSI could be defined, this does not imply that a higher dose is unsafe, but simply that insufficient data are available to determine precise dose-response relationships. Further discussions on specific recommendations for each supplement can be found in the individual chapters.

The committee agreed that in general, when assessing an animal dietary supplement, the minimum amount of data that might be offered as evidence of safety of a compound is that which demonstrates the lack of adverse events when the product, as manufactured, is administered to the target animal at reasonable magnitudes of increased dose or duration of recommended use. This might be accomplished by determining a NOAEL in the target population. If the active ingredient is not known for certain, safety can still be reasonably assessed if the data are generated for the product as manufactured and dosed based on that which is recommended on the product label. Similar data might be expected in populations that have been identified at risk because of the unique properties of the proposed active ingredient.

The next level of data that might support safety assessment of a compound would be information regarding its effect or the body's response to the compound (what the compound does to the body, e.g., pharmacodynamics) and information regarding its disposition (that is, what the body does to the compound, e.g., pharmacokinetics).

Provision of effect or response data would facilitate the identification of signals of adversity. Provision of disposition (pharmacokinetic) data ideally would minimally provide information regarding the movement of the presumed active ingredient into (absorption) and out (excretion) the body such that the following can be either determined or reasonably predicted: (1) Time to steady-state, that is, the time that must elapse from the first dose until the maximum concentration of the compound will be achieved with multiple dosing; and (2) elimination or disappearance half-life such that appropriate dosing intervals might be determined and, should adversities occur, the time to elimination of the adverse compound might be known. For selected compounds, identification of target tissues for which concentrations of the active (beneficial or toxic) ingredient are highest (e.g., organs of excretion and sites of preferential distribution) might allow a reasonable prediction of signals of adversity.

In addition to assessing safety in normal, healthy animals, pharmacokinetic and pharmacodynamic data for the purported active ingredient might also provide a basis for comparison between the healthy animal and, once the compound is in widespread use, those animal populations that might emerge as "at-risk" due to physiologic (e.g., age, gender, or species differences) or pathologic (e.g., renal or liver disease) changes, or due to pharmacologic–nutrient interactions. The more complex the compound (e.g., the number of purported active ingredients or variability in preparations), the more foreign the compound to the animal, and the greater the anticipated exposure of the animal to the compound (e.g., higher doses, longer durations or exposure to extracted and concentrated preparations as opposed to natural form), the greater the need, particularly for pharmacokinetic and pharmacodynamic data.

For all products, postmarket surveillance is strongly encouraged to ensure that a method exists to detect, assess, and report potential adverse events to animal dietary supplements.

Lutein

Summary of Findings

A number of limitations mark the safety assessment of lutein in target animals. The impact of processing, food matrix, concentration of lutein, and concentration of other carotenoids necessitates some basic level of information. Reaching consensus among studies also is limited by differences in the proportion of free vs. esterified lutein, the different sources, the impact of esterification on disposition, and the relevance of data from one type of product (i.e., protein-bound or free lutein, mono- vs. diesterified lutein, or free (extracted) crystalline lutein). Formulation (e.g., suspended in oil vs. directly applied to food) may profoundly impact results. Clear guidance on the impact of processing, and specifically differences in products in regards to oral bioavailability, is paramount. They include, but are not necessarily limited to, the impact of light on oxidation status, isomeric conversion to less biologically active forms, the appropriateness of standardization of lutein content based on color, and the risk of microbial, pesticide, herbicide, and heavy metal contamination. Pharmacokinetic studies, including dose-concentration relationships that would have facilitated cross-correlations between studies, have not been performed. The lack of a standard, which has limited previous studies, may have been rectified with the generation of a USP lutein monograph. However, analytical methods must be standardized and should include specifications to ensure that lutein and metabolites are not detected as one.

Although lutein seems to be safe, understanding species differences in the disposition of the compound are important not only to demonstrate safety, but also to establish a minimum recommended dose for efficacy. Scientific studies and review of lutein, particularly earlier studies, tended to originate from countries in which lutein was often used empirically and whose sources of lutein were not limited by patent rights. Often xanthophylls (including zeaxanthin) or metabolites are included as lutein in analytical methods, so care must be made to discriminate what actually is measured. Exposure of tissue samples post-collection to light, oxygen, and temperature differences impact lutein measurements.

The committee established a number of research needs. Analytical methods must be standardized and validated in each target population. Methods should distinguish between parent compound and metabolites. Methods should include directives that minimize lutein-containing solutions' (whether "stock" analytical solutions or lutein-containing tissue samples) exposure to UV light or variations in temperature.

General guidelines should be promulgated regarding the impact of processing and differential sources of lutein on its bioavailability and safety. Safety should include rate of exposure to lutein, but more importantly risk of exposure to unintended contaminants.

Recommendations should be offered regarding safe levels of lutein intake when included as part of the food or as a supplement, with recommendations varying with the type of product offered (i.e., extracted vs. nonextracted).

Data should be promulgated to ensure maintenance of potency when stored according to labeled recommendations. As such, standards should be promulgated to define optimum storage conditions, with a focus on impact of UV light, environmental oxygen, and storage temperatures.

Manufacturers should be directed to label ingredients with the amount of total lutein in mg/weight of unit dose or per unit weight of food and to cite the state of lutein (e.g., crystalline or esters).

Feline susceptibility to retinal toxicity with fluorquinolones suggests marked species differences in retinal physiology that predispose the cat to adversity. As such, special considerations should be made in assessing the role of lutein in feline vision.

Presumed Safe Intake

A number of considerations support the safety of lutein intake as a supplement. Although a carotenoid, multiple authors and review bodies have noted that side effects typical of provitamin A or vitamin A compounds should not occur with lutein because mammals do not have the enzymatic capability of converting it to retinol. In target species, history of safe use is supported by the lack of any apparent adverse effects in association with ingestion of diets containing lutein at a content that results in an approximate daily intake (mg/kg BW) of up to 8.3, 0.45, and 0.85 in horses, dogs, and cats, respectively. Studies provided by the Pet Food Institute support safe use in cats at 3.6 mg/kg BW for 8 weeks and 0.94 mg/kg BW for 2 years, and in dogs at 0.89 mg/kg BW for 8 weeks. Although the perceived risk remains low, the possibility of gestationally related adverse events in cats warrants further consideration. Finally, studies focusing on the impact of lutein on immune function reported no adverse events in dogs or cats receiving lutein at a rate of 1.9 mg/kg BW and 7.0 mg/kg BW for 12 weeks, respectively. In the horse, the PSI of lutein is 8.3 mg/kg BW when eaten as forage or natural sources; no data exist to support recommendations regarding supplements. In the dog, the PSI of lutein is 1.8 mg/kg BW with an HSI of 0.45 mg/kg BW. In the cat, the PSI of lutein is 7.2 mg/kg BW with an HSI of 0.85 mg/kg BW.

Evening Primrose Oil

Summary of Findings

Scientific data available to make a proper risk assessment are lacking. Most studies utilized products from a single manufacturer, in spite of the fact that EPO is a natural product that contains multiple components that vary by source and processing methods. The two fatty acids most commonly associated with the biological activity of EPO are linoleic acid and γ-linolenic acid (GLA). The fatty acid composition of an animal's diet may influence activity, yet these data are rarely available when assessing EPO safety. Evening primrose oil is often given in combination with other oils (e.g., fish oil), which further confounds safety assessment of EPO alone. Because of the central role that such fatty acids have in an animal's metabolism, short-term feeding trials are not representative of the potential biological effects that may be seen with long-term (or even lifetime) EPO supplementation after a steady state has been achieved. Data on long-term exposure do not exist. The majority of dog and cat EPO supplementation data are from animals with skin disorders. As with most of the supplements studied, data were not collected in trials specifically designed to assess safety. Data describing EPO supplementation during pregnancy, lactation, growth, and strenuous exercise in the target species have not been published.

Presumed Safe Intake

To the committee's knowledge, comprehensive study on the safety of EPO supplementation in horses has never been completed. The longest period of EPO supplementation in horses documented in the literature is 24 weeks; therefore, effects of chronic supplementation in the horse are unknown. Despite lack of data, the committee's consensus is that EPO supplementation at levels in common use in other species (50–400 mg/kg BW) is likely to be relatively safe in horses. This decision is based primarily on the relative safety of the fatty acids in EPO, as well as its reported use in other species without significant adverse events. Linoleic acid, found in the highest quantities in EPO, is found in almost all feedstuffs that are routinely included in equine diets. In addition, this fatty acid predominates in vegetable oils (e.g., corn oil and soybean oil) that may be added to the equine diet. In contrast to linoleic acid, GLA does not seem to be found in measurable quantities in common feedstuffs fed to horses. Nonetheless, this fatty acid is an intermediate compound in the metabolism of ω-6 fatty acids and can presumably be synthesized in the horse from linoleic acid. The committee has set the PSI in horses at 400 mg EPO/kg BW. When adding EPO to the equine diet, other sources of dietary fat must be adjusted to accommodate the upper level of dietary fat tolerated by the individual horse.

Based on history of safe use and long-term clinical efficacy trials, the committee concluded that the dose of EPO typically administered in clinical trials (i.e., 42–424 mg EPO/kg BW or 4–36 mg GLA/kg BW) is well tolerated when fed long term to dogs. All of these trials were conducted with dogs that had skin disorders; however, the committee believes that similar levels of supplementation would be not harmful to normal, healthy dogs. The committee has set the PSI for dogs at 424 mg/kg BW, which is the upper level used in clinical trials. Most likely the upper safe intake for EPO is quite a bit higher than this in dogs.

The committee has set the PSI for cats at 391 mg/kg BW; however, it is likely that cats could tolerate higher levels of EPO. Because EPO does not contain adequate amounts of all the essential fatty acids (particularly arachidonic acid, α-linolenic acid, EPA and DHA) and the cat has limited Δ5- and Δ6-desaturase activities, the main concern when feeding high concentrations of EPO (particularly above the PSI level) is a deficiency of essential fatty acids.

Garlic

Summary of Findings

Garlic is a plant and thus variability on what is used or measured is great. Processing and preparation (whole, cut, processed) is crucial to defining what active substances garlic actually contains. Of the three supplements studied by this committee, garlic is most likely to be contaminated. The USP has taken a lead on defining standards for different garlic preparations. This committee is not convinced that a single marker such as allicin is representative of the biological activity of different garlic preparations. Compounds such as S-allylcysteine have different absorption, distribution, metabolism, and excretion properties across the target species, making it difficult to extrapolate garlic dose-response relationships. Manufacturer recommendations for garlic usage rates are broad and in some cases nebulous resulting in widely varying usage rates. There is a lower level used as a flavor additive that has been used for decades. The lower levels are generally assumed to be safe by other bodies examining this topic, although specific endpoints of toxicity were not evaluated in a controlled setting. However, more recently higher levels have been used for specific indications that exceed this common level.

Many garlic preparations are available on the market and these preparations differ in their constituents and pharmacological properties. Most of the work on garlic has been carried out in humans and rodents, but it seems that the major toxicity or safety issues that affect other species such as the dog, cat, and horse may not be as apparent in these studies due to differing sensitivities of cells to processes such as oxidative damage. This means that while potential side effects detected in other species may be useful to consider for companion animals, safety limits can not necessarily be set based on the available data in rodents or humans. Metabolism of the main sulfur components of garlic also differ considerably between species (e.g., S-allyl-l-cysteine (SAC) has a half-life of ≈ 10 hours after oral administration in dogs but only 0.77 hours in mice). Its pharmacokinetics do not seem to be known in horses or cats. Unfortunately there is a lack of safety data in target species and non-clinically apparent adverse events may not be noticed during certain trials due to the design or other factors.

Because of the variability in the nature of garlic and garlic preparations and the lack of standardization of commercial garlic preparations, it is difficult to determine a realistic LOAEL (lowest observed adverse effect level) for either short- or long-term administration for any species based on the literature currently available for garlic as a generic material. Problems and concerns do arise due to intrinsic toxicity, contamination, mistaken labeling, potential unfavorable garlic-drug interactions, and lack of standardization, among other concerns. Above certain intake levels, which will vary according to the garlic preparation (including processing) being fed as well as the individual animal being fed, the committee believes that garlic administration will result in an adverse event in horses, dogs, and cats. However, at low levels of administration, garlic can be fed safely to such animals. Microscopic evaluation of blood smears is not currently required as a component of AAFCO testing protocols to establish nutritional adequacy, and most modern laboratories use automatic hematology analyzers. Therefore, the committee could not assume that garlic-flavored pet foods having passed an AAFCO trial for nutritional adequacy are necessarily suitable to assess safety, with respect to the increased presence or otherwise of Heinz bodies, for that level of garlic intake. Additional supportive data are required.

The committee recommends that ideally, due to the complexity and variability within garlic preparations, safety evaluations should be undertaken for each type of product, especially if fed above the levels recommended below. Because of the high potential for biological activity of garlic and because garlic-derived compounds that can be either beneficial or detrimental, further work is required to define more accurately the safe, efficacious dose of specific garlic preparations with known levels of core active ingredients. Standardization of preparations based on agreed active compound(s) is essential. However, clarification as to what should be considered an adverse event and over what period of time any trial should be undertaken (e.g., half-life of the red blood cells [RBC]) is required initially in order for the most benefit to be gained from this work.

The committee established a number of research needs. Due to the wide use and easy availability of garlic, further research should be conducted to determine the safety and quality of garlic preparations, especially if they are to be fed above the levels recommended. In the future, in reports of garlic administration in any species, including humans, more complete information is required with respect to the nature and type of garlic provided and time of administration as well as a more complete evaluation of potential adverse effects. These effects should ideally include the more commonly recognized adverse events, as well as, where applicable, potential consequences such as exacerbation of any gastric ulceration in horses, particularly in racehorses, where > 90 percent may suffer from some level of gastric ulceration. Adverse effects of garlic on microflora within the equine gastrointestinal tract should be considered given that the horse is a herbivore that utilizes microflora as part of the normal digestive process.

It may be important in future safety or efficacy studies to clearly define what would constitute an adverse event or overt toxicity for any particular substance. With respect to garlic, this poses a number of questions including: Is "anemia" the adverse event or is it the finding of an increased percentage of Heinz bodies? Does the animal have to become clinically anemic before a study would be reported as showing an adverse event? At what RBC/Heinz body level would it be considered an adverse event? And is this or does it have to be of any clinical significance? What would be reported if, for example, the RBC decreased but did not reach the predefined level? If no anemia were seen but no specific check of the level of Heinz bodies had been made, can the paper report no adverse events? Should an increase in the percentage of Heinz bodies be considered an adverse event, whereas clinical anemia represents toxicity?

The committee believes that available human- or rodent-based safety data may not be appropriate to guarantee safety in dogs, cats, or horses. It was not possible for the committee to provide values for whole garlic or aged garlic for horses, dogs, or cats because of the lack of published or historical data.

Presumed Safe Intake

There are two studies that have confirmed that garlic administration above a certain amount will cause Heinz body hemolytic anemia in horses and another report suggesting that, in certain individual animals, skin reactions may occur. The committee is also concerned that there is the potential for the putative antibacterial action of garlic to have an adverse consequence on the horse, due to effects on the microfloral balance of the gastrointestinal tract. Although more data are needed, the committee believes that intake levels of 15 mg/kg BW/day on a long-term basis of dried garlic powder are unlikely to result in a risk of an adverse event in horses under normal circumstances and that levels up to 90 mg/kg BW/day may not be associated with any adverse events in healthy, nonexercising, nonoxidatively stressed adult horses. The threshold level above which the risk of an adverse event will increase significantly is likely to be between 15 and 200 mg/kg BW of dried garlic and most probably between 90 and 200 mg/kg BW potentially depending on the health and oxidative status of the individual horse involved.

Allium species are associated with toxicoses and adverse events in dogs, but have also been used for a long time as flavorings and health supplements. While most reports of toxicity concern ingestion of onions (*Allium cepa*), a number of reports of adverse effects of garlic in dogs are also available. Toxic effects included gastrointestinal disturbances when applied directly to the gastric mucosa and hemolytic anemia (Heinz bodies, methemoglobenimia, and hemoglobinuria). Garlic has a long history of safe use as a supplement, with mean levels of ≈ 22 mg/kg BW being reported with apparently no serious adverse events. This level is similar to the 0.1 percent level used without any overt adverse events in long-term AAFCO trials and has therefore been given as the historical use level. Levels of up to 56 mg/kg BW of garlic powder or garlic oil seem to have been included in foods for dogs with no apparent adverse events being reported.

The cat, like the horse, lacks sufficient data to support a generic recommendation that covers all the types of garlic preparations. Mean intake levels of 17 mg/kg BW have been reported with apparently no serious adverse events, which is similar to the levels recommended for long-term use with no apparent problems. Currently, however, there seems to be less supportive data for the long-term feeding of cats with garlic-supplemented feeds above this level. This, coupled with the potential for an increased susceptibility in cats, means that more data are needed to support the safety of inclusion of garlic at levels above those historically used as a flavor. For these reasons, the committee was unable to establish a PSI for cats.

Appendixes

Appendix A

Committee Statement of Task

A committee will collect and examine data related to the safety of three dietary supplements offered for horses, dogs, and cats, whether in feed or separately. During its review of the data for each of the three supplements, the committee will reflect on whether the compounds raise unique issues for safety and on their implications for general and specific considerations that need to be taken into account in determining supplement safety. In a report to the FDA, the committee will describe its findings and conclusions about the safety of the three supplements and provide recommendations for factors to consider in future analyses. Although not meant to be comprehensive, these considerations will help form the basis of a more general framework for evaluating supplement safety.

Appendix B

Abbreviations and Acronyms

A	Absorption
AAFCO	Association of American Feed Control Officials
ABC	ATP-binding cassette
ADI	Acceptable daily intake
ADME	Absorption, distribution, metabolism, and excretion
AGE	Aged garlic extract
AHC	American Horse Council
AMD	Age-related macular degeneration
AMS	Allyl methyl sulfide
APPMA	American Pet Products Manufacturers Association
ASPCA	American Society for the Prevention of Cruelty to Animals
ATP	Adenosine tri-phosphate
AUC	Area under the curve

BROD	Benzyloxyresorufin-O-dearylation
BW	Body weight

CAR	Constitutive androstane receptor
CDER	Center for Drug Evaluation and Research (FDA)
CFR	Code of Federal Regulations
cfu	Colony forming unit
Cl	Clearance
CMT-13	Canine mammary tumor cell
CVM	Center for Veterinary Medicine (FDA)
CYP 450	Cytochrome P450

D	Distribution
DADS	Diallyl disulfide
DAS	Diallyl sulfide
DAT	Diallyl trisulfide
DDG	Dried distillers' grains
DGLA	Dihomo-γ-linolenic acid
DHA	Docosahexaenoic acid
DM	Dry matter
DP50	Degree of polymerization 50
DRV	Daily reference value
DSHEA	Dietary Supplement Health and Education Act

E	Excretion
EBM	Evidence-based medicine
ED	Effective dose
ED_{50}	Median effective dose
EPA	Eicosapentaenoic acid
EPO	Evening primrose oil

FAO	Food and Agriculture Organization of the United Nations
FDA	Food and Drug Administration
FDG	Freeze-dried garlic
FFDCA	Federal Food, Drug, and Cosmetic Act

GC	Gas chromatography
GIT	Gastrointestinal tract
GLA	γ-Linolenic acid
GMO	Genetically modified organism
GMP	Good manufacturing practice
GNPD	Global New Products Database
GO	Garlic oil
GRAS	Generally recognized as safe
GSH	Glutathione
GST	Glutathione-S-transferase
GT	Garlic-treated

HB	Heinz body
HCT	Hematocrit
HIS	Historical safe intake
HPLC	High-performance liquid chromatography
HSCCC	High-speed, counter-current chromatography
HSUS	Humane Society of the United States

i.p.	Intraperitoneal

i.v.	Intravenous
IgE	Immunoglobulin E
IHC	International Harmonization Conference
ILSI	International Life Sciences Institute
IOM	Institute of Medicine
IU	International unit
IUB	International Union of Biochemistry
IUPAC	International Union of Pure and Applied Chemistry
JECFA	Joint Expert Committee on Food Additives
LD_{50}	Median lethal dose
LOAEL	Lowest observed adverse effect level
M	Metabolism
MCH	Mean corpuscular hemoglobin
MCHC	Mean corpuscular hemoglobin concentration
MCV	Mean corpuscular volume
MDRP1	Multidrug resistance protein
ME	Metabolizable energy
MRT	Mean residence time
NAHMS	National Animal Health Monitoring System
NASC	National Animal Supplement Council
NDF	Neutral detergent fiber
NEFA	Non-esterified fatty acid
NIH	National Institutes of Health
NOAEL	No observed adverse effect level
NRC	National Research Council
NRCS	Natural Resources Conservation Service (USDA)
Nrf2	Nuclear factor E2-related factor 2
NSAID	Nonsteroidal anti-inflammatory drug
NSFI	National Sanitation Foundation, International
NSRC	National Standard Research Collaboration
NTP	National Toxicology Program
OECD	Organisation for Economic Co-operation and Development
OEI	Office of Evaluations and Inspections
OFAS	Office of Food Additive Safety
OSL	Observed safe level
OTC Med	Over-the-counter medicine
OTSC	Office of the Texas State Chemist
P	Post
PAF	Platelet activating factor
PAN	Pesticides Action Network
PCV	Packed cell volume
PETP	Peptide export transport protein
PFI	Pet Food Institute
PMN	Polymorphonuclear neutrophil
PSI	Presumed safe intake
PVB	Purple viper's bugloss
QR	Quinone reductase
RBC	Red blood cell
RDI	Reference daily intake
ROS	Reactive oxygen species
s.c.	Subcutaneous
SAC	S-Allyl cysteine
SAMC	S-Allyl mercaptocysteine
SD	Standard deviation
SER	Smooth endoplasmic reticulum
SUL	Safe upper limit
$t_{1/2}$	Half-life
TMPT	Thiopurine methyltransferase
TRP	Transient receptor potential
U.S. EPA	United States Environmental Protection Agency
UL	Upper limit
USDA	United States Department of Agriculture
USP	United States Pharmacopeia
v/v	Volume/volume
Vd	Volume of distribution
VLDL	Very low-density lipoprotein
V_{max}	Maximal velocity
w/w	Weight/weight
WBC	White blood cell
WHO	World Health Organization

Appendix C

Glossary of Terms

Adverse event: harm in an animal administered a compound (supplement), but not necessarily caused by the compound; any untoward medical occurrence that may present during treatment with a (pharmaceutical) product, but which does not necessarily have a causal relationship with this treatment (International Conference on Harmonization, as reviewed by Nebeker et al., 2004). (See also "medication error" and "adverse reaction".)

Adverse drug event: harm caused by a drug or the inappropriate use of a drug; adverse drug event is a regulatory term.

Adverse event to dietary supplements: any health-related event associated with the use of a dietary supplement that is adverse (http://www.fda.gov/cvm/nadaappr.htm.).

Adverse event, "serious": an adverse event that results in death, a life-threatening experience, inpatient hospitalization, a persistent or significant disability or incapacity, or a congenital anomaly or birth defect; or requires, based on reasonable medical judgment, a medical or surgical intervention to prevent an outcome described above (www.fda.gov/cvm/nadaappr.htm.).

Adverse reaction: in medicine and pharmacology, the development of a deleterious, usually unintended effect (Lewis, 1998). Committee use: a noxious and unintended (harmful) response to a compound (including animal dietary supplement) that occurs at doses recommended for the intended use. The term "adverse drug reaction" is a regulatory term (Nebeker et al., 2004). An adverse reaction differs from an adverse event in that a causal relationship between the drug (compound) and adverse event exists, meaning, the reaction is in response to the drug and reflects its inherent properties.

Type A (I) adverse reactions: related to concentration of the compound at the tissue site, and occur in a sufficiently large proportion of the populations if the conditions of risk are met. As such, Type A, "augmented" adverse drug reactions are often avoidable if actions are taken to accommodate for patient factors.

Type B (II) adverse reactions: reactions caused by a compound that are unrelated to the concentration of the drug, occur in a small population of patients, and as such, may not be evident until very large numbers of patients receive the medication. Examples of Type B, "bizarre" reactions include idiosyncratic reactions, which may reflect genetic polymorphisms, or allergic responses.

Animal dietary supplement: a substance for oral consumption by horses, dogs, or cats, whether in/on feed or offered separately, intended for specific benefit to the animal by means other than provision of nutrients recognized as essential or for provision of essential nutrients for intended effect on the animal beyond normal nutritional needs, but not including legally defined drugs (Committee definition).

Antinutrient: an undesirable substance that can inhibit nutrient metabolism or absorption (Committee definition).

Bioavailability: the degree to which, or rate at which, a compound is absorbed or becomes available at the site of physiologic activity after administration. For the purposes of this committee, the site of physiologic action is generally the plasma. Absolute bioavailability of a compound, particularly xenobiotics, is often determined by comparing the area of the plasma concentration curve (AUC) of the compound of interest after intravenous administration (thus assuring 100 percent of the compound enters the blood stream) to the AUC after administration via the route of interest. For animal dietary supplements, the route is generally oral (Committee definition).

Botanical drug: a botanical drug product is intended for use in the diagnosis, cure, mitigation, treatment, or prevention of disease in humans. A botanical drug product consists of vegetable materials, which may include plant materials, algae, macroscopic fungi, or combinations thereof. A botanical drug product may be available as (but not limited to) a solution (e.g., tea), powder, tablet, capsule, elixir, topical, or injection. Botanical drug products often have unique features, for example, complex mixtures, lack of a distinct active ingredient, and substantial prior human use. Fermentation products and highly purified or chemically modified botanical substances are not considered botanical drug products (http://www.fda.gov/Cder/Offices/ODE_V_BRT/botanicalDrug.htm).

Clearance: the hypothetical volume of tissue (e.g., blood or plasma) that can be freed of a specified constituent in a specified time by any number of pathways of removal (e.g., renal, hepatic, or others) (Ritschel and Kearns, 1999; Merriam-Webster, 2008).

Cold press: to press (as olives) without applying heat from an external source; also: to extract (oil) by cold-pressing (Merriam-Webster, 2008).

Compound feed: see "feed."

Cook: to heat in the presence of moisture to alter chemical and/or physical characteristics or to sterilize (AFIA, 2005).

Crush: see "roll."

Cytochrome P450: A heme enzyme that catalyzes the insertion of one atom of O_2 into substrates; found in animal, plant, and bacterial species, it has important roles in biosynthetic and detoxification pathways in mammalian liver, adrenal cortex (steroid), and other tissues (Morris, 1992).

Diet: feed ingredients or mixture of ingredients, including water, which is consumed by animals (AAFCO, 2007).

Dietary ingredient: see "feed ingredient" (AAFCO, 2007).

Dietary supplement (animal use): see "animal dietary supplement."

Dietary supplement (human use): this term was codified in the Dietary Supplement Health and Education Act of 1994, as displayed in Box 1-2 (http://www.cfsan.fda.gov/~dms/dietsupp.html).

A product taken by mouth that contains a dietary ingredient intended to supplement the diet. The dietary ingredients in these products may include: vitamins, minerals, herbs or other botanicals, amino acids, and substances such as enzymes, organ tissues, glandulars, and metabolites. Dietary supplements can also be extracts or concentrates, and may be found in many forms such as tablets, capsules, softgels, gelcaps, liquids, or powders. Dietary supplements can also take other forms, such as a bar. If they do, information on their label must not represent the product as a conventional food or a sole item of a meal or diet (http://www.fda.gov/Cder/Offices/ODE_V_BRT/botanicalDrug.htm).

Disposition: the act or the power of disposing or the state of being disposed. In the context of animal health, the term is used to refer to the behavior of a compound in the body, including its absorption, distribution, metabolism, or excretion (Merriam-Webster, 2008).

Drug: (as defined by FDA as applied to feed) a substance (a) intended for use in the diagnosis, cure, mitigation, treatment, or prevention of disease in man or other animals or (b) a substance other than food intended to affect the structure or any function of the body of man or other animals (AAFCO, 2007) (http://www.fda.gov/opacom/laws/fdcact/fdcact1.htm).

Dry: to remove water or other liquids from materials (AFIA, 2005).

Effective concentration 50 (EC_{50}): the concentration of a substance that causes a response that is 50 percent of the maximum (Lewis, 1998).

Effective dose 50 (ED_{50}): the median effective dose (Lewis, 1998).

Enantiomer: either of a pair of chemical compounds whose molecular structures have a nonsuperimposable mirror-image relationship to each other (Merriam-Webster, 2008).

Endogenous: produced or synthesized within the organism or system (Merriam-Webster, 2008).

Ergogenic agents: a substance that can be used to improve performance by (1) improving physiological capacity directly, (2) removing physiological constraints to physiological capacity or (3) providing a mechanical advantage specific to the sport (Williams, 1983).

Excipient: a usually inert substance (as gum arabic or starch) that forms a vehicle (as for a drug) (Merriam-Webster, 2008).

Exogenous: introduced from or produced outside the organism or system; specifically: not synthesized within the organism or system (Merriam-Webster, 2008).

Extrude: to press or push feed through constrictions under pressure (AFIA, 2005).

Feed (also known as compound feed): edible materials(s) which are consumed by animals and contribute energy and/or nutrients to the animal's diet (usually refers to animals rather than man) (AAFCO, 2007).

Feed additive: an ingredient or combination of ingredients added to the basic feed mix or parts thereof to fulfill a specific need. Usually used in micro quantities and requires careful handling and mixing (AAFCO, 2007).

Feed concentrate: a feed used with another to improve the nutritive balance of the total and intended to be further diluted and mixed to produce a supplement or a complete feed (AAFCO, 2007).

Feed ingredient: a component part or constituent of any combination or mixture making up a commercial feed. (Primary feed ingredients are usually intended to provide nutrients or serve as a source of dietary energy.) (AAFCO, 2007.)

Feed supplement: a feed used with another to improve the nutritive balance or performance of the total and intended to be: (1) fed undiluted as a supplement to other feeds, (2) offered free choice with other parts of the ration separately available, or (3) further diluted and mixed to produce a complete feed (AAFCO, 2007).

Feedstuff: see "feed" (AAFCO, 2007).

First-order kinetics: a reaction whose rate is dependent on the concentration of substrate (Morris, 1992).

Food additive *[note this definition is distinct from feed additive]*: a food additive is defined in Section 201(s) of the Food, Drug, and Cosmetic Act as any substance the intended use of which results or may reasonably be expected to result, directly or indirectly, in its becoming a component or otherwise affecting the characteristic of any food (including any substance intended for use in producing, manufacturing, packing, processing, preparing, treating, packaging, transporting, or holding food; and including any source of radiation intended for any such use); if such substance is not generally recognized as safe or sanctioned prior to 1958 or otherwise excluded from the definition of food additives (http://www.cfsan.fda.gov/~dms/opa-def.html).

Food(s): when used in reference to animals, is synonymous with feed(s) (AAFCO, 2007).

Formula feed: two or more ingredients proportioned, mixed, and processed according to specifications (AAFCO, 2007).

Functional (or designer) feed: any modified feed or feed ingredient that may enhance physiological performance or provide a health benefit beyond the nutrients it contains (Adapted from Wildman, 2001).

> **Functional food:** any food or food ingredient that may provide a health benefit beyond the traditional nutrients it contains (Food and Nutrition Board, Institute of Medicine).
>
> **Designer food:** processed foods that are supplemented with food ingredients naturally rich in disease-preventing substances. This may involve genetic engineering of food (Crane et al., 2000).

GRAS: abbreviation for the phrase "Generally Recognized as Safe." A substance which is generally recognized as safe by experts qualified to evaluate the safety of the substance of its intended use (AAFCO, 2007).

Grazed or browsed material: represents the aerial portion of grass or herbage or the small stems, leaves and/or flowers and fruits of shrubs, trees, or woody vines that are harvested and consumed by animals (Committee definition).

Grind: to reduce particle size using a hammermill or roller mill (AFIA, 2005).

Half-life ($T_{1/2}$): the average period of time during which the mass, concentration, or activity of a substance decreases to one-half of the initial value in a given system (e.g., a living organism, the atmosphere, a population, community) under specified conditions (Lewis, 1998).

Hazard: the qualitative nature of the adverse effect resulting from a particular toxic chemical, physical effect, or inappropriate action. For example, carcinogenesis is a hazard, as is asphyxiation (Hodgson et al., 1988).

Herbs: includes herbaceous perennials, trees, shrubs, annuals, vines, and more primitive plants, such as ferns, mosses, algae, lichens, and fungi. They are valued for their flavor, fragrance, medicinal and healthful qualities, economic and industrial uses, pesticidal properties, and coloring materials (dyes) (Brown, 2001).

Lethal dose 50 (LD_{50}): the amount of a toxicant or other infective agent estimated to kill 50 percent of a test population that is exposed to the agent for a specified period of time (Lewis, 1998).

Mean residence time: average length of time a molecule remains in the body; the time when 63.2 percent of an intravenous dose of a compound has been eliminated from the tested system (Ritschel and Kearns, 1999).

Medical food: a food which is formulated to be consumed or administered enterally under the supervision of a physician and which is intended for the specific dietary management of a disease or condition for which distinctive nutritional requirements, based on recognized scientific principles, are established by medical evaluation (http://www.cfsan.fda.gov/~dms/medfood.html).

Medicated feed: any feed which contains drug ingredients intended or presented for the cure, mitigation, treatment, or prevention of diseases of animals other than man or which contains drug ingredients intended to affect the structure or any function of the body of animals other than man. Antibiotics included in a feed growth promotion and/or efficiency levels are drug additives and feed containing such antibiotics are included in the foregoing definition of "medicated feed" (AAFCO, 2007).

Medication error: a preventable event that may cause or lead to inappropriate medication use or patient harm while the medication is in the control of the health care professional, patient, or consumer. Medication errors might result from miscommunication, confusion regarding packaging, improper dose or interval, the wrong product, or any variety of errors made on the judgment of the caregiver or, in the case of animals, the animal owner (Committee definition).

Microbiome: the collective microbial genome of a region (adapted from Egert et al., 2006).

Microbiota: the microscopic living organisms of a region (Blood et al., 2007).

Mill: to grind into flour, meal, or powder (Merriam-Webster, 2008).

NOAEL (no-observed-adverse-effect-level): greatest concentration or amount found by experiment or observation, which causes no detectable adverse alteration of morphology, functional capacity, growth, development, or life span of the target organism under defined conditions (IUPAC Compendium of Chemical Terminology—the Gold Book; http://goldbook.iupac.org/index.html).

Novel food: foods and food ingredients consisting of, or containing, chemical substances not hitherto used for animal consumption to a significant extent in the locality in question (including microorganisms, fungi, or algae and substances isolated from them, and organisms obtained using genetic modification techniques). A food or ingredient to which has been applied a process not currently used for food manufacture or which has not been previously marketed and which gives rise to changes that affect its nutritional value or safety (Bender, 2006).

Nutraceutical (coined by Stephen DeFelice in 1989): any substance that is a food or a part of a food and provides medical or health benefits, including the prevention and treatment of disease. Such products may range from isolated nutrients, dietary supplements and specific diets to genetically engineered designer foods, herbal products, and processed foods such as cereals, soups and beverages (http://chemistry.about.com/library/glossary/bldef575.htm).

Any substance that may be considered a food or part of a food and provides medical or health benefits, including the prevention and treatment of disease (Committee definition).

Nutrient: (1) a chemical compound used in an organism's metabolism or physiology. The primary nutrients are carbohydrates, amino acids, fatty acids, minerals, vitamins, and water. Oxygen, although essential for life, is not normally classified as a nutrient for animals (Committee definition); (2) an essential dietary factor such as a vitamin, mineral, amino acid, and fatty acid (Bender, 2006).

Pellet: to agglomerate feed by compacting and forcing it through die openings by a mechanical process; the product resulting from this process (hard pellet) (AAFCO, 2007).

Pharmaceutical: see "drug."

Pharmacodynamics: the study of what a drug (compound) does to the body; the study of the biochemical and physiological effects of a drug (compound) on the body, the mechanisms of its action and the relationship between its concentration in the body and effect (Committee definition).

Pharmacokinetics: the study of what the body does to a drug (compound); the study of changes of the concentration of a compound (e.g., xenobiotic) across time following administration into a dynamic system (Committee definition).

Pharmafood: foods or nutrients that claims medical or health benefits, including the prevention and treatment of disease (Crane et al., 2000).

Phytochemical: a chemical compound derived from a plant, including fruits and vegetables (See USDA database at http://www.pl.barc.usda.gov/home.cfm.).

Substances found in edible fruits and vegetables that may be ingested by people daily in gram quantities and that exhibit a potential for modulating human metabolism in a manner favorable for cancer prevention (Crane et al., 2000).

Poison (toxicant): any substance that causes a harmful effect when administered to a living organism. Due to the popular connotation that poisons are, by definition, fatal in their effects and that their administration is usually involved with attempted homicide or suicide, most toxicologists prefer the less prejudicial term "toxicant" (Hodgson et al., 1988).

Polypharmacy: the practice of administering many different medicines especially concurrently for the treatment of the same disease (Merriam-Webster, 2008).

Prebiotic: a nondigestible feed ingredient that beneficially affects the host by selectively stimulating the growth and/or activity of one or a limited number of bacteria in a compartment of the gastrointestinal tract of the host. (Adapted from Schrezenmeir and De Vrese, 2001). Experts in this field are still using the following definition: nondigestible food ingredients that beneficially affect the host by selectively stimulating the growth and/or activity of one or a limited number of bacterial species already established in the colon, and thus in effect improve host health (Gibson and Roberfroid, 1995).

Presumed safe intake (PSI): amounts that will not impair animal health or production efficiency (Committee definition).

Probiotic: a preparation of or a product containing viable, defined microorganisms in sufficient numbers, which alter the microflora (by implantation or colonization) in a compartment of the host and by that exert beneficial health effects in this host. (Schrezenmeir and De Vrese, 2001). Live microorganisms which when administered in adequate amounts confer a health benefit on the host (WHO, 2006).

Retort: a vessel or chamber in which substances are distilled or decomposed by heat: to treat by heating in a retort (Merriam-Webster, 2008).

Risk, toxicological: the probability that some adverse effect (e.g., cancer) will result from a given exposure to a chemical; it is the estimated frequency of occurrence of an event in a population. Risk may be expressed in absolute terms (e.g., one in one-million or 10^{-6}) or in terms of relative risk (the ratio of the risk in an exposed population to that in an equivalent unexposed population) (Hodgson et al., 1988).

Risk/benefit ratio: a measure of the acceptability of an adverse reaction and is based on importance, frequency and duration of either the therapeutic benefit or the adverse reaction (Committee definition).

Roast: to cook by exposing to dry heat (Merriam-Webster, 2008).

Roll: to change the shape and/or size of particles by compressing them between rollers, sometimes involving conditioning (AFIA, 2005).

Safe upper limit (SUL): the maximal concentration or amount of a nutrient that has not been associated with adverse effects (NRC, 2006).

Saponification: the process whereby esters are hydrolyzed under basic conditions to form an alcohol and the salt of the carboxylic acid. If sodium hydroxide is used as the base, a hard soap is formed whereas potassium hydroxide yields a soft soap. For triglycerides, saponification frees the fatty acid from the glycerol (Committee definition).

Side effect: a usually predictable or dose-dependent effect of a drug that is not the principal effect for which the drug was chosen; the side effect may be desirable, undesirable, or inconsequential. The difference between adverse events (including adverse reactions) and side effects reflects the level of harm sustained in the use of a product (Nebeker et al., 2004).

Steady state: a state of equilibrium in which the input and output of a compound from the system (e.g., body) are equivalent. Steady state occurs with multiple dosing of a compound and reflects the amount that the compound will accumulate in the body (Ritschel and Kearns, 1999).

Synbiotic: a product that contains both probiotics and prebiotics. Because the word alludes to synergism, this term should be reserved for products in which the prebiotic compound selectively favors the probiotic compound (Schrezenmeir and De Vrese, 2001).

Toxicant: see "poison."

> **Direct:** toxicant that injures the cells with which it comes in contact.
>
> **Indirect:** toxicant that acts by injuring a group of cells that subsequently precipitate injury to others.

Toxic response: any deleterious response of a cell or organism due to exposure to a toxicant (Lewis, 1998).

Toxicity: the state or quality of being poisonous; the capacity to poison living systems; having a toxic or poisonous quality (Lewis, 1998); the quantitative amount or dosage of a poison or toxicant that will produce a defined effect (Osweiler, 2006).

Acute toxicity: the capacity of a biologically active agent to cause serious harm, injury, or death to a living system following a single dose or a single brief exposure during a 24-hour period (Lewis, 1998; Osweiler, 2006).

Subacute toxicity: any toxic effects that becomes apparent between 1 week and 30 days after exposure to a toxicant.

Subchronic toxicity: toxicity due to exposure to quantities of a toxicant that do not cause an evident acute toxicity for a time period that is extended, but is not so long as to constitute a significant part of the lifespan of the species in question. In subchronic toxicity tests using mammals, a 30–90 day period is considered appropriate (Hodgson et al., 1988; Osweiler, 2006).

Chronic toxicity: the capacity of a biologically active agent to produce toxic effects following long-continued, or numerous brief exposures (Lewis, 1998). Effects of a toxicant after exposure of 90 days or longer (Osweiler, 2006).

Toxin: a toxicant produced by a living organism (Hodgson et al., 1988); poisons that originate from biological sources biotoxin (Osweiler, 2006).

Treat: a food given as source of special delight or pleasure (Committee definition).

Volume of distribution: a theoretical volume of fluid that would be required to dissolve the total amount of a compound to yield the same concentration as that found at the test site (e.g., plasma). It is a proportionality constant that relates the amount of compound in the body to the measured concentration in the biological fluid (Ritschel and Kearns, 1999).

Xenobiotic: a compound that is foreign to a living organism. Principal xenobiotics include: drugs; carcinogens; and various compounds that have been introduced into the environment by artificial means (IUPAC Compendium of Chemical Terminology—the Gold Book; http://goldbook.iupac.org/index.html). This definition ignores compounds that are "natural," but just not to a specific animal.

Any substance, harmful or not, that is foreign to the animal's biological system (Blood et al., 2007).

Xenobiotic interactions: occur whenever the action of one xenobiotic is modified by the presence of another, concurrently administered xenobiotic. Interactions can occur during the pharmaceutical phase, before the compound is absorbed; the pharmacokinetic phase, during which one xenobiotic alters the disposition of another; or the pharmacodynamic phase, during which one compound alters the response to another (Committee definition).

Zero-order reaction: a chemical reaction in which the rate of the reaction does not depend on the concentration of the individual reactants.

REFERENCES

AAFCO (Association of American Feed Control Officials). 2007. Official Publication. Oxford, IN: Association of Official Feed Control Officials.

AFIA (American Feed Industry Association). 2005. Feed Manufacturing Technology V. Arlington, VA: American Feed Industry Association.

Bender, D. A. 2006. Benders' Dictionary of Nutrition and Food Technology 8th ed. Boca Raton, FL: CRC Press.

Blood, D. C., V. P. Studdert, and C. C. Gay. 2007. Saunders Comprehensive Veterinary Dictionary. 3rd ed. New York: Elsevier.

Brown, D. 2001. The Herb Society of America New Encyclopedia of Herbs and Their Uses. New York: Dorling Kindersley.

Crane, S. W., R. W. Griffin, and P. R. Messent. 2000. Introduction to commercial pet foods. Pp. 111–126 in Small Animal Clinical Nutrition., M. S. Hand, C. D. Thatcher, R. L. Remmillard, and P. Ruoudebush, eds. Topeka, KS: Mark Morris Institute.

Egert, M., A. A. De Graaf, H. Smidt, W. M. De Vos, and K. Venema. 2006. Beyond diversity: Functional microbiomics of the human colon. Trends Microbiol. 14:86–91.

Gibson, G. R., and M. B. Roberfroid. 1995. Dietary modulation of the human colonic microbiota: Introducing the concept of prebiotics. J. Nutr. 125:1401–1412.

Hodgson, E., R. B. Mailman, and J. E. Chambers. 1988. Dictionary of Toxicology. New York: Van Nostrand Reinhold Company.

Lewis, R. A. 1998. Lewis' Dictionary of Toxicology. Boca Raton, FL: Lewis Publishers.

Merriam-Webster. 2008. Online Dictionary. Online at: www.m-w.com. Accessed January 31, 2008.

Morris, C. 1992. Academic Press Dictionary of Science and Technology. New York: Academic Press.

Nebeker, J. R., P. Barach, and M. H. Samore. 2004. Clarifying adverse drug events: A clinician's guide to terminology, documentation, and reporting. Ann. Intern. Med. 140:795–801.

NRC (National Research Council). 2006. Nutrient Requirements of Dogs and Cats. Washington, DC: The National Academies Press.

Osweiler, G. D. 2006. General toxicological principles. Pp. 2–17 in Small Animal Toxicology, M E. Peterson and P. A. Talcoott, eds. St. Louis, MO: Elsevier Saunders.

Ritschel, W. A., and G. L. Kearns. 1999. Handbook of Basic Pharmacokinetics 5th ed. Washington, DC: American Pharmaceutical Association.

Schrezenmeir, J., and M. De Vrese. 2001. Probiotics, prebiotics, and synbiotics—Approaching a definition. Am. J. Clin. Nutr. 73:361S–364S.

WHO (World Health Organization). 2006. Probiotics in Food: Health and Nutritional Properties and Guidelines for Evaluation. FAO Food and Nutrition Paper 85. Rome, Italy: World Health Organization-Food and Agriculture Organization.

Wildman, R. E. C. 2001. Nutraceuticals: A brief review of historical and teleological aspects. Pp. 1–12 in Handbook of Nutraceuticals and Functional Foods, R. E. C. Wildman, ed. Boca Raton, FL: CRC Press.

Williams, M. H. 1983. Ergogenic Aids in Sport Human Kinetics. Champaign, IL: Publishers, Inc.

Appendix D

Contributors

The Committee on Examining the Safety of Dietary Supplements for Horses, Dogs, and Cats and staff appreciate the contributions of several individuals and organizations to the work of the committee. Some of these contributions were in person at an open session of the committee; others occurred later during the data collection and writing.

Greg Aldrich
Pet Food & Ingredient Technology, Inc.

Clare Barfoot
Mars Horsecare UK, Ltd

Sharon A. Benz
Center for Veterinary Medicine, Food and Drug Administration

Kristen Blanchard
Nutramax Laboratories

Bill Bookout
National Animal Supplement Council

George A. Burdock
Burdock Group

Paul M. Coates
National Institute of Health

Nancy K. Cook
Pet Food Institute

Ian F. DeVeau
United States Pharmacopeia

Alex Dugdale
Faculty of Veterinary Science
University of Liverpool, UK

Daniel Fabricant
Natural Products Association

Gabriel I. Giancaspro
United States Pharmacopeia

Jarrod H. Kersey
American Feed Industry Association

William D. Price
Center for Veterinary Medicine, Food and Drug Administration

Jennifer Radosevich
Kemin Industries

Richard S. Sellers
American Feed Industry Association

Emanuela Valle
University of Veterinary Medicine
Grugliasco, Italy

Appendix E

Committee Member Biographies

Jim E. Riviere *(chair)* is the Burroughs Wellcome Fund Distinguished Professor of Pharmacology and director, Center for Chemical Toxicology Research and Pharmacokinetics, College of Veterinary Medicine, North Carolina State University. He is an elected member of the Institute of Medicine of the National Academies and serves on its Food and Nutrition Board. From 2001 to 2003, he served on NRC's Subcommittee I on Meat and Poultry. He is the editor of the *Journal of Veterinary Pharmacology and Therapeutics*, and cofounder and codirector of the USDA Food Animal Residue Avoidance Databank (FARAD) program. He has served as an officer in various Specialty Sections of the Society of Toxicology, on the Science Board of the Food and Drug Administration, and on the editorial boards of various toxicology, pharmacology, and veterinary journals. His honors include the 1999 O. Max Gardner Award from the Consolidated University of North Carolina, the 1991 Ebert Prize from the American Pharmaceutical Association, the Harvey W. Wiley Medal and FDA Commissioner's Special Citation, and the Lifetime Achievement Award from the European Association of Veterinary Pharmacology and Toxicology. Dr. Riviere received his B.S. (summa cum laude) and M.S. degrees from Boston College and his D.V.M. and Ph.D. in pharmacology from Purdue University.

Dawn M. Boothe is a professor and director of the Clinical Pharmacology Laboratory at Auburn University's College of Veterinary Medicine. She is a member of the American Veterinary Medical Association, the American College of Veterinary Internal Medicine (ACVIM), the American Association of Clinical Pharmacology, and the American Academy of Veterinary Pharmacology and Therapeutics. She is a diplomate in the ACVIM. Additionally she was certified by the ACVIM in 1985 and the American College of Veterinary Clinical Pharmacology in 1991. Dr. Boothe is an expert in veterinary pharmacology and therapeutics, including antimicrobial therapy, antimicrobial resistance, antibiotic use in the surgical patient, evidence-based medicine in small animal therapeutics, cardiovascular drug therapy, and anticonvulsant therapy. Dr. Boothe received the Distinguished Achievement Award in Teaching (University Level) and the Merck AgVet Award for Creativity in Teaching. She received her B.S. degrees in zoology and veterinary medicine, D.V.M degree, M.S. degree in physiology, and Ph.D. in veterinary physiology, all from Texas A&M University.

Gail L. Czarnecki-Maulden is a senior research nutritionist at Nestle Purina PetCare PTC, where she is responsible for development of innovative nutritional concepts for implementation in pet food products. Before moving to Nestle Purina in 1990, she spent six years as an assistant, and then associate, professor in the Department of Animal Sciences and Division of Nutritional Sciences at the University of Illinois. There she helped develop the graduate program in Companion Animal Nutrition. She is a member of the American Society for Nutrition, the Comparative Gastroenterology Society, and the American Society of Animal Sciences. From 1990 to 1994 she helped set nutrient standards for dog and cat foods in the United States by serving on the Association of American Feed Control Officials' Canine and Feline Nutrition Experts Subcommittees. She has also served on the American Society of Animal Science Companion Animal Committee (2000–2003) and the University of Illinois External Advisory Committee (2000–2006; chair 2003–2004). Dr. Czarnecki-Maulden has reviewed numerous publications, among them the *Mineral Tolerance of Animals* (NRC, 2005), as well as papers for the *Journal of Nutrition*, *American Journal of Clinical Nutrition*, and *Journal of Animal Science*. In 1985, she was awarded the American Society of Animal Science's Hoffmann-LaRoche Outstanding Research Paper Award. Dr. Czarnecki-Maulden received her B.S. in animal science from Cornell University and her M.S. and Ph.D. in animal nutrition from the University of Illinois.

David A. Dzanis is owner of Dzanis Consulting and Collaborations, which provides postproduct development consulting services on matters related to veterinary nutrition and regulation, including services regarding interpretation of state and federal laws and regulations as they pertain to labeling and marketing compliance issues. Prior to beginning full-time work as a consultant in 1998, Dr. Dzanis spent eight years as a veterinary nutritionist in the Food and Drug Administration's Center for Veterinary Medicine of the Department of Health and Human Services. He served as a member (2000–2004) of the NRC's Committee on *Nutrient Requirements of Dogs and Cats*. Dr. Dzanis is currently a contributing editor of *Petfood Industry* and an adjunct professor for the Regulatory Science Program in the University of Southern California School of Pharmacy. He has served as chairman of the Association of American Feed Control Officials' Canine and Feline Nutrition Expert Subcommittees. Dr. Dzanis has also served as chairman of the American College of Veterinary Nutrition (Diplomate 1990) and president of the American Academy of Veterinary Nutrition. Awards and honors received include the Pet Food Regulatory Workshop Recognition Award in 2001, Association of American Feed Control Officials' Distinguished Service Award in 1994, FDA Commissioner's Special Citation in 1992, FDA Commendable Service Award in 1991, and the ALPO/American Veterinary Medical Association Foundation's Fellowship in Veterinary Nutrition in 1984. He has published numerous articles and given many presentations for both scientific and lay audiences. Dr. Dzanis received his D.V.M. from Purdue University and his Ph.D. from Cornell University.

Patricia A. Harris is senior equine nutritionist at Waltham Centre for Pet Nutrition, the director of equine science at Effem Equine, Ltd, and an adjunct professor of equine studies at Virginia Polytechnic Institute and State University. Before moving to Waltham, she became the head of the Clinical Chemistry and Hematology Laboratories as well as her own Metabolic Lameness Research group. She served as president of the British Equine Veterinary Association in 1999 and as executive board director of the *Equine Veterinary Journal* from 1999–2006. In 2002, she was awarded Diplomate status of the European College of Veterinary Clinical and Comparative Nutrition. Dr. Harris lectures worldwide on nutrition as it affects the health, welfare, behavior, and performance of the horse. She is the author or coauthor of numerous lay publications, scientific papers, abstracts, and book chapters. She was a reviewer of the NRC's 2007 publication *Nutrient Requirements of Horses*. Dr. Harris received an M.A., a VetMB/MRCVS, and a Ph.D., all from Cambridge University.

Wouter H. Hendriks is head and chair of the Animal Nutrition Group at Wageningen University and head of the Nutrition group at the Faculty of Veterinary Medicine at Utrecht University in the Netherlands. Before this appointment, he held concurrent positions as head of the Department of Animal Nutrition and Physiology of the Institute of Food, Nutrition and Human Health, director of the Centre for Feline Nutrition, and codirector of the AgResearch Centre for Pastoral Food Research, all at Massey University in New Zealand. In these capacities, he managed and directed active research programs that examined aspects of general mammalian and avian nutrition and physiology, as well as specialized nutrition of nonruminants (including cats, dogs, pigs, and poultry) and ruminants. The research included nutritional requirements, palatability, forage utilization, protein metabolism, and the interaction between nutrients and the gastrointestinal tract. Hendriks was a reviewer of the NRC's 2006 publication *Nutrient Requirements of Dogs and Cats*. He is an expert in companion animal nutrition, digestive physiology, and feline physiology. Dr. Hendriks received an Ingenieur degree in animal nutrition from Wageningen University and Ph.D. in monogastric nutritional physiology from Massey University.

Claudia A. Kirk is an associate professor in the Department of Small Animal Clinical Sciences at the University of Tennessee. She spent nine years (1994–2003) as a nutritionist and senior scientist for Hill's Pet Nutrition, Inc. She is a Diplomate of the American College of Veterinary Nutrition and of the American College of Veterinary Internal Medicine. From 2001 to 2002, she served as chair of the American College of Veterinary Nutrition and currently serves as examination chair. She is also a member of the American College of Veterinary Internal Medicine, American Veterinary Medical Association, American Society for Parenteral and Enteral Nutrition, American Academy of Veterinary Nutrition, American Institute of Nutrition, and Society for Comparative Endocrinology. She has been honored with the Chairman's Award (2002), the Max Kleiber Research Award (1999), ACVIM (Society for Comparative Endocrinology) Award for Outstanding Resident Abstract (1989), and The Animal Medical Center's Intern of the Year Award (1987). Dr. Kirk received her D.V.M. and Ph.D. in nutrition and endocrinology from the University of California, Davis.

Lori K. Warren is an assistant professor in the Department of Animal Sciences at the University of Florida. From 2000 to 2002, she worked as provincial horse specialist for Alberta Agriculture, Food and Rural Development in Edmonton, Alberta. She is a member of the American Society of Animal Science, the Equine Science Society, and the American Registry of Professional Animal Scientists. Dr. Warren currently serves on the board of directors of the Equine Science Society and the Horse Industry Association of Alberta. She has reviewed articles for the *Equine Veterinary Journal*, the American Society of Animal Science Annual Meeting, and the Equine Nutrition and Physiology Symposium's Production & Management Section. Her current research interests include the effect of omega-3 fatty acid supplementation on immune function and dietary modifications that help to reduce the nutrient content of horse waste. Dr. Warren received her B.S. in animal sciences from the University of Wyoming and her M.S. and Ph.D. in animal sciences and equine nutrition and exercise physiology from the University of Kentucky.

HORSES, DOGS, AND CATS OF COMMITTEE MEMBERS AND STAFF

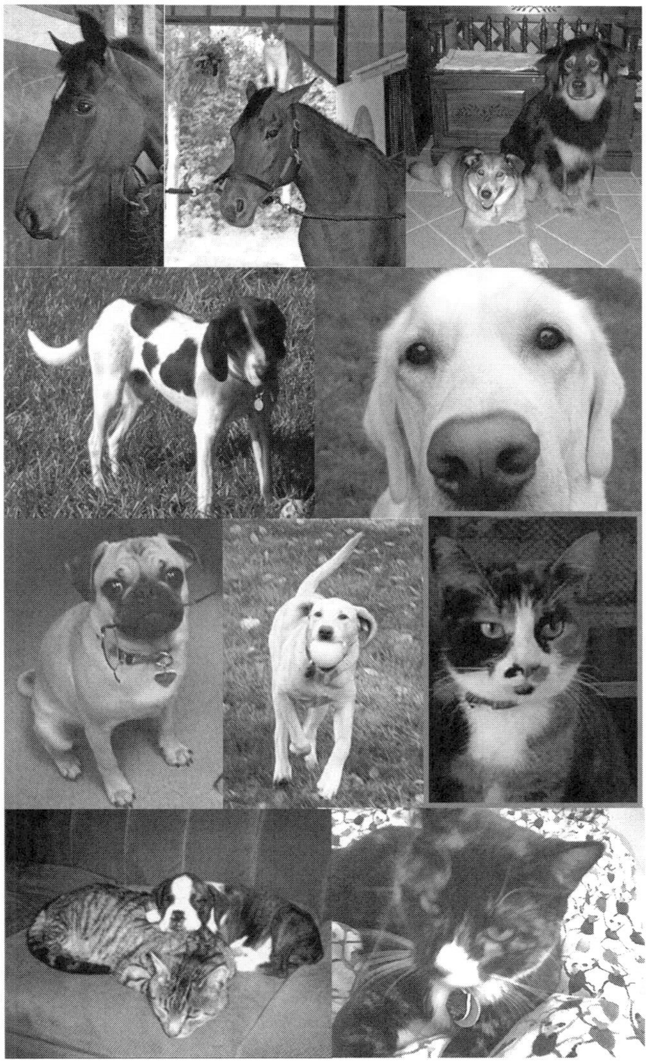

Appendix F

Recent Publications of the Board on Agriculture and Natural Resources

POLICY AND RESOURCES

Achievements of the National Plant Genome Initiative and New Horizons in Plant Biology (2008)
Agricultural Biotechnology and the Poor: Proceedings of an International Conference (2000)
Agriculture, Forestry, and Fishing Research at NIOSH (2008)
Agriculture's Role in K-12 Education (1998)
Air Emissions from Animal Feeding Operations: Current Knowledge, Future Needs (2003)
Animal Biotechnology: Science-Based Concerns (2002)
Animal Care and Management at the National Zoo: Final Report (2005)
Animal Care and Management at the National Zoo: Interim Report (2004)
Animal Health at the Crossroads: Preventing, Detecting, and Diagnosing Animal Diseases (2005)
Biological Confinement of Genetically Engineered Organisms (2004)
California Agricultural Research Priorities: Pierce's Disease (2004)
Changes in the Sheep Industry in the United States: Making the Transition from Tradition (2008)
Countering Agricultural Bioterrorism (2003)
Critical Needs for Research in Veterinary Science (2005)
Designing an Agricultural Genome Program (1998)
Diagnosis and Control of Johne's Disease (2003)
Direct and Indirect Human Contributions to Terrestrial Carbon Fluxes (2004)
Ecological Monitoring of Genetically Modified Crops (2001)
Emerging Animal Diseases: Global Markets, Global Safety: Workshop Summary (2002)
Ensuring Safe Food: from Production to Consumption (1998)
Environmental Effects of Transgenic Plants: The Scope and Adequacy of Regulation (2002)
Exploring a Vision: Integrating Knowledge for Food and Health (2004)
Exploring Horizons for Domestic Animal Genomics (2002)
Frontiers in Agricultural Research: Food, Health, Environment, and Communities (2003)
Future Role of Pesticides for U.S. Agriculture (2000)
Genetically Engineered Organisms, Wildlife, and Habitat: A Workshop Summary (2008)
Genetically Modified Pest-Protected Plants: Science and Regulation (2000)
Global Challenges and Directions for Agricultural Biotechnology (2008)
Incorporating Science, Economics, and Sociology in Developing Sanitary and Phytosanitary Standards in International Trade (2000)
National Capacity in Forestry Research (2002)
National Research Initiative: A Vital Competitive Grants Program in Food, Fiber, and Natural-Resources Research (2000)
Predicting Invasions of Nonindigenous Plants and Plant Pests (2002)
Professional Societies and Ecologically Based Pest Management (2000)
Publicly Funded Agricultural Research and the Changing Structure of U.S. Agriculture (2002)
Safety of Genetically Engineered Foods: Approaches to Assessing Unintended Health Effects (2004)
Scientific Advances in Animal Nutrition: Promise for a New Century (2001)
Scientific Criteria to Ensure Safe Food (2003)
Status of Pollinators in North America (2007)
The National Plant Genome Initiative (2002)
The Scientific Basis for Estimating Emissions from Animal Feeding Operations: Interim Report (2002)
The Scientific Basis for Predicting the Invasive Potential of Nonindigenous Plants and Plant Pests in the United States (2002)
The Use of Drugs in Food Animals: Benefits and Risks (2000)

ANIMAL NUTRITION PROGRAM—NUTRIENT REQUIREMENTS OF DOMESTIC ANIMALS SERIES AND RELATED TITLES

Mineral Tolerance of Animals: Second Revised Edition (2005)
Nutrient Requirements of Beef Cattle, Seventh Revised Edition, Update (2000)
Nutrient Requirements of Dairy Cattle, Seventh Revised Edition (2001)
Nutrient Requirements of Dogs and Cats (2006)
Nutrient Requirements of Horses: Sixth Revised Edition (2007)
Nutrient Requirements of Nonhuman Primates, Second Revised Edition (2002)
Nutrient Requirements of Small Ruminants: Sheep, Goats, Cervids, and New World Camelids (2007)
Nutrient Requirements of Swine, Tenth Revised Edition
Scientific Advances in Animal Nutrition: Promise for a New Century (2001)
The First Seventy Years 1928-1998: Committee on Animal Nutrition (1998)
The Scientific Basis for Estimating Emissions from Animal Feeding Operations: Interim Report (2002)

Further information and prices are available from the National Academies Press website at http://www.nap.edu/. To order any of the titles above, go to http://www.nap.edu/order.html or contact the Customer Service Department at (888) 624-8373 or (202) 334-3313. Inquiries and orders may also be sent to the National Academies Press, 500 Fifth Street, NW, Lockbox 285, Washington, DC 20055.

Index

A

B

C

D

G

H

T

U

V

W

X

Z